NEW INSIGHTS INTO THE PREVENTION AND TREATMENT OF BULIMIA NERVOSA

Edited by **Phillipa Hay**

New Insights into the Prevention and Treatment of Bulimia Nervosa
Edited by Phillipa Hay

Published by InTech

Janeza Trdine 9, 51000 Rijeka, Croatia

Publishing Process Manager Sandra Bakic

Technical Editor Teodora Smiljanic

Cover Designer InTech Design Team

Additional hard copies can be obtained from orders@intechopen.com

New Insights into the Prevention and Treatment of Bulimia Nervosa, Edited by Phillipa Hay
p. cm.
ISBN 978-953-307-767-3

For EU product safety concerns:
IN TECH d.o.o., Prolaz Marije Krucifikse Kozulić 3, 51000 Rijeka, Croatia,
info@intechopen.com or visit our website at intechopen.com.

Meet the editor

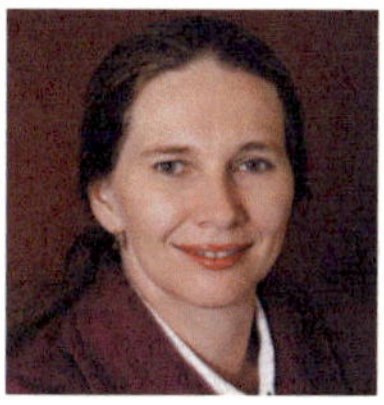

Professor Phillipa Hay is Foundation Chair of Mental Health at the UWS School of Medicine, Senior Psychiatrist at the Macarthur Eating Disorder Clinic in Campbelltown and Adjunct Professor at James Cook University. She is immediate Past-President of the Australian and New Zealand Academy for Eating Disorders and is Co-Chair of the Sisterhood, Affiliates and Chapters Committee of the International Academy for Eating Disorders. Her early seminal work was in analytic epidemiologic studies and community burden of bulimic eating disorders. Her current research program includes treatment trials, public health interventions and meta-analytic studies of efficacy. Professor Hay has been invited to give scientific addresses at meetings in every continent and she has written over 100 peer reviewed scientific papers.

Contents

Preface

Bulimia nervosa and eating disorders are a common cause of distress and health related burden for young women and men. First described over three decades ago by Russell as an "ominous variant of anorexia nervosa" and Boskind-Lodahl and colleagues as "bulimarexia", there have since then, been rapid advances in treatment and understanding of bulimia nervosa phenomenology and determinants. The early terminology reflected the origin of the diagnosis in the context of anorexia nervosa, the first eating disorder to be delineated. Since then links with other problems of binge eating have been clarified and specific psychotherapies trialled and are now in widespread use. However, for many patients treatment comes late in the course of the illness and may incompletely address complex psychopathology and co-morbidities. The present book thus brings timely and contemporary understandings of the illness to aid in current thinking regarding prevention and treatment.

The first chapter describes interpersonal therapy for bulimia nervosa. It is based on interpersonal therapy for depression and used as a control therapy for specific psychotherapy in bulimia. However, the relationship of bulimia nervosa symptoms to interpersonal function are specifically now addressed. Medical and physical aspects of the illness are reviewed in a chapter by Francavilla et al. and the role of exercise in maintenance of illness in a chapter by Bratland-Sanda et al. and other new approaches by Torres-McGehee et al.

How to help people earlier access therapy is discussed in a chapter describing two randomized controlled trials of targeted prevention for bulimia nervosa based around adaptations of health literacy and self-help that can be applied in community and primary care settings. Guidance for early detection is also provided in a chapter on practical screening methods. Eating disorders arise in adolescence and early adult years and a book would be incomplete without attention to this. This book is no exception and a fresh look at adolescents and body dissatisfaction is found in the chapter by Souza-Kaneshima et al.

Mood disorders are one of the most important co-morbidities and Mario et al. review and discuss the role of depressive features in the maintenance of bulimia nervosa. Further maintaining and predisposing features are discussed in chapters on personality and coping by Tomaz et al. and a comprehensive review of by Ignacio et al. Untested approaches that may address intra and inter personal deficits using psychodrama and object relations and further dynamic understanding are discussed over two chapters by Izydorczyk et al.

This book will be read by therapists interested in enhancing their current approaches and those interested in earlier and more effective prevention and closing the gap between illness onset and accessing treatment. They will find practical guidance but also new ideas and ways of thinking about the bulimia nervosa and the illness experience in this book.

Phillipa Hay
University of Western Sydney,
Australia

Part 1

Developments in Treatment

1

Interpersonal Problems in People with Bulimia Nervosa and the Role of Interpersonal Psychotherapy

Jon Arcelus[1,2], Debbie Whight[1] and Michelle Haslam[2]
[1]Leicestershire Partnership NHS Trust, Leicester,
[2]Loughborough University Centre for Research into Eating Disorders (LUCRED),
Loughborough University,
UK

1. Introduction

The term 'interpersonal' encompasses not only the patterns of interaction between the individual and significant others, but also the process by which these interactions are internalised and form part of the self-image (Sullivan, 1953). Interpersonal functioning is considered crucial to good mental health. According to Klinger (1977), when people are asked what makes their lives meaningful, most will mention their close relationships with others. Being involved in secure and fulfilling relationships is perceived by most individuals as critical to wellbeing and happiness (Berscheid & Peplau, 1983).

Maladaptive interpersonal functioning is considered central to several psychiatric disorders, such as depression (e.g. Petty, et al, 2004), anxiety (e.g. Montgomery et al, 1991), schizophrenia (e.g. Sullivan & Allen, 1999) and autistic spectrum disorders (e.g. Travis & Sigman, 1998). Interpersonal skill deficits may cause vulnerability to developing mental health problems and may also play a role in maintaining it. This is the chicken and egg question: are interpersonal problems vulnerability factors for the development of a psychiatric disorder or are they the result of this disorder?

2. Interpersonal problems and eating disorders

Considering that unhealthy interpersonal functioning is central to several mental health problems, it is not surprising that evidence suggests this is also the case in eating disorders. Walsh et al (1985) demonstrated a high frequency of affective disorder, particularly major depression, among patients with bulimia nervosa (BN), which may explain the strong correlation found between this disorder (BN) and interpersonal problems (Hopwood et al, 2007). Research in this area have found that people suffering from BN were more likely to display domineering, vindictive, cold, socially avoidant, non-assertive, exploitable, overly nurturing, or intrusive characteristics than non-BN (Hopwood et al, 2007).

Social support and social networks have also been studied in people with BN. Grisset and Norvell (1992) found that people with BN reported receiving less emotional and practical support from friends and family. They argue that this inadequate support creates a vulnerability towards developing eating disorder symptoms as a coping mechanism. Eating disordered individuals are also less likely to utilise support from others, particularly due to a negative attitude towards emotional expression (Meyer et al 2010). In terms of relationship satisfaction, women with eating problems report more discomfort with closeness and have been described to fear intimacy with a partner (Evans & Wertheim, 1998; Pruitt et al, 1992). Therefore in view of the correlation between interpersonal problems and BN, it is not surprising that a specific therapy aimed at helping patients with interpersonal problems (IPT) was considered as a treatment of this disorder.

3. The development of Interpersonal Psychotherapy (IPT)

IPT was developed for the treatment of depression and originates from theories in which interpersonal functioning is recognised to be a critical component of psychological wellbeing. The work of 1930's psychiatrist Harry Sullivan first suggested that patients' mental health was related to their interpersonal contact with others. Challenging Freud's psychosexual theory, Sullivan emphasized the role of interpersonal relations, society and culture as the primary determinants of mental health (Sullivan, 1968). Sullivan's work was further developed by Gerald Klerman and Myrna Weissman in the 1980's, who studied depression treatments using the interpersonal approach. Whilst studying the efficacy of antidepressants, alone or paired with psychotherapy, it was found that 'high contact' counselling was effective, leading to the further development of the therapy which was renamed interpersonal psychotherapy (Klerman et al, 1984). These positive results led to the inclusion of IPT in the NIMH Treatment of Depression Collaborative Research Program, which compared this therapy with antidepressants, placebo and Cognitive Behavioural Therapy (CBT) for depression (Elkin et al., 1989). As a part of this study the original IPT manual, Interpersonal Psychotherapy for Depression, was published as a manual for the research project (Klerman et al, 1984). Patients in all conditions showed significant reduction in depressive symptoms and improvement in functioning, those having the antidepressant Imipramine plus clinical management generally doing best, the two psychotherapies second best, and placebo plus clinical management worst. There was no significant difference between the two psychotherapies.

Since then, there have been several systematic reviews of studies investigating the efficacy of IPT for depression (Jarrett & Rush, 1994; Klerman, 1994; Feijo de Mello et al., 2005). They concluded that IPT was superior to placebo in nine of thirteen studies and better than CBT overall. However IPT plus medication was no more effective than medication alone. The researchers also found that several factors were associated with good therapy outcome, including the ability to engage in more than one perspective and to take responsibility for actions, empathy for others, a desire to change, good communication skills, and a sense of cooperation and willingness to engage with the therapist.

Feske et al (1998) examined predictors of outcome in 134 female patients with major depression, and found that those who did not improve experienced higher levels of anxiety and were also more likely to meet diagnostic criteria for panic disorder. In addition, they found that poor outcome was associated with greater vocational impairment, longer duration of episode, more severe illness, and surprisingly, lower levels of social impairment. Other authors have found that despite comparable efficacy between IPT and CBT, IPT was more affected by personality traits and therefore less suitable for those with personality disorders (Joyce et al. 2007).

4. The development of IPT for Bulimia Nervosa

Since the conception of IPT, the original manual has been updated (Weissman et al, 2000; Weissman et al, 2007) and several manuals have been written concerning modifications of IPT, including those for depressed adolescents (Mufson et al, 2004), the elderly (Hinrichsen & Clougherty, 2006), perinatal women (Weissman et al, 2000), HIV patients (Pergami et al 1999), bipolar disorder (Frank, 2005), social phobia (Hoffart et al., 2007), dysthymic disorder (Markowitz, 1998) and finally bulimia nervosa (IPT-BN; Fairburn, 1993).

IPT-BN was not developed systematically through an adaptation from IPT for depression, but instead was discovered to be effective when used as a control treatment for CBT during a randomised controlled trial for individuals with BN (Fairburn et al., 1991). IPT was not adapted specifically for BN in the treatment trial, and beyond limited initial psychoeducation, eating problems were not addressed during the treatment. It was hypothesised that as IPT shared some non-specific factors with CBT, its inclusion in the trial would highlight the benefits of cognitive behavioural techniques in CBT that were not present in IPT. However, while CBT was considered most effective, IPT also resulted in the improvement of eating disorder symptoms. This discovery led to the further development of IPT-BN as a viable treatment option, and it was manualised in 1993 (Fairburn, 1993).

Since its conception, IPT has been compared to CBT, the current treatment of choice, with equally positive results in both individual and group settings (Fairburn, 1997; Fairburn et al, 1993; Fairburn et al., 1991; Fairburn et al, 2000; Roth & Ross, 1988; Wilfley et al., 2003; Wilfley et al., 1993). Agras et al (2000) found that CBT was superior to IPT at the end of treatment however there was no significant difference between the two treatments at one year follow-up. Based on these findings, the NICE guidelines for eating disorders in the UK (NICE, 2004) recommends IPT as an alternative to CBT for the treatment of BN but patients should be informed that it could take longer that CBT to achieve comparable results.

The efficacy of IPT in patients with BN has been explained by Fairburn (1997). He claimed that IPT might work through several mechanisms. Firstly, IPT helps patients to overcome well established interpersonal difficulties, for example when focusing on interpersonal 'role transitions' this can be helpful for those patients who have missed out on the interpersonal challenges of early adulthood as a result of their eating disorder. Secondly, IPT can open up new interpersonal opportunities and as a result patients learn to rely more on interpersonal functioning for self evaluation instead of focusing wholly on eating, weight and shape. Finally, IPT gives patients a sense that they are capable of influencing their interpersonal lives and therefore may lessen their need to control their eating, weight and shape.

5. Modification of IPT-BN

The IPT Team in Leicester (UK) adapted IPT-BN further by bringing back the original components of IPT (psycho-education, directive techniques, problem solving, modelling, role play and symptom review) and modifying the treatment for individual with BN where the eating disorders problems are taken into consideration. Although they have been using this model of treatment for BN for more than 15 years, only recently they have manualised it (Whight et al, 2010). This new modified version of IPT for BN is called IPT-BNm in this chapter to differentiate it from the IPT-BN developed by Fairburn.

IPT-BNm uses a time frame of 12-20 weekly sessions. The usual number of sessions is 16, which roughly breaks down into three areas: 4 assessment sessions, 10 middle sessions and 2 termination sessions. There is also a pre-treatment session (Session 0) where the patient and therapist agree goals for treatment and the model is explained. Therapy may be extended to up to 20 sessions if this is felt to be clinically appropriate, however this should be agreed with the patient close to the start of therapy and not towards the end of therapy as this can affect the potency of the termination sessions. The number of sessions may also be reduced if felt to be appropriate for the patient, but again should be agreed near the beginning of treatment.

5.1 Overview of IPT-BNm

5.1.1 Early sessions: sessions 0-4

Broadly speaking the initial sessions are as detailed in the original IPT manual for depression (Klerman et al 1984) but specific for eating disorders. The aims of these sessions are to get a clear picture of the current problems along with a history of previous difficulties and interpersonal events. This enables the therapist and patient to identify areas of current difficulty, agree realistic treatment goals and to establish a focus for therapy. Areas for assessment include mood, interpersonal network, historical events (timeline) and eating disorder symptomatology. The main task of the therapist is to help the patient gain some understanding of the inter-relatedness of their presenting difficulties and to establish a specific focus for treatment dependent on their individual situation. As a part of this process and what makes this therapy specific for patients with BN is the use of psycho education related to eating. Throughout the therapy patients will be encouraged to complete food diaries that will be used to regulate patients eating. Psycho-education is a fundamental part of therapy.

By the end of session 4 the therapist will have a good understanding of whether or not the patient is able to work within the IPT model. The model is not suitable for everybody therefore if IPT is felt to be inappropriate other treatment options may be considered with the patient. IPT is primarily an outpatient treatment, but the early sessions could be started as an inpatient if needed, with the understanding that the patient would be discharged before treatment ended. This would enable them to practise skills between sessions and to build their interpersonal networks, which may be more difficult to achieve as an inpatient.

5.1.1.1 The role of the therapist

The therapist needs to engage the patient in therapy. A non-pejorative approach and an empathic understanding of the patient's distress can be crucial in gaining the trust - and therefore the commitment - of the patient. The therapist also needs to be clear about the boundaries of therapy. The sessions are weekly and commitment to regular sessions is an important part of therapy. Weekly therapy helps to maintain the intensity of the treatment whilst also giving the patient time to practice tasks between sessions. It is helpful to count down each session, letting the patient know where they are in therapy and how many sessions are left - for example "We are on session 2. We have 14 sessions left". This helps to start the process of termination but also emphasises the short-term nature of the therapy. This in turn acts as an incentive for the patient to make changes in therapy as they are aware of what time they have got from the beginning. It is also important for the therapist to stick to the boundaries of therapy - start on time, finish on time and always state the date and time of the next appointment at the end of each session. It can be very helpful to have the dates of all the sessions agreed as this avoids any confusion.

The role of the therapist in the early sessions is of active participation. The therapist is tasked to gather information on the patient's history, presenting problems, interpersonal world and expectations of treatment. He/She is also helping the patient to make links between their difficulties and their interpersonal issues. This can be difficult, particularly as secrecy is so often an issue with patients with BN.

5.1.1.2 The role of the patient

The patient needs to be actively involved in therapy throughout. The more they put into therapy the more they will get out of it. Initially the patient should be willing to share their difficulties and be able to listen to the therapist, working with them at making sense of the current difficulties and identifying realistic goals. The patient needs to be able to attend all planned sessions and to focus on any agreed tasks between sessions. Patients are also expected to track their symptoms each week and to bring to the session any relevant information about the agreed focus area. Changes in symptoms can often be markers of interpersonal events, so helping to link these changes to the agreed interpersonal focus area is an important skill for the patient to master.

5.1.1.3 Interpersonal focus area

The main task of session 4 is in helping the patient to choose a focus area to work on during the middle sessions of therapy. As in the original manual for IPT for depression, there are 4 clear focus areas:

- *Interpersonal Role Disputes:* Difficulties occur when the patient has non-reciprocal expectations from a significant other. This could be an overt or covert dispute and often there is a pattern of difficult relationships around the patient. It is important to focus on one key relationship that is current and where the patient feels that change is possible.
- *Interpersonal Role Transitions:* Difficulties occur when the patient has difficulty adjusting or adapting to changes in their life. This could be changes at work, in living situation, in relationships, in financial status or any other area. What is key is that the patient has not adapted well to the changes and this is linked to their illness onset or deterioration.
- *Interpersonal Deficits:* Difficulties occur when patients had problems making or sustaining relationships with people. There are often repeated patterns of broken or failed relationships and the patient may be socially isolated. The patient may be highly sensitive to their difficulties so it can be very helpful to use role play in the session to help them practice new skills.
- *Complicated Bereavement:* Difficulties can occur when a patient is not able to resolve the death of a significant figure. This is often a partner or a family member, but can be the death of a friend or even a pet. The key feature is that the patient is not able to complete a grieving process and this impacts on their eating disorder and mood. The nature of the attachment with the deceased is an important consideration when considering grief as a focus area.

The task of the therapist is to find the most appropriate focus with their patient. All the information gained so far is assessed by the therapist, who by session 4 usually has an idea of what interpersonal issues are central to the patient's problems. IPT does not seek to understand the dynamics behind the eating disorder/depression but rather to help the patient make changes to their life now. The formulation for IPT is therefore simple, pragmatic and collaborative. Using the patient's words and a summary of the identified problem areas that have been highlighted over the previous 3 sessions, the therapist may suggest an area to focus on in therapy.

5.1.2 Middle sessions: Sessions 5-14

The middle sessions follow a similar format to each other, with the patient being asked to bring in their own material from the week to work within therapy. The therapist helps the patient to link the changes in the symptoms to the focus area, then works with the patient at active problem solving, contingency planning or practising new skills as appropriate.

The therapist maintains a hopeful and realistic stance on the patient's ability to make changes and to recover. All attempts at change should be praised as it can help to enhance the patient's feelings of self worth and their confidence at trying something new. It also helps to keep them engaged in therapy and to feel that the therapist is on their side working with them. This also needs to be balanced with the patient's capacity to change so it is important to be realistic.

All patients will have some difficulties with changing their way of eating, bingeing and vomiting. It is important to review the symptoms each week to maintain the focus and to identify change, but lack of change is also an issue. Some patients find it more difficult to make changes to their eating patterns and can really struggle to do things differently. It is part of the therapist's role to continue to encourage and support them whilst also being open and frank about change. Because the therapy is time limited this helps to motivate people to change, but lack of progress should not be ignored. Enquiring about what difficulties the patient is experiencing and helping them to develop problem-solving strategies to enhance their abilities to put therapy into practise can enable the patient to feel more attended to and can address feelings of having failed or worthlessness. As these can be key features of both eating disorders and depression they are important issues to address. Feeling attended to and supported can help the patient to stay engaged in therapy.

Half way through IPT (session 8) therapy is reviewed. This review is planned from the beginning. It is highlighted as a time to see how things have progressed thus far, ensuring that the right focus area is being worked on and allowing room for change if needed by the patient or the therapist.

5.1.3 Termination sessions: 15-16

The end of therapy should not come as a surprise to the patient; the therapist will have been counting down sessions and will have planned the dates of the final session with the patient. However it can still can come as a shock. The final 2 sessions are explicitly about ending therapy, about recognising and maintaining changes made, acknowledging that which has not changed and exploring feelings about ending. This can feel very positive for a patient who has recovered or more anxiety provoking for one who has not. It is important to end after the agreed number of sessions.

5.2 Efficacy of IPT -BN(m)

Arcelus et al (2009) conducted a case series evaluation of 59 patients and found that by the middle of therapy there had been a significant reduction in eating disordered cognitions and behaviours, alongside an improvement in interpersonal functioning and depressive symptoms. The authors found that although patients did improve significantly after eight sessions, their symptomatology did not continue to improve in the same way within the last eight sessions. This may suggest that there was something in the first sessions that facilitates change, which is lost in the last sessions. This could be explained by the impetus of the initial sessions; targeting symptoms, an opportunity to change and exploring the interpersonal context and maintenance of the eating disorder. Perhaps this sets the ground for facilitating change and the setting of interpersonal goals can instill hope. Although the use of a case series was considered appropriate given the exploratory nature of the study, it is important to remember that these preliminary findings should be interpreted within the limitations of a case series design. Although there is incidental evidence from clinicians and patients of the effectiveness of this modified version of IPT for BN, there is a lack of research evidence which can only been achieved by a control Trial.

6. New modifications of IPT for patients with eating disorders

In recent months, a new theoretical model of IPT for eating disorders has been proposed (Reiger et al., 2010). This model suggests that eating disorders are triggered by negative feedback regarding an individual's social worth due to its negative effect on self-esteem and associated mood. Eating disordered behaviours often begin because of this negative social evaluation, and over time such behaviours may become a more reliable source of self esteem and mood regulation than social interactions. The aim of IPT then is to help the patient to develop positive, healthy relationships, which replace the eating disorder in the attainment of positive esteem and affect. This newly proposed model also includes the monitoring of eating disorder symptoms and other elements, which were taken out of the original IPT-BN to make it comparable with CBT. However, this new therapeutic model has not yet been supported by empirical studies and does not differentiate between the treatment of anorexic and bulimic disorders.

7. Conclusion

Interpersonal difficulties are both vulnerability factors and consequences of several psychiatric disorders, including Bulimia Nervosa. Over the last several years a growing number of research studies have demonstrated the efficacy of IPT as a treatment for several conditions. Within the field of eating disorders, IPT has been shown to be effective for patients with BN, although it appears to work slower than CBT. In order to make this treatment more effective several authors in different countries have modified this treatment further. In spite of the modification that IPT has gone through, the core elements of the therapy have been retained. Throughout IPT, therapists aim to help patients to identify the interpersonal difficulties maintaining the eating disorders symptoms in order to work through them. Although IPT has been used successfully over a number of years, research evidence for the new modified versions is still required.

8. Acknowledgement

We would like to acknowledge the IPT team in Leicester: Mrs Lesley McGrain, Ms Lesley Meadows, Dr Jonathan Baggott and Mr Chris Langham.

9. References

Agras, W.S., Walsh, T., Fairburn, C.G., Wilson, G.T., and Kraemer, H.C (2000) A multicenter comparison of cognitive-behavioral therapy and interpersonal psychotherapy for bulimia nervosa. *Archives of General Psychiatry*, 57, 5, 459-66

Arcelus, J., Whight, D., Langham, C., Baggott, J., McGrain, L., Meadows. L., & Meyer, C. (2009). A case series evaluation of a modified version of interpersonal psychotherapy (IPT) for the treatment of bulimic eating disorders: A pilot study. *European Eating Disorders Review*, 17, 260-268.

Berscheid, E., & Peplau, L. A. (1983). The emerging science of relationships. In *Close relationships,* H. H. Kelley, E. Berscheid, A. Christensen, J. H. Harvey, T. L. Huston, G. Levinger et al. (Eds.) pp. (1-19), W.H.Freeman & Co Ltd, 978-0716714439, New York.

Elkin, L., Shea, T., Watkins, J. T., Imber, S. D., Sotsky, S. M., Collins, J. F. (1989). National Institute of Mental Health Treatment of Depression Collaborative Research Program: General effectiveness of treatments. *Archives of General Psychiatry, 46,* 971-982.

Evans, L., & Wertheim, E. H. (1998). Intimacy patterns and relationship satisfaction of women with eating problems and the mediating effects of depression, trait anxiety and social anxiety. *Journal of Psychosomatic Research*, 44, 355–365.

Fairburn, C.G. (1993). Interpersonal psychotherapy for bulimia nervosa. In *New applications of interpersonal therapy,* G.L. Klerman & M.M. Weissman (Eds.), pp. (278–294), American Psychiatric Press, 978-0880485111, Washington DC

Fairburn, C.G. (1997). Interpersonal psychotherapy for bulimia nervosa. In *Handbook of treatment for eating disorders,* D.M. Garner & P.E. Garfinkel (Eds.), pp. (278–294). Guilford Press, 978-1572301863, New York.

Fairburn, C. G., Wilson, G. T., & Kraemer, H. C. (2000). A multicenter comparison of cognitive-behavioural therapy and interpersonal psychotherapy for bulimia nervosa. *Archives of General Psychiatry*, 5, 459-466.

Fairburn, C. G., Jones, R., Peveler, R. C., Carr, S. J., Solomon, R. A., O'Connor, M. E., Burton, J., & Hope, R. A. (1991). Three psychological treatments for bulimia nervosa: A comparative trial. *Archives of General Psychiatry,* 48, 463-469.

Fairburn, C. G., Jones, R., Peveler, R. C., Hope, R. A., & O'Connor, M. (1993). Psychotherapy and bulimia nervosa: longer term effects of interpersonal psychotherapy, behavior therapy and cognitive behaviour therapy. *Archives of General Psychiatry*, 50, 419-428.

Feijo de Mello, M., de Jesus Mari, J., Bacaltchuk, J., Verdeli, H., & Neugebauer, R. (2005). A systematic review of research findings on the efficacy of interpersonal therapy for depressive disorders. *European Archives of Psychiatry and Clinical Neuroscience*, 255, 75-82.

Feske, U., Frank, E., Kupfer, D. J., Shear, K., Weaver, E. (1998). Anxiety as a predictor of response to Interpersonal psychotherapy for recurrent major depression: an exploratory investigation. *Depression and Anxiety*, 8, 135–141.

Frank, E. (2005). *Treating Bipolar Disorder: A Clinician's Guide to Interpersonal and Social Rhythm Therapy,* Guilford, 978-1593854652, New York

Grissett, N.I. and Norvell, N.K. (1992). Perceived social support, social skills, and quality of relationships in bulimic women. *Journal of Consulting Clinical Psychology*, 60, 293–299.

Hinrichsen, G.A., & Clougherty, K.F. (2006). *Interpersonal psychotherapy for depressed older adults,* American Psychological Association, 978-1591473619, Washington, DC

Hoffart, A., Abrahamsen, G., Bonsaksen, T., Borge, F.M., Ramstad, R., Lipsitz, J., & Markowitz, J.C. (2007). *A Residential Interpersonal Treatment for Social Phobia.* New York, Nova Science Publishers Inc.

Hopwood, C., Clarke, A., Perez, M. (2007). Pathoplasticity of Bulimic Features and Interpersonal Problems. *International Journal of Eating Disorders*, 40, 652 - 658.

Jarrett, R. B., & Rush, A. J. (1994). Short term psychotherapy of depressive disorders: current status and future directions. *Psychiatry*, 57, 115-132.

Joyce, P. R., McKenzie, J. M., Carter, J. D., Rae, A. M. Luty, S. E., Frampton, C. M. A., Mulder, R. T. (2007). Temperament, character and personality disorders as predictors of response to interpersonal psychotherapy and cognitive-behavioural therapy for depression. *The British Journal of Psychiatry*, 190, 503-508.

Klerman, G.L., DiMascio, A., Weissman, M.M., Prusoff, B.A., & Paykel, E.S. (1974). Treatment of depression by drugs and psychotherapy. *American Journal of Psychiatry*, 131, 186-191.

Klerman, G.L.,Weissman, M.M., Rounsaville, B.J., & Chevron, E.S. (1984). *Interpersonal psychotherapy of depression*. Basic Books, 978-1568213507, New York.

Klinger, E. (1977). *Meaning and void: Inner experience and the incentives in peoples lives.* University of Minnesota Press, Minnesota

Markowitz, J. C. (1998). *Interpersonal Psychotherapy for Dysthymic Disorder.* American Psychiatric Press, 978-0880489140, Washington, D.C.

Meyer, C., Leung, N., Barry, L., & De Feo, D. (2010). Brief Report. Emotion and Eating Psychopathology: Links with Attitudes Toward Emotional Expression Among Young Women. *International Journal of Eating Disorders*, 43, 2, 187-189

Montgomery, R. L., Haemmerlie, F. M., & Edwards, M. (1991). Social, personal, and interpersonal deficits in socially anxious people. *Journal of social behaviour and personality*, 6, 859-872.

Mufson, L., Dorta, K.P., Moreau, D., & Weissman, M.M. (2004). *Interpersonal Psychotherapy for Depressed Adolescents*, Guildford press, 978-1609182267, New York.

National Institute of Clinical Excellence (NICE) (2004). *Core interventions in the treatment and management of anorexia nervosa, bulimia nervosa and related eating disorders.* British Psychological Society/RCPsych Publications, 978-1854333988, London

Petty, S. C., Sachs-Ericsson, N., & Joiner, T. E. (2004) Interpersonal functioning deficits: temporary or stable characteristics of depressed individuals? *Journal of Affective Disorders*, 81, 115-122.

Pruitt, J.A., Kappius, RE. & Gorman, P.W. (1992). Bulimia and fear of intimacy. *Journal of Clinical Psvchology*, 48, 472-476.

Reiger, E., Van Buren, D. J., Bishop, M., Tanofsky-Kraff, M., Welch, R., & Wilfley, D.E. (2010). An eating disorder specific model of interpersonal psychotherapy (IPT-ED): causal pathways and treatment implications. *Clinical Psychology Review*, 4, 400-410.

Roth, D.M. & Ross, D. R. (1988). Long-term cognitive-interpersonal group therapy for eating disorders. *International Journal of Group Psychotherapy*, 38, 491-510.

Sullivan, H. (1968). *The interpersonal theory of psychiatry*. W. W. Norton & Company.

Sullivan, R. J., & Allen, J. S. (1999).Social deficits associated with schizophrenia defined in terms of interpersonal Machiavellianism. *Acta Psychiatrica Scandinavia*, 99, 148- 54.

Travis, L. I., & Sigman, M. (1998). Social deficits and interpersonal relationships in autism. *Mental Retardation and Developmental Disabilities Research Reviews*, 4, 65–72.

Walsh, T., Roose, S. P., Glassman, A. H., Gladise, M., Sadik, C. (1985). Bulimia and Depression. *Psychosomatic Medicine*, 47, 123-131.

Weissman, M. M., Markowitz, J. C., & Klerman, G. L. (2000). *Comprehensive guide to interpersonal psychotherapy*. Basic Books, 978-0465095667, New York.

Weissman, M. M., Markowitz, J. C., & Klerman, G. L. (2007). *Clinicians quick guide to interpersonal psychotherapy*. Oxford University Press, 978-0195309416, USA.

Whight, D., McGrain, L., Langham, C., Baggott, J., Meadows, L. & Arcelus, J. (2010). *A new version of interpersonal psychotherapy for bulimic disorders*. The manual, LPT, Retrieved from www.wix.com/leicesteript/ipt-leicester

Wilfley, D. E., Agras, W. S., Telch, C. F., Rossiter, E. M., Schneider, J. A., Cole, A.G., Sifford, L., & Raeburn, S. D. (1993). Group cognitive-behavioral therapy and group interpersonal psychotherapy for the nonpurging bulimic individual: A controlled comparison. *Journal of Consulting and Clinical Psychology*, 61, 296-305.

Wilfley, D., Stein, R., & Welch, R. (2003). Interpersonal Psychotherapy. In J. Treasure, U. Smith & E. van Furth (2003). *Handbook of eating disorders*. John Wiley and Sons.

2

Application of Psychodrama and Object Relations Psychotherapy – An Integrated Approach to the Treatment of Bulimia Nervosa Based on Selected Elements of the Theory and the Author's Own Experience

Bernadetta Izydorczyk
Department of Clinical and Forensic Psychology, University of Silesia in Katowice, Poland

1. Introduction

Bulimia nervosa is an eating disorder characterized by self-destructive behaviours which gradually affect the sufferer's mental well-being and lead to body emaciation. The results of the scientific research conducted in the past few decades point to a multitude of determinants of this disorder, including biological, familial, socio-cultural and individual factors [Mikołajczyk, Samochowiec, Kent,Waller, Dagnan, Hartt, Wonderlich , Rorty, Yager, Rossotto, Lacey, Evans].

Chronic stress and traumatic events which the person experiences in his or her life (e.g. acts of violence or sexual abuse) are considered to be significant triggering factors for bulimia nervosa [Mikołajczyk, Samochowiec, Kent, Waller, Dagnan, Hartt, Wonderlich, Rorty, Yager, Rossotto]. Traumatic experiences which bulimia sufferers are exposed to, and their emotional deficits affect the recovery process. In the therapeutic process, the patient needs to develop a cognitive and emotional insight into psychological mechanisms underlying the disorder which he or she suffers from, and to undergo a corrective emotional experience in the contact with the other person. This points to the significance of an "encounter with the other person and establishing a positive emotional bond (the therapeutic alliance) with this person". Thus, psychodrama is the therapeutic method which allows to intensify reactive actions and facilitates positive changes in the emotional structure of the patient's personality, and proves to be an effective technique of reducing bulimic symptoms.

Eating disorders belong to the category of psychopathology which is characterized by various levels of personality dysfunctions which range from neurotic disorders to psychosis. The choice of diagnostic and therapeutic interventions applied in the process of treatment should then be determined by the kind of a personality disorder identified in the given individual. Developing insight into psychological mechanisms underlying eating disorders, as well as establishing a therapeutic bond, constitute a crucial element of therapeutic interactions which can be supported by such methods as psychodrama and object relations technique.

Integrating psychodrama, which allows to gain insight into psychological mechanisms underlying bulimia nervosa, with the approach that focuses on corrective interactions in emotional relationships with significant others (objects), proves to be an effective method of reducing destructive symptoms of this eating disorder. I witness this in my own therapeutic work. The effectiveness of various psychological therapies applied in the treatment of anorexia and bulimia nervosa has been discussed in the subject literature[Hay, Bacaltchuk, Byrnes, Claudino, Ekmeijan, Yong, Bahar, Latzer, Kreitler, Berry].Psychoanalytic and psychodynamic psychotherapies, which include therapeutic interventions based on the theoretical assumptions of classical psychoanalysis, object relations theory and psychology of the self [Bahar, Latzer, Kreitler ,Berry], are regarded as the most significant in the process of treatment. They prove to be effective especially in the long-term treatment of personality disorders in adult patients. Similarly, it has been demonstrated that application of psychodynamic therapy in the treatment of eating disorders can give positive effects [Bruch, Glickauf- Hughes , Wells, Hay , Bacaltchuk, Byrnes, Claudino, Ekmejian, Yong]. As viewed in psychological literature cognitive therapy as well as the therapy based on eclectic approach which involves integrating various theoretical elements, can be used in the treatment of anorexia and bulimia nervosa. However, application of artetherapy and psychodrama, combined with psychoanalytic and psychodynamic psychotherapy (based on object relations theory) in the treatment of eating disorders has not been thoroughly discussed in subject literature [Levens, Jay]. It applies mainly to Polish references.

According to early psychoanalytical conceptions concerning the origins of an eating disorder, bulimia nervosa is a psychosomatic illness [Bruch]. Conversion symptoms have primitive symbolic significance (e.g. oral fantasies where the mouth is symbolically equated with vagina, and eating is accompanied by the fear of "oral impregnation") [Bruch]. The etiology of eating disorders is also related to such factors as the person's psychopathological personality structure and disturbances in the process of solving internal conflicts by the bulimia sufferer. The conflicts are predominantly related to destabilization occurring during such processes as development and emotional experiencing of sexuality, and accepting one's own femininity (in case of female patients). Bulimia sufferers attempt to solve the conflicts by distorting their body image and making a cognitive interpretation of their body stimuli [Bruch]. An appropriate relationship between a caregiver (a mother) and a child (which means that a caregiver adjusts to the child's experiences) is considered to have a significant impact on the development of pathological mechanisms which underlie the aforementioned dysfunctions. Thus, eating disorder symptoms, including bulimic patterns, constitute a substitute of affect regulation.

Broadly defined object relations theories represent a significant contribution to a new understanding of eating disorder psychopathology, viewed from the perspective of the significance of object relations and the characteristics of internal object representations developed in the later stages of the person's mental life [Glickauf- Hughes, Wells].On the basis of the subject literature [Bruch, Izydorczyk] as well as my own experience, gathered in the course of therapeutic work with bulimic patients, I can state that these individuals resort to certain "external measures", or activities (such as eating) in order to cope with their internal emotional conflicts. The specific life experiences which bulimia sufferers (predominantly women) tend to report in an anamnestic interview include:

1. Playing the role of the so called "responsible child", who takes over the parents' duties such as taking care of younger siblings or running the house. The child learns how to recognize and satisfy other people's needs, which consequently leads to suppressing his or her own needs. Such childhood experience usually takes its toll on the life of a female who finds it difficult in her adult life to accept the feeling of anger in her relationship

with parents, who "cast" her in the role of "a responsible child". The anger is directed mainly towards the mother, who the person, as a child, was trying to protect against experiencing negative emotions.

2. Playing the role of "a good child", causing no troubles, thereby meeting expectations set by parents who encourage the desired behaviour and reward the child for it. This gradually hinders the child's ability to express alternative feelings and pursue behaviours which their parents regard as "bad=wrong" and "needy". The child feels he or she is a disappointment to the parents. A child lives, as it were, in the world which is merely "good" or "bad", and this bipolar view of the world affects his or her self-perception. As a result, the child denies the "bad", "needy" aspect of his ore her personality to gain his or her parents' approval. In this respect, bulimia nervosa can serve as a means of externalizing (e.g. through eating) and_denying undesirable aspects of personality. However, despite the fact that eating is considered to be an "external activity", it has a direct impact on the feelings and emotions which bulimic individuals have towards themselves. When a bulimic has a good day, because she or he has eaten only "good" food, the individual feels good. Such a condition lasts until the bulimia suffer decides to consume "bad" food, which results in reversing the process of self-evaluation. It proves that self-assessment is influenced by external factors. When talking to my female patients suffering from bulimia nervosa, I notice that they often use such expressions as: "I should" or "I shouldn't". The need for approval, which goes hand in hand with failure to comply with self-set standards, makes it difficult for bulimia sufferers to establish social relationships. When selecting partners, bulimics oscillate between individuals who need to be taken care of and those who need to take care of others. Due to their low self-esteem bulimia sufferers find it difficult to acknowledge that their partners perceive them as attractive. The fact that bulimic individuals disapprove of and reject their own bodies triggers problems in the sexual sphere. Alcohol and drug abuse turns out to be a common coping strategy.

Recent scientific research demonstrates that the pathomechanisms underlying eating disorders, particularly bulimia nervosa, develop in response to such difficult life experiences as acts of violence or sexual abuse, which an individual is exposed to either during childhood or adult life [Mikołajczyk, Samochowiec, Kent, Waller, Dagnan, Hartt, Wonderlich , Rorty, Bruch, Izydorczyk]

A number of personality profile studies conducted on bulimia sufferers prove that they display the following personality disorders: borderline and histrionic personalities, impulse control disorders, impulsivity, or an obsessive-compulsive disorder. Bulimics tend to be quick-tempered, and have low frustration tolerance and frequent dysphoric moods. They also display a tendency to withdraw and to get depressed [Mikołaczyk, Samochowiec].

Lacey and Evans defined the notion of a "Multi-Impulsive Personality Disorder" and specified its characteristic behaviours (such as psychoactive substance abuse, repeated self-harm, compulsive dozing of substances, shoplifting and gambling), placing bulimia nervosa among them [Lacey, Evans]. Inadequate impulse control, present in bulimic patients, leads to regular episodes of binge eating, vomiting, using drugs, drinking alcohol, compulsive smoking, repeated self-harm and indulging in a variety of impulsive, tension-releasing behaviours._Such behaviours are frequently accompanied by the feelings of self-loathing and disgust towards one's own body, guilt and shame. By contrast with patients suffering from anorexia nervosa, who tend to deny their illness, bulimic individuals go through their illness accompanied by pain and the feeling of shame. They are filled with great remorse for their behaviour towards themselves as well as others, their nearest and dearest. That is why it happens quite frequently that they do not reveal their illness for a long time. The need for control plays an important role in the life of a bulimic, who makes attempts to keep control of food intake (the person controls the quality and quantity of food, performs compulsive eating rituals, etc.), weight, as well as his or her internal experiences and external behaviours. A bulimic individual finds it difficult to accept the fact that he or she is not able to control all aspects of his or her life. In order to become aware of it, the person has to undergo psychotherapy, which is aimed at unblocking the bulimia sufferer's creativity and spontaneity.

Exposure to social situations provokes anxiety in patients with bulimia nervosa, since it triggers the fear of loss of control, or reveals its lack. Once a bulimia sufferer realizes that he or she is unable to control his or her impulses or compensatory behaviours, or even other reactions in the person's life, the individual becomes frustrated and tends to experience intense emotional states (e.g. depression), which the person wishes to avoid. This implies that patients suffering from bulimia nervosa find it difficult to ask for help and seek psychological support. Making a decision to participate in psychotherapy might be the first step in strengthening the bulimic's motivation for introducing changes into his or her life.

Theoretical fundamentals of psychoanalytic and psychodynamic psychotherapy point to the fact that the development of these impulsive (psychopathological) symptoms is underlain by incorrect (destructive) psychological (unconscious) mechanisms which function within the structure of the bulimic individual's personality.

An object relations approach to psychotherapy emphasizes great significance of_human relations which play a key role in the recovery process and replace drives as the main determinant of the person's mental development. The approach focuses on the possibility of making changes within these relations [Mikołajczyk, Samochowiec, Kent, Waller, Dagnan]. Object relations theories are based on an assumption that the patterns of relationships with significant others (objects) formed during early childhood (the early interactions between a child and the most important objects such as the mother, father, or a caretaker) significantly affect the individual's adult relationships and the person's social and emotional functioning (the phenomenon of transference) [Mikołajczyk, Samochowiec, Kent, Waller, Dagnan, Glickauf- Hughes, Wells]. This correlation seems to relate the object relations theory to Moreno's concept of psychodrama, according to which the key to understanding the genesis of the person's emotional problems should be sought in psychological background related to social_relationships, which engenders dysfunctions in the sphere of an individual's reactions and behaviours. Hence integrating the approach which utilizes the corrective influence of "good" object relations therapy with psychodrama techniques such as surplus reality, might prove to be an effective method in the treatment of eating disorders, including bulimia nervosa.

Based on a review of subject literature, and drawing from my own experience gained in the course of individual and group therapy conducted on patients suffering from bulimia nervosa, I wanted to stress in this paper the importance of integrative approach to diagnosis and treatment of bulimia nervosa. My intention was to demonstrate the basic similarities between psychodrama and the object relations theory, and point to the fact that these two therapeutic approaches may complement each other.

2. The psychopathology of bulimia nervosa – as viewed from the perspective of the object relations theory and J.L. Moreno's psychodrama

In my psychotherapeutic work with patients suffering from bulimia nervosa, I refer to a psychoanalytic and psychodynamic paradigm of the psychopathology of this disorder, grounded on the concepts of object relations. Taking into account the psychodynamic principles and the structure of the therapeutic process (e.g. conducting the unconscious input analysis; applying verbal therapeutic interventions including clarification, confrontation and interpretation; taking into consideration the significance of insight, developing a therapeutic relationship, and conducting transference analysis), I have applied Moreno's psychodrama in individual and group therapy which I have been conducting for several years.

According to the fundamental assumptions of psychoanalytically oriented therapies for bulimia nervosa, which underpin the classical psychoanalytic theories based on Freudian concepts, this eating disorder is a biologically determined condition. An object relations approach to the origins of the illness is slightly different. Although the major theoreticians who employ this approach belong to various schools such the British Object Relations School (Klein, Fairbairn, Guntrip, Winnicott), the American Object Relations School (Mahler, Kernerg, Kohut), and the American School of Interpersonal Relations (Sullivan), they put forward unanimous views on the issue of the etiology of eating disorders. They maintain that the origins of the eating disorder psychopathology lay in the person's traumatic life experiences, emotional deficits and patterns (the matrix) of internalized, emotionally destructive interactions of an individual with significant objects, especially the relationships established during childhood, which are "replicated" in all social interactions in the later stages of the person's life [Glickauf- Hughes, Wells]

Identification of this internal pattern of relationships with a caregiver (object) facilitates the process of psychotherapy. A therapist is able to recognize and better understand the client's interpersonal behaviours, as well as modify the internal structure of the individual's personality (object representations, self-representations, feelings). The object relations theory is considered to be in opposition to Freud's classical theory of psychoanalysis, since the person's need for emotional relationships with other people is seen as replacing sexual drive and aggressive impulses as the original motivational system for human behaviour. Focusing on social interactions as a significant element in the development of a human being, the object relations theory resembles a psychodrama approach to an emotional difficulty and an illness symptom in the process of psychotherapy [Glickauf- Hughes, Wells].

In my diagnostic and therapeutic work with patients suffering from bulimia nervosa I refer to the fundamental assumptions of the object relations theory which provide a basis for psychotherapy for this kind of disorder. Whenever I try to diagnose bulimic symptoms (such as episodes of binge eating, self-induced vomiting or purging), I attempt to identify the current as well as the past pattern of the bulimic's relationships with a caregiver (a significant object). Most frequently, I focus on my patient's relationship with his or her mother, not disregarding the significance of the father-patient relationship [Glickauf-Hughes, Wells]. The infant-mother pattern of relationship, formed during infancy and early childhood, related to breastfeeding, proves to be an important factor determining the development of an eating disorder in the later stages of an individual's life. This can be confirmed by many years' research and clinical experiments conducted by Hilda Bruch and other authors [Bruch]. It can be stated that the object relations school emphasizes the significance and dominance of interpersonal and emotional relationships over drives in the process of mental development of an individual [Waller, Kauffman, Teutsch]. Similarly, the major therapeutic and diagnostic assumptions of psychodrama refer to a dominant role of psychological-and-social underpinnings of an individual's behaviour and reactions. In psychodrama the main stress is put on an individual's potential rather than on the specific psychopathology. However, symptoms of the pathology are not disregarded in the therapeutic work on the stage.

In both of the aforementioned therapeutic approaches, considerable significance is attached to the concept of an encounter, interpreted in psychodrama as the phenomenon of "being together; a reciprocal encounter; empathy and sharing; mutual understanding; intuitive insight" [Glickauf- Hughes, Wells, Jay, Blatner, Goldmann, Morrison]. Such an interpretation corresponds to the role that an encounter plays in psychodynamic psychotherapy, which relies on empathy and the so called "authentic patient-therapist relationship", as well as on the therapist's intuition used to develop insight and to take corrective action aimed at establishing an emotional relationship. Thus, the concept of encounter is considered to be equally significant in both therapeutic approaches.

3. Characteristics of psychodrama applied in psychodynamic psychotherapy for patients suffering from bulimia nervosa – a psychological diagnosis of the self-image and self-feelings

Some of the core psychodrama techniques, applied to investigate bulimic symptoms and psychological mechanisms of this disorders include role reversal, role training, doubling, mirroring and surplus reality.

In role reversal, the protagonist reverses his or her role with another person (an auxiliary ego) on the psychodrama stage. This gives the patient-protagonist a chance to enact particular situations, inner thoughts, behaviours or other states from his or her life which are related to the significance of food, body parts and feelings in the patient's life. Thus, role reversal allows the individual to increase his or her self-awareness, and gain insight into how the person reacts in such life situations as feeding, eating, or the mother-child interaction. Role reversal provides invaluable experiential insight through seeing oneself from the perspective of another. The auxiliary ego helps the protagonist explore his or her unconscious conflicts. The role of an auxiliary ego (in monodrama the role is assigned to an object or a director) is to "give voice" to inner thought and feelings the protagonist does not yet feel able to express. It is through a dialogue with the auxiliary ego, accompanying the further role reversals, that the protagonist explores his or her unconscious mind and is able to make corrections to the dysfunctional behaviours. The protagonist enters into a dialogue with him/herself on the psychodrama stage. Reversing roles with his or her stomach or other important body part, a bulimia sufferer has a chance to find out about the unconscious feelings towards these parts, and recognize the destructive behaviours the person tended to engage in. Consequently, as a result of this powerful confrontation technique, the patient is able to introduce positive changes into his or her bahaviour.

The mirror technique involves another member of the group mirroring the protagonist's postures, gestures, and words as they appeared in the enactment. The protagonist observes his or her own bahaviour as reflected by another person, watches the enactment of him/herself from outside, adopts the so called metaposition of an audience member, an observer, and his or her role on the stage is acted out by a double. The mirror and double techniques prove to be effective therapeutic instruments in the process of releasing the repressed feeling of rebellion (anger) or other emotions which a young patient fears or does not notice. Doubling occurs when a member of the group - the therapist-director - takes on the physical stance of the protagonist and attempts to enter his or her internal world by speaking the person's inner thoughts and feelings. Thus, the director is referred to as the unconscious or "inner voice" of the protagonist who might prefer to keep "hidden" [Bruch, Blatner, Goldmann, Morrison]. The technique allows a bulimic patient to become more aware of buried and partially obscured and hidden negative emotions which very often include the feelings of shame for their weakness, and an intense fear of gaining weight.

Doubling is the technique which is designed to support the protagonist (it stimulates the protagonist's response); it involves confrontation (provokes the patient to express his or her feelings and thoughts), and reveals the protagonist's ambivalent feelings (contradictory emotions, thoughts and conflicts). The director is able to express the protagonist's unvoiced thoughts and emotions (e.g. the hidden feeling of anger, the fear of maturity, responsibility and separation), thereby helping the patient deepen insight into psychological mechanisms underlying the bulimic symptoms which the individual suffers from.

A surplus reality technique, frequently applied in psychodrama, provides a patient with corrective emotional experience which the person desired in his or her life but did not have a chance to get due to his or her emotional family deficits (the individual's fundamental needs are not satisfied in the family environment).

Psychodrama techniques may be applied in the preliminary stages of individual psychodynamic psychotherapy, when a therapist builds therapeutic alliance with a client. In this phase, props (objects) assume the role of an auxiliary ego. Reversing roles with the auxiliary ego, the patient explores his or her unconscious emotions. It applies also to the preliminary stage of psychodrama - the so called warm-up phase. The warm-up technique applied in the early phase of individual psychodynamic therapy is a dialogue with a patient. During an early individual session, the client is asked such questions as: "How are you today?", "How is it going?", "What would you like to talk about today?". Such exploratory questions and therapeutic interventions prepare the patient for further stages of psychodramatic work aimed at exploring the person's feelings, attitudes, beliefs, and social relationships. Since the warm-up phase of the individual psychodynamic therapy session involves verbal communication, and lasts for a relatively short period of time, it is difficult for the patient to get prepared for the role of a protagonist. A protagonist, who displays certain characteristic personality traits (which was scientifically proven), uses a variety of defence mechanisms which include emotional blockage, dissociation, denial, rationalization, cognitive distortions concerning body image and self-assessment [Kent ,Waller, Dagnan].

The techniques and exercises which a therapist employs in the warm-up phase of the session, must be carefully selected, since they are designed to develop a sense of safety, a foundation of trust, which would facilitate the process of self-exploration. The techniques applied in the therapy for bulimia sufferers, who regard their bodies as "bad objects which should be destroyed", should facilitate the gradual process of making the patient acquainted with work on the stage (it refers both to group and individual therapy), and making it easier for him or her to get accustomed to physical contact, through teaching the individual how to touch various body parts. If the techniques are applied to fast, it might result in deepening the patient's trauma, especially if the person had experienced body boundary violation before. Taking into account the psychological profile of a bulimic, I seldom employ typical protagonist games. Applying the game therapy might be particularly risky in case of patients who reveal symptoms of personality pathologies such as psychosis, impulsive personality disorder or borderline personality disorder.

It is a frequent occurrence that when bulimic patients start their treatment, their first and primary objective is to eliminate the uncomfortable compensatory behaviours that they exhibit (such as regular cycles of binge eating and purging, self-induced vomiting, or taking laxatives), which very often cause embarrassment, guilt and even self-disgust. During the very early stage of treatment, when I try to develop a therapeutic alliance with the patient, and establish a contract which specifies the goals and procedures concerning the verbal dialogue and the treatment of psychopathology, based on theoretical assumptions of psychodynamic psychotherapy, I usually apply such psychodramatic techniques as role reversal and the mirror. The psychodrama stage is not only the physical space in which the patient-protagonist enacts situations from his or her life, but it also represents symbolically the client's internal world of feelings and emotions which the individual experiences when coming for therapy.

In the first-contact sessions I tend to use visualization and the technique which involves setting up particular scenes on the stage. If a patient resists participating in psychodrama work on the stage (e.g. the person is silent or flatly refuses to act on the stage), I resort to therapeutic dialogue with the person, trying to identify the source of the patient's resistance. In the next phase, I suggest that the patient should try to set up a scene without getting up from his or her chair. I encourage the individual to create certain scenes from his or her life, to show on the stage what hindered his or her decision to take up treatment and seek therapist's help earlier. At this stage, I introduce an auxiliary ego, whose task is to take on the so called symbolic roles (e.g. the roles of the props chosen by the patient to represent symbolically the elements of the scene he or she is attempting to create). The props used in the session include sheets of colourful paper, or scarves, and help the resistant, silent, or impulsive patient who is often full of self-disgust, describe what he or she really sees, or even feels. However, the person is not encouraged to judge his or her experiences as "good" or "bad", which makes the patient feel that he or she is engaged in setting up his or her own scene.

The interview the therapist-director conducts with the patient-protagonist prior to the therapeutic game, when the individual is sitting on the chair, describing what he or she sees and feels, setting up his or her scene using symbolic objects, allows the therapist to prepare the next phase of the session which is aimed at identifying the factors affecting the patient's motivation for treatment, and discovering the genesis of the illness (the therapist explores the patient's repressed feelings, and internal conflicts which underlie the symptoms of the illness). Once the patient becomes more active (i.e. he or she responds to the director's questions, chooses props and arranges them in such a way that helps the person visualize what he or she sees or feels), I usually invite the individual-protagonist to stand up and analyze the sequence of scenes set up on the stage. The realism of the scene setting promotes maximum opportunity for warming up, for expression of actions, thoughts and feelings. The scenes created by the protagonist bring out the reasons of the person's delayed decision to approach a therapist, the obstacles which the individual had to overcome in order to start therapy, and the current inner world of the patient's feelings and emotions. It is frequently at this stage that the patient reveals his or her self-feelings, concerns over body image, and his or her approach to an illness. The therapeutic technique I usually apply in this situation is the use of symbols, which is designed to help the patient work through the aforementioned issues.

From subject literature as well as my own clinical experience, it appears that patients (especially females) with bulimia nervosa very often bring up the issue of negative (auto-destructive) feelings they have towards their bodies such as self-disgust, embarrassment, anger, anxiety, and a desire to overcome those feelings [Lacey, Evans]. If the issue of self-disgust, which is related to the problem of binge eating and self-induced vomiting, occurs during the therapy, I often encourage the patient to use one of the props (e.g. one of the colourful scarves) to represent his or her self-disgust. When holding an object which is a symbol of the person's self-disgust, the bulimic patient is able to take a closer look at it as well as feel it, and the therapist-director can enquire about the person's experience (the therapist tries to find out whether it is intense, overwhelming, or strong, and to identify its length, structure and genesis, etc). Thus, the patient has a chance to overcome his or her resistance and to identify the self-feelings the person experiences, whereas the therapist is able to make a preliminary diagnosis of psychological factors determining the bulimic symptoms the patient suffers from.

When the patient-protagonist talks about his or her feelings (e.g. he or she says: "I feel ashamed and terrified"), I ask the individual to enact a scene which would represent the person's embarrassment and extreme fear. I encourage my patient to use objects (props) to show the feelings of embarrassment and terror which he or she experiences. Afterwards, I suggest that the patient should reverse roles with some chosen elements of the scene he or she has just created.

The patient-protagonist, encouraged by the therapist-director's enquiries, is thus able to reveal his or her inner contradictory thoughts and feelings concerning various aspects of the person's self (e.g. the reasons behind the patient's imprecise motivation for taking up treatment). The therapist-director interviews the patient-protagonist who is in the role of self-disgust or terror, asking him or her the following questions: "How strong and intense are you?", "When did you originate?", "What is your colour?", "What is your main characteristic feature?", and others. This allows the individual to show, using symbols, the source of his or her fear or shame.

Another feeling reported by a bulimic patient at this stage of therapy is anger. The protagonist is encouraged to reverse roles with anger and asked to answer the director's questions such as: "What is your origin?", "When_did you originate?", "How strong are you?", "Who are you directed at?", "Who do you serve?", "Are you the protagonist's friend or enemy?", and others. The technique is instrumental in increasing the patient's awareness of the feeling of anger directed towards him/herself as well as towards others. Once I discover that the feelings which the patient exhibits are intense and have been lasting for a long period of time, and I find out that the person is under pressure from his or her family to recover quickly and fully from an illness, I understand why the patient-protagonist's attitude to an illness and his or her own body is dominated by the feelings of resistance, shame, anger and anxiety.

The therapeutic method which involves portraying on the stage auto-destructive feelings exhibited by the patient- protagonist, who is supported and understood by a therapist-director, allows to strengthen the bulimia sufferer, stimulate his or her greater spontaneity, and encourages the person to design possible scenarios of overcoming such pathological impulsive behaviours as binge eating or self-induced vomiting. While interviewing the psychodrama participant, the director is able to bring out the negative aspects of the patient's feelings which he or she seems to be unaware of. The therapist supports and guides the bulimic individual during the process of making a decision concerning taking up treatment, as well as in coping with the aforementioned bulimic symptoms and destructive feelings (especially the feeling of guilt) which the person suffers from in everyday life. Application of the mirror technique allows the protagonist to observe his or her own bahaviour as reflected by another person, and watch the enactment of him/herself from outside. The patient adopts the so called metaposition of an audience member, and his or her role on the stage is acted out by a double. Taking on the role of an observer helps the protagonist adopt a less emotional approach to stage enactment, fosters self-reflection, and provides the person with a cognitive and intellectual insight into the factors underlying his or her bulimic symptoms.

4. Application of monodrama in individual psychotherapy aimed at investigating compensatory behaviours and bulimic symptoms

When I manage to establish a successful therapeutic relationship with my bulimic patient, he or she gradually starts to reveal the negative, repeatedly accumulating life experiences, and uncomfortable disease symptoms the sufferer has to cope with. At this stage, the patient is frequently very reluctant to accept the fact that bulimia nervosa is a recurrent disease. A bulimic person often suffers from abnormally low self-esteem, which usually determines the individual's negative (auto-destructive) view of oneself and the surrounding world ("I am nobody, I am nothing").

When bulimics approach a therapist, seeking his or her help, they frequently talk about the feelings of pain, remorse, anxiety and shame, which are related to the compensatory behaviours that they engage in, such as binge eating or self-induced vomiting. I recall the words of my bulimic patients who tend to complain: "It is so hard for me; I didn't make it again; I went on a binge again; I'd rather disappear than live this kind of life", or they say: "I cried over myself; I could feel pain all over my body just after the binge; I stuffed myself like a pig; It won't work; I'm a looser; Each time I do it, I promise myself that it is going to be the last time, but it doesn't make sense." Other female patients often confess: "After the binge I feel like scrubbing everything out, wash and clean everything, I always wash myself after the binge to cover up all the tracks, to forget…; I have never felt such self-disgust before, I feel I am nothing when I do it, I puke, I stink and I don't know what is going to happen next". I realize that in the context of auto-destructive thoughts reported by my patients, and their denial of body image, I should make an attempt at integrating monodrama with such therapeutic approaches as a therapeutic dialogue and psychodynamic psychotherapy which focuses on conducting transference analysis and developing cognitive and emotional insight by means of verbal therapeutic interventions such as clarification, confrontation and interpretation. Monodrama is a psychodramatic technique in which there is only one participant - a protagonist, who is asked by a director to select a group of props (e.g. objects, scarves), which take on the role of an auxiliary ago. If I receive my patient's consent, I start investigating his or her bulimic symptoms (I place special emphasis on the cycle: binge eating-vomiting- the feeling of guilt), employing such monodrama techniques as role reversal, mirroring, doubling, or surplus reality. In the last of the aforementioned techniques, the director invites the protagonist to enact the unreal, "imaginary" scenes from his or her life, to act out what had never happened, but what the person would have liked to happen, to "undo" what was done, and to do what needs to be done. Thus, surplus reality helps transcend the boundaries of the "real world" of the protagonist; it is reenactment of a traumatic situation in which the protagonist can take corrective action [Tomalski,

Izydorczyk]. Below I present a short scenario of a monodrama applied in individual therapy for bulimia nervosa.

4.1 Monodrama dynamics – clinical case description

A 23 year old patient, a single woman with no children, brought up in a two-parent family, an only child, who has been suffering from bulimia nervosa for several years. The first bulimic symptoms (such as binge eating and self-induced vomiting) appeared at the age of 17 as a consequence of desperate attempts at losing weight, and prior symptoms of anorexia nervosa. For the first time, the patient decided to undergo therapy when the number of binge eating episodes incresed to more than a dozen a day. This led to physical as well as mental health deterioration (symptom worsening, stomach ache, collapse, fainting, or depression). Worsening of symptoms, accompanied by ambivalence about undertaking treatment, drove the woman's decision to approach a doctor and a psychotherapist. She did it because she was in fear for her life.

The monodrama scenario - a preliminary phase: warm- up

During the early phase of one of the sessions of psychodynamic psychotherapy (conducted on a weekly basis), when talking about what happened between the previous visit and the current session, the bulimic patient brought up the issue of shame and guilt, the feelings she had experienced two day before, when she had a binge of eating and vomiting. Sitting on a chair, the woman confessed that she felt as if she was "in the grasp of something", and complained that she felt stomach ache, and that she did not respect her own body. When I prompted her to explain what she had meant, the patient replied that she was in the grasp of emotions she had mentioned before, and added that she did not understand it. The woman openly admitted that it was hard for her to talk about what she had done and that she was ashamed of it. She added that she found it difficult to reveal her feelings and emotions which she was scared and ashamed of. When talking about disrespect for her body, the patient was sitting on a chair and clutching her stomach. I asked the woman to take notice of that fact and encouraged her to describe the feelings she was experiencing at that moment. I directed the patient's attention to that particular body part because it was the stomach that the woman touched and focused her attention on. Through direct physical contact with her stomach, the patient had a chance to feel it. I regarded this part of the therapy as a warm-up designed to prepare the patient for the further work aimed at investigating her bulimic symptoms (episodes of binge eating and self-induced vomiting). I continued the individual therapy session and received the patient's consent to apply the technique involving stage acting. Performing the role of a director, I encouraged the woman to describe the feelings she experienced when touching her stomach. She replied that she felt guilt, anger and shame. I suggested setting up a scene.

Scene I: "The patient's feelings of guilt, anger and shame"

As a director, I encouraged the patient to choose some colourful scarves to symbolize her feelings. The woman spread three scarves out on the stage: a red one - to represent shame, a black scarf symbolizing anger, and a grey one which was supposed to be the symbol of guilt. Asked about the title of the scene, the woman replied that she didn't know what it was. The patient was unable to name certain things, but the choice of symbolic colours which she had made, proved that the woman was trying to express something in a non-verbal way. Red might have symbolized intensity and ambivalence of the protagonist's feelings. It could have represented the intensity of the feeling of shame as well as be a symbol of life (red is the colour of blood). Black might have stood for the patient's tendency towards depression, the person's sense of helplessness and aggression. Grey seemed to symbolize repressed feelings and a sense of helplessness and uncertainty.

When the patient set up the scene, I suggested that she should reverse roles with the feelings symbolized by the scarves. She refused to do so. At that moment, I realized it was too soon for the patient to confront the feelings, and the woman was not warmed up enough and needed more time. That is why I employed another technique - the mirroring. I introduced an object -a prop (a white scarf chosen by the patient-protagonist) which was supposed to take on the role of an auxiliary ego (the double), and be a component of the scene set up by the protagonist, who placed it in the middle of the stage (in the middle between shame and the feelings of anger and guilt). The protagonist had a chance to watch the scene from the perspective of the audience, which fostered her self-reflection and emotional responsiveness. The woman used the following words to comment on what she had seen: "This is my internal world, dominated by the feelings of guilt, anger and shame". Thus, the patient was able to name the unvoiced feelings which she had experienced.

Finally, I asked the woman to let the objects which she had chosen step out of the roles they were acting out. During the phases of sharing and identification feedback, the patient talked about the experienced feelings of guilt and shame which accompanied her bulimic symptoms ("now I feel ashamed of myself and of my symptoms, it is the feeling of shame that dominates my entire life"). In the final stage of the session I empowered the patient to reduce the feeling of guilt for her bulimic symptoms, and I supported her courageous decision to make an attempt to overcome her illness. I also encouraged the woman to acknowledge the feeling of guilt. I, as it were, gave my client "permission" to feel guilty, since the feeling had already occurred.

During the next few sessions of individual psychotherapy, the patient reported improvements in her mental condition (e.g. a decreased tendency towards depression, less intense feelings of guilt and shame following the cycles of binge eating and self-induced vomiting). However, the woman still suffered from bulimic episodes, occurring twice or three times a day.

At the beginning of one of the further sessions, clutching her stomach, the woman complained: "I've got enough of it, I did it again, I stuffed myself like a pig and I was throwing up. Now, I feel pain all over my body, and I have a terrible burning in my stomach". I asked her to focus on what she was feeling when touching her stomach (I also suggested that she should close her eyes in order to strengthen the body sensations). After a moment of silence, with closed eyes and her hand resting on the stomach, the patient confessed: "I can hear my stomach bubbling, I feel pain in it, and I wish I could tell my stomach that I feel awful doing this to it, but I just can't stop it". Afterwards, I asked my patient to open her eyes and participate in monodrama stage acting.

4.2 Dynamics of the action stage of a monodrama focusing on the theme of a "stomach" (description of the process)

The patient placed a brown scarf on the stage and "cast" it in the role of a stomach. Then, she stood opposite it, taking on the part of a protagonist. Holding the role of a director, I encouraged the participant to reverse roles with her stomach. Once the protagonist took on the part of her stomach, I asked the patient (her stomach): "Ms N. was throwing up

yesterday, do you know anything about it?". Performing the role of the stomach, the patient-protagonist replied: "Yes, I know. That's why I feel so much pain." In the further stages of the session I was interviewing the protagonist in the role of her stomach. The main aim of the psychodrama interview in role reversal was to provide the patient with the opportunity to see the situation from the point of view of the other body part. The protagonist had a chance to explore the feelings and sensations which her own body part (a stomach) was forced to experience when she tormented it with binge eating and self-induced vomiting. Thus, the patient was able to experience ambivalent feelings: pain and suffering of her stomach, and a sense of relief following the episode of vomiting.
Once the protagonist in the role of her stomach admitted that she had lost control over binge eating and vomiting ("I don't know why I'm doing this, I am afraid of something"), I decided, holding the role of a director, to interview my patient in the role of her stomach:

DIRECTOR: "It is anxiety or vomiting that Ms N. suffers from. And what about you, stomach? What about your pain?"
PROTAGONIST-STOMACH: "Well, I will manage to put up with it, it will pass".
DIRECTOR: "Are you helping her overcome anxiety?"
PROTASGONIST-STOMACH: "She feels relieved, so that's how I help her".
DIRECTOR: "Do you consider yourself to be her friend or enemy?"
PROTAGONIST-STOMACH: "Well, I want to make her feel relieved."
DIRECTOR: "But do you think she feels relieved if she feels pain?"
PROTAGONIST-STOMACH: "At least she doesn't feel tense or anxious, which is better than feeling pain. What is more, she maintains her weight. She is afraid of feeling anxious and being fat, which is worse than the feeling of pain."
DIRECTOR: "Worse? Do you mean more dangerous than pain?"
PROTAGONIST-STOMACH: "Yes. She is also scared of what is going to happen to her."
DIRECTOR: "What do you mean? Could you be more specific?"
PROTAGONIST-STOMACH: "You know, she is afraid of being fat, ugly and bad. Now, I'm empty and safe, and she is safe, too. She will not put on weight; she can eat whatever she wants and feel relieved".
DIRECTOR: "Is it only relief that she can feel? You have mentioned also some other feelings ..."
PROTAGONIST-STOMACH: "Well...maybe she feels a bit guilty and she has some pain."
DIRECTOR: "You are saying that you help her. How do you do it?"
PROTAGONIST-STOMACH: "She is not fat and can calm down and feel relaxed, that's how I help her."
DIRECTOR: "Do you think there is any other way to reduce the feeling of guilt and anxiety which she experiences?"
PROTAGONIST-STOMACH: "I don't know. Throwing up is stronger, I can't control it. She would have to get her feet on the ground."
DIRECTOR: "What do you mean?"
PROTAGONIST-STOMACH: "She would have to feel safe and regain self-confidence."
DIRECTOR: "How could she do it? What would you like to tell Ms N.?"
After a moment of silence:
PROTAGONIST-STOMACH: "You destroy me when you throw up, cut it off, think something up."

In the next phase, I asked the protagonist to step out of the role of her stomach and become herself again, and listen to the message which her own stomach passed along to my patient (I gave voice to my patient's stomach, repeating what the protagonist had said in the role of her stomach). The protagonist listened carefully. She seemed nervous (emotionally moved), and finally said with a raised voice:

PROTAGONIST: "Damn throwing up, again! It is disgusting! I want to get rid of this habit, but I don't know how to do it, I can't control it!"
DIRECTOR: "Would you like to get to know what makes you vomit?"
After a while the patient replied:
PROTAGONIST: "It seems to be a good idea. Now I know that vomiting must denote something, but I don't what exactly. Yes, I do want to know the reason behind my throwing up, perhaps it has something to do with my unsettled affairs…"
DIRECTOR: "What affairs?"
PROTAGONIST: "I have to take a closer look at what happened four years ago, that is what gets me down, it was then that I started binge eating."

I reinforced the patient's readiness for further therapeutic work, and asked if we could complete the session. She agreed.

The final phase of monodrama –sharing

In the final phase of monodrama, I asked the patient to let the props which she had chosen, "step out" of their auxiliary ego roles. We completed the sharing phase (the stage during which the patient shared her thoughts and emotions that she had experienced during our therapeutic session) and discussed identification feedback which I gathered from the patient. The woman, having reflected upon the therapeutic work she had been involved in, declared her readiness to "encounter" her habit of vomiting and binge eating on the stage. We scheduled our next session, planning a monodrama whose main theme was supposed to be "the patient's encounter with her habit of vomiting", and we finished the session.

The author's comments on the dynamics of the psychotherapeutic process and the patient's monodrama.

During advanced stages of a therapeutic process, when the relationship between a therapist and a bulimic patient is established, the therapist's role is to focus on the patient's physical symptoms, the individual's internal conflicts and the introjected patterns of relationships with significant others, as well as on correcting developmental deficits. The psychodynamic psychotherapy which I conducted in the bulimic patient whose case I described above was aimed at bringing out the patient's internal conflicts; diagnosing and changing the pathological strategies the patient adopted in order to cope with her internal conflicts; and at interpreting the phenomenon of transference. The monodrama techniques, which utilize symbolic representation, were applied in the therapy for binge eating and self-induced vomiting, frequently followed by a sense of guilt, increasing tension and self-disgust. The method proved to be instrumental in identifying the patient's emotional conflicts and her "here and now" experiences, as well as in exploring the person's accumulated tensions and emotions (especially the negative ones), which she tended to "release" unconsciously, adopting the compulsive, unhealthy compensatory strategies. It proves that the therapy which involves stage acting "weakens" the protagonist's control and defence mechanisms. Monodrama, when applied in the advanced stages of the aforementioned individual therapy, triggers the patient's "emotional catharsis" and leads to the release of tension. This safe and controllable method of tension reduction contributed to diminishing the number of destructive symptoms of an illness. As a result, the person's constructive schemes of perception and cognitive functioning, based on senses, intuition and feelings were developed.

In the further stages of the therapy, the protagonist agreed to experience an encounter with her compulsive habit of vomiting. The purpose of this element of therapy was to encourage the patient to find some alternative ways of coping with her bulimic symptoms. The therapeutic interventions which I undertook at that stage of treatment process were aimed at finding an alternative to the habit of self-induced vomiting which the patient regarded as a way of coping with her destructive feelings. My intention was to evoke in the_bulimia sufferer the feeling of emotional ambivalence toward her symptoms. Setting up a scene on the psychodramatic stage shortly after a period of binge eating and self-induced vomiting (which was the case of my patient), allows a thorough, step-by-step analysis of the bulimic episode, facilitates identifying specific alarm signals which proceed the episode, and provides the protagonist with an opportunity to try out alternative strategies which the person might use in the future to cope with binge eating and self-induced vomiting. Encouraged by the therapist to reverse roles with the particular aspects of the situation proceeding a bulimic episode (ambivalent feelings which occur prior to the episode, situational stress, or interpersonal conflicts) as well as with her self-feelings and bulimic symptoms (binge eating or vomiting), my patient had a chance to unearth some unknown aspects of her personality. The role reversal helped the protagonist realize how destructive it was to try to control her body by engaging in bulimic compensatory behaviours. The technique proved to be useful in stimulating the patient to assume proper control over her own drives, impulses, feelings and needs.

5. Characteristics of group therapy for bulimia patients – application of selected elements of psychodrama

The first sessions of the psychodynamic psychotherapy conducted in a group which is heterogeneous in terms of gender and the character of mental disturbances (neurotic and personality disturbances), are usually aimed at establishing a patient-therapist contract (under which both parties are obliged to maintain confidentiality and participate in all sessions), as well as at building a patient-therapist alliance, which allows to set boundaries and strengthens the individual's sense of security. Patients with bulimia nervosa usually adopt a characteristic attitude to therapy. They seek guidance, assistance and structure, and wish a therapist could lift the burden of emotional discomfort (impulsiveness, the feeling of shame and guilt about their bulimic symptoms) from their shoulders as soon as they take up therapy. The issue which bulimic patients usually bring up during therapy sessions is a relationship with mother and a desire to have the so called "good mother". They tend to project this desire onto a group therapist [Lacey, Evans, Levens ,Jay].

In advanced stages of psychodynamic group therapy aimed at developing the patients' insight into psychological mechanisms underlying the eating disorder they suffer from, individual bulimia sufferers tend to focus on their own problems and difficulties related to their compensatory bulimic symptoms. They concentrate less on the problems of other therapy group members, which is followed by the feeling of guilt they report in the further phase of the therapy. What characterizes a psychodrama group is the fact that as a result of working on the stage in the role of a protagonist, its participants experience an incresed feeling of guilt once they realize that they "have taken up other participants' time, focusing other group members' attention on their own problems". Thus they repeat a pattern of a bulimic cycle: obsessive compulsive eating and vomiting followed by a sense of guilt [Jay]. However, in the early stages of group therapy, the similar diagnostic background (the problems and difficulties related to eating disorders) of its participants allows to create a sense of group identification and build mutual trust among group members. A common feeling among group therapy members, especially when a group is just starting, is that of being isolated, unique, and apart from others. Enormous relief accompanies the recognition that they are not alone, which is a special benefit of group therapy. The phenomenon of sharing experiences among group members, which Yalom refers to as "universality", is a major therapeutic factor which helps group therapy participants overcome their sense of isolation.

It is a common case that people suffering from bulimia nervosa spend their energy on satisfying others. The therapy group, watching the protagonist acting out the roles he or she chooses (e.g. the role of "a loving sister", "a loyal friend", or "a diligent student"), provides supportive witnessing and helps the individual get in touch with the denied, "needy" aspects of him/herself, as well as acknowledge those aspects of his or her personality which the person regards as satisfactory. Thus, a patient has a chance to build a more complete self-image, which is, as it were, contrary to the "bad/poor" bulimic self-representation [Jay]. Group members need the therapist's assistance when the therapy proceeds from the preliminary stage of identification into the phase of establishing the relationships which are not related to the sphere of eating. There are certain structured exercises that the therapist might employ as an effective tool to facilitate the aforementioned process. An example might be an exercise in which the therapy participants' task is to follow the therapist's instruction: "Put eating aside for a while and think about two feelings which you often experience. Take on the roles of these feelings and introduce yourselves to your partners." This exercise helps to increase group identification [Levens]. Spontaneous behaviour is regarded by bulimic patients as irresponsible and reckless, and is usually followed by a sense of guilt. Hence it is necessary for the therapist to prepare clients for such spontaneous reactions by means of exercises aimed at increasing the participants' self-esteem and building up mutual trust within the group [Lacey, Evans, Jay]. The more structured the exercises are, the more relaxed the group becomes. As the therapy proceeds, the level of tolerance increases and it makes it possible for the therapist to gradually abandon the structured exercises. Prior to feeling accepted by other group members, the therapy participant feels he or she must take on the role of a protagonist and act out the particular bulimic aspects of his or her life, very often using symbols (e.g. a fridge, favourite food consumed during the episode of binge eating). Role reversal proves to be an effective technique aimed at facilitating the patient's understanding of the symbolic context, which in turn allows the person to explore his or her problems concerning the issue of relationships. A bulimia sufferer has a chance to encounter his or her despair, inner emptiness, denied needs and repressed anger. The patient finds it difficult to acknowledge the fact that he or she "is given to" by others, which is followed by a sense of guilt. "Being given to", as opposed to "giving", is what bulimics feel uncomfortable about. According to Yalom, altruism is an important healing factor in group therapy [Yalom]. It fosters unconditional satisfaction of needs, which in turn, in case of therapy for bulimia nervosa, facilitates therapeutic investigation, e.g. it leads to discovering the roots of guilt which follows the act of "getting" something from others. Psychodramatic techniques can considerably improve the process of investigating bulimic symptoms.

6. Summary

Since psychodrama is a method which utilizes a universal concept of time (the past, the present and the future), place and a scene, as well as the so called surplus reality, it can support psychodynamic psychotherapy applied in the treatment of bulimia nervosa.
Psychodrama is a therapeutic method which takes into account a variety of aspects which include social relationships, personality features, internal conflicts, attitudes and beliefs. Thus, the technique provides an opportunity to intensify and accelerate the process of developing emotional and cognitive insight into the mechanisms underlying an eating disorder. Through role playing and spontaneous behaviour, psychodrama triggers constructive feedback from a patient who discovers effective problem solving strategies to replace old destructive ones, and thus finds an alternative to his or her disease symptoms. Spontaneity and creativity in the here and now, which are focused on in psychodrama sessions, allow the participant to explore his or her internal conflicts which the person tends to "transfer" onto his or her body. This proves that psychodrama is an effective therapeutic method, which can be combined with the fundamental principles of psychodynamic psychotherapy, based on the patient-therapist relationship. It can be concluded that the core idea which underpins both of the aforementioned therapeutic approaches is the patient-therapist encounter aimed at accomplishing the objective specified in the therapy contract.

7. References

[1] Mikołajczyk E., Samochowiec J., Cechy osobowości u pacjentek z zaburzeniami odżywiania. Psychiatria Via Medica 2004; vol.1, no. 2, 91-95

[2] Kent A., Waller G., Dagnan, D., A greater role of emotional than physical or sexual abuse in predicting disordered eating attitudes: the role of mediating variables. Int. J. Eat Disord.1999, vol. 25, 2, p.159-67

[3] Hartt J. Waller G., Child abuse, dissociation and core beliefs in bulimic disorders. Child Abuse .Neglect.Sep.2002, vol.26, 9, p.923-38

[4] Wonderlich SA., et al. Eating disturbance and sexual trauma in childhood and adulthood. Int. J Eat Disord.2001, vol. 30, 4, p.401-12

[5] Rorty M., Yager J., Rossotto E., Childhood sexual, physical and psychological abuse in bulimia nervosa. Am. J Psychiatry, 1994, vol. 151, 8, p.1122-26

[6] Kent A., Waller G., Childhood emotional abuse and eating psychopathology. Clinical Psychology Rev.2000, vol. 20, 7, p.887-903

[7] Lacey, J.H., Evans, C.D.H., The impulsivist: A Multi - Impulsive Personality Disorder. British Journal of Addition, 81, 641-649

[8] Bruch H., Death in Anorexia Nervosa, "Psychosomatic Medicine", 1971; 33, no.2

[9] Bruch H., Psychotherapy in primary anorexia nervosa, in: The psychiatric treatment of adolescents, (ed.) H.A. Esman "Int. Universities Press", New York, 1983

[10] Hay PJ, Bacaltchuk J, Byrnes RT, Claudino AM, Ekmejian AA, Yong PY. Individual psychotherapy in the outpatient treatment of adults with anorexia nervosa. Cochrane Database of Syst. Rev 2003, Issue 4. CD003909.DOL:101002/14651858.CD003909.If 4.6UPDATED 2008

[11] Bahar E, Latzer Y, Kreitler S, Berry EM. Empirial comparison of two psychological therapies. Self psychology and cognitive orientation in the treatment of anorexia and bulimia. Journal of Psychotherapy and Practice Research 1999;8:115-28
[12] Glickauf- Hughes Ch., Wells M., Object Relations Psychotherapy. An Individual and Integrative Approach to Diagnosis and Treatment. Jason Aronson, Inc.1997
[13] Waller JV, Kauffman R.M, Teutsch F., Anorexia nervosa: a psychosomatic entity? Psychosomatic Medicine 1940, vol. 2, p.3-16
[14] Tomalski R., Dysocjacja i aleksytymia u chorych z bulimią i zespołem gwałtownego objadania się, niepublikowana praca doktorska, Śląski Uniwersytet Medyczny, Katowice, 2009
[15] Glickauf- Hughes Ch., Wells M., Object Relations Psychotherapy. An Individual and Integrative Approach to Diagnosis and Treatment. Jason Aronson, Inc.1997
[16] Izydorczyk B. Psychodrama w leczeniu anoreksji psychicznej, [in:] Psychodrama. Elementy teorii i praktyki, in: A. Bielańska, ed. Eneteia, Warszawa, 2009
[17] Levens M. Art Therapy and Psychodrama with Eating Disordered patients In: Fragile Board Arts Therapies and Clients with Eating Disorders, Jessica Kingsley Publishers, London and Philadelphia, 2000, p.159 -174
[18] Jay S. The Use of Psychodrama in the Field of Bulimia. In: Fragile Board Arts Therapies and Clients with Eating Disorders, Jessica Kingsley Publishers, London and Philadelphia, 2000, p. 177-189
[19] Blatner. A., Foundations of Psychodrama: History, Theory and Practice. New York: Springer Publishing. Co, 1988
[20] Goldmann E.E., Morrison D.S., Psychodrama. Experience and process. Dubinque, Iowa: Kendall/Hunt Publishing, Co, 1984
[21] Yalom I. Leszcz M. Psychoterapia grupowa – teoria i praktyka. Kraków, Wydawnictwo Uniwersytetu Jagiellońskiego, 2006

3

Gastrointestinal Aspects of Bulimia Nervosa

Elena Lionetti[1], Mario La Rosa[1],
Luciano Cavallo[2] and Ruggiero Francavilla[2]
[1]*University of Catania*
[2]*University of Bari*
Italy

1. Introduction

Eating disorders are an important cause of physical and psychosocial morbidity in adolescent girls, young adult women, and to lesser extent in men. In the diagnostic and statistical manual of mental disorders fourth edition (DSM-IV), three broad categories of eating disorders are delineated: anorexia nervosa, bulimia nervosa, and eating disorder not otherwise specified (American Psychiatric Association, 1994). The international classification of diseases tenth revision (ICD-10) also reported three categories of eating disorders: anorexia nervosa, bulimia nervosa, and atypical eating disorder (World Health Organization, 1992). In detail, anorexia nervosa is characterised by extremely low bodyweight and a fear of its increase; bulimia nervosa comprises repeated binge eating, followed by behaviour to counteract it. The category of eating disorder not otherwise specified encompasses variants of these disorders, but with sub-threshold symptoms (e.g., menstruation still present despite clinically significant weight loss, purging without objective binging) (Treasure et al., 2010).

The main feature that distinguishes bulimia nervosa from anorexia nervosa is that attempts to restrict food intake are punctuated by repeated binges (episodes of eating during which there is an aversive sense of loss of control and an unusually large amount of food is eaten). The amount consumed in these binges varies, but is typically between 4.2 MJ (1000 kcals) and 8.4 MJ (2000 kcals) (Fairburn & Harrison, 2003). In order to prevent weight gain, self-induced vomiting and excessive exercise, as well as the misuse of laxatives, diuretics, thyroxine, amphetamine or other medication, may occur. The combination of under-eating and binge eating results in bodyweight being generally unremarkable, providing the other obvious difference from anorexia nervosa. There is some controversy concerning whether those who binge eat but do not purge should be included within this diagnostic category. The ICD-10 criteria stress the importance of purging behaviour on the grounds that vomiting and laxative misuse are considered pathological behaviours in our society in comparison to dieting and exercise. The DSM-IV criteria agree about the importance of compensatory behaviour but distinguish between the purging type of bulimia nervosa in which the person regularly engages in self-induced vomiting or the misuse of laxatives, diuretics or enemas, from the non-purging type in which other inappropriate compensatory behaviours such as fasting or excessive exercise occur but not vomiting or laxative misuse (National Collaborating Centre for Mental Health, 2004).

It is noteworthy that bulimia may be suspected also in patients undergoing bariatric surgery. Indeed, this kind of surgery, also named weight loss surgery, includes a variety of procedures performed on people who are obese. Weight loss is achieved by reducing the size of the stomach with an implanted medical device (gastric banding) or through removal of a portion of the stomach (sleeve gastrectomy or biliopancreatic diversion with duodenal switch) or by resecting and re-routing the small intestines to a small stomach pouch (gastric bypass surgery). When determining eligibility for bariatric surgery, psychiatric screening is critical.

Bulimia nervosa may lead to significant morbidity and mortality. The diagnosis depends on obtaining a history supported, as appropriate, by the corroborative account of a parent or relative. This will require an empathic, supportive, non-judgemental interview style in which the person is enabled to reveal the extent of his or her symptoms and behaviours. Although those with bulimia nervosa generally have fewer serious physical complications than those with anorexia nervosa, they commonly report more physical complaints when first seen (National Collaborating Centre for Mental Health, 2004). The gastrointestinal tract is the site of most acute and chronic medical complications of the disease (Table 1). Identification of any of the gastrointestinal aspects may aid in establishing an early diagnosis, which has been shown to increase the likelihood of recovery.

Effects of bulimia
Dental erosion
Dental caries
Oral dryness
Parotid and salivary glands enlargement (raised serum amylase)
Dysphagia
Esophagitis/oesophageal ulcers
Vomiting
Hematemesis (rare)
Increased gastric capacity
Delayed gastric empting
Gastric rupture (rare, but high letality)
Bloating
Abdominal pain
Diarrhoea
Constipation
Volvulus (rare)
Rectal prolapse (rare)

Table 1. Common adverse effects of bulimia nervosa on the gastro-intestinal tract.

Many changes in gastrointestinal physiology are associated with bulimia nervosa. Some of these are particularly interesting because they may favour the maintenance or even an increase in eating disorder symptoms and so militate against recovery. Some gastrointestinal complications are due to unrelenting abuse of the alimentary canal occurring over the course of years. Others occur in an acute form in a severely ill patient and may require urgent attention.

In this chapter we provide a systematic review of the existing literature on the gastrointestinal involvement in patients affected by bulimia nervosa. We searched the Medline databases for articles on bulimia nervosa published since 1980. The key words used were eating disorders, bulimia nervosa, bulimia, binge eating, gastro-intestinal tract, oesophagus, stomach, oral cavity, and bowels. Only articles written in English were reviewed.

2. Oral cavity

Oral pathology plays a crucial role in the diagnosis of bulimia, often providing the vital link between the patient and medical intervention. The acidic contents of the regurgitated in patients with bulimia nervosa causes erosion of the deciduous and permanent dentition. The erosion particularly affects the posterior teeth and the palatal aspects of the upper anterior teeth; both the deciduous and the permanent dentitions can be affected. Erosions generally occur after six months of vomiting behaviour, and severity of erosions increases with time. The erosion of enamel of the teeth exposes the underlying dentin, producing acute contact and thermal hypersensitivity (pain on eating hot or cold meals).

Dental caries are a further oral feature of bulimia nervosa, and are related either to the cariogenicity of the diet or to the lowering pH sustained by vomiting. To protect teeth from the effects of chronic vomiting, regular dental review is highly recommended; patients should be given appropriate advice on dental hygiene, which should include avoid brushing teeth after vomiting as it may increase tooth damage, mouth rinsing after vomiting with water and sodium bicarbonate (or other non-acid mouth wash) in order to neutralise the acid environment, use of fluoride mouth rinses and toothpastes which may be helpful for desensitisation, reduce intake of acidic foods (fruit, fruit juice, carbonated drinks, pickled products, yoghurt and some alcoholic drinks), finishing meals with alkaline foods (e.g. milk or cheese), avoiding habits such as prolonged sipping, holding acidic beverages in the mouth and "frothing" prior to swallowing, chewing sugar-free gum after meals to stimulate salivary flow (although this may cause increased gastric secretions).

Painless bilateral enlargement of salivary glands (especially the parotid gland, but occasionally the submandibular salivary glands) are a frequent finding in bulimia nervosa, and are a useful indicator in diagnosing and monitoring the disease, avoiding unnecessary tests. Possible explanations for enlarged parotid glands include nutritional deficiencies, excessive starch consumption, re-feeding after starvation, and functional hypertrophy associated with repeated episodes of binge eating. Therefore, increase amylase secretion is characteristic of bulimia nervosa, and it may be useful in monitoring the degree of compliance to therapeutic programs (Anderson et al., 1997).

Oral dryness may also be a sign of bulimia nervosa; although no differences between patients with bulimia nervosa and controls has been found in the salivary flow rates and fluid secretory capacity for parotid and submandibular glands, oral dryness may be related to surface mucosal alteration and to a change in ability to perceive moisture adequately (Anderson et al., 1997).

3. Oesophagus

Pharyngeal and velar gag reflex may be impaired in bulimia nervosa. This was believed to be a learned response and a form of desensitization from years of gastric purging. Loss of the gag reflex facilitates self-induced vomiting by making it less aversive. Abnormal oesophageal motility has also been found frequently in patients with bulimia. Initially, patients need to provoke the gag reflex using their fingers or another object, whereas in advanced stages, physical means may not be necessary. Reflux of gastric contents into the lower oesophagus may cause relaxation of the lower oesophageal sphincter; loss of sphincter control may be sufficient to induce vomiting.

Vomiting is the main symptom suggestive of bulimia. It may be induced by medications such as ipecac, hypertonic saline, or other emetogenic substances. It may be a result of self-induced gagging, as mentioned above; therefore, calluses on the back of the hand may be found (Russell's sign), suggesting the use of the hand to stimulate the gag reflex and induce vomiting. It may also be promoted by forceful abdominal muscle contraction during spontaneous lower oesophageal sphincter relaxations associated with belching. This characteristic is sometimes useful in manometrically discriminating the patient with bulimia from the patient with gastro-oesophageal reflux. These patients often vomit surreptitiously.

Vomiting and subsequent electrolyte disturbances may lead to cardiac and metabolic effects out side the alimentary canal, such as dehydration, hypokalaemia and cardiac dysrhythmias and hypochloremic alkalosis. When electrolyte disturbance is detected, it is usually sufficient to focus on eliminating the behaviour responsible. In the small proportion of cases where supplementation is required to restore the patient's electrolyte balance, oral rather than intravenous administration is recommended, unless there are problems with gastrointestinal absorption (National Collaborating Centre for Mental Health, 2004).

Dysphagia, esophagitis, oesophageal erosions, ulcers and bleeding occur frequently in patients who practise self-induced vomiting. However, it has been suggested that psychiatric diagnosis is often mistaken and that many patients thought to have eating disorders may well be suffering primarily from oesophageal disorders such as achalasia. Therefore, bulimia nervosa should be considered in the diagnostic work-up of patients referred for suspect gastro-oesophageal reflux disease, but a 24-h oesophageal multichannel intraluminal impedance, endoscopy and/or manometry should be always performed to excluded an organic cause of symptoms.

Hematemesis may result from a mucosal tear of the lower end of the oesophagus during vomiting (Mallory-Weiss Syndrome) or from haemorrhagic esophagitis due to acid reflux. The initial evaluation of any patient with upper gastrointestinal bleeding must include a brief history followed by a rapid assessment of the physical condition, with particular attention to the vital signs and the patient's level of consciousness. If the bleeding is severe, therapy may need to begin before the location of the bleeding can be ascertained. Significant gastrointestinal bleeding will be initially manifest by tachycardia, whereas hypotension occurs later, an ominous signal of impending cardiovascular collapse. Immediate therapy is aimed at correction of volume loss and anaemia, which should include aggressive fluid and blood resuscitation. If the patient remains unstable after receiving a blood transfusion of approximately 85 mL/kg or greater, emergency exploratory surgery is indicated. Surgical consultation is mandatory in any case of severe upper gastrointestinal bleeding.

Small amounts of red blood in vomitus may be due to the fingernails injuring the pharynx and the history and examination will generally clarify this.

4. Stomach

Gastric capacity increases in bulimia nervosa, presumably as a result of repeated large volume binge-eating episodes. This may be associated with an absence of satiety signals until a large amount of food has been ingested. A decrease in gastric emptying rate is also been found in bulimic patients, as well as lower amplitude of antral contractions.
Acute gastric dilation has rarely been reported in bulimia nervosa. It is usually accompanied by pain and discomfort. Stomach (or oesophageal) perforation is a complication, which has a high mortality, and occurs in two situations. Firstly, it may occur in a patient with unrecognized acute gastric dilatation who continues to eat or binge. The thin gastric wall continues to dilate and eventually tears. The result may be an acute abdomen with sub-diaphragmatic air observed on an erect abdominal or chest X-ray. Alternatively, there may be a relatively silent oesophageal tear with air observed in the mediastinum on the chest X-ray. The condition is an acute surgical emergency requiring immediate laparotomy and repair. Secondly, it may occur in a patient, who may be of normal weight, who is unable to vomit following a binge-eating episode and suffers a gastric or oesophageal (Mallory-Weiss) tear. The cause appears to be strenuous attempts to vomit, which expose the stomach to extreme strain and rupture.

5. Bowels

Bulimic patients often abuse laxatives; indeed, patients believe that laxatives prevent absorption, having observed solid food appear in their stools, although it has been showed that laxatives have no detectable effect on the absorption of liquid nutrients. Stimulant laxatives are most frequently used, because they are fast-acting and reliable way to produce watery diarrhoea; therefore the effects of laxative abuse include diarrhoea, steatorrhea, and general malabsorption of nutrients. Irritable bowel syndrome type symptoms may be present. Colonic damage is mainly the result of prolonged abuse of laxatives, which have been shown to cause degeneration of the colonic autonomic nerve supply. The urgent presentations of colonic dysfunction are due to the weak, atonic cathartic colon. This can present as volvulus, prolapse of the rectum through the anus and intractable constipation. Any of these problems, if severe enough, can require surgery and sometimes colectomy. Mouth to caecum and total gut transit times are significantly prolonged, as is colonic transit time. This slowing, in addition to gastric delay, may also contribute to prolonged satiety by producing long-lasting feelings of general abdominal fullness.
Constipation is extremely common, mainly due to dehydration. Recommended treatment to avoid constipation is regular food intake, adequate fluids and exercise.
Laxative abuse carries also the acute complication of electrolyte and fluid disturbances and can be particularly dangerous in low weight individuals. Abrupt cessation of laxatives in those who are taking them regularly can result in reflex fluid and sodium retention, and consequent weight gain, and oedema. This can increase patient anxiety and reluctance to curtail the use of laxatives. To avoid this effect a gradual reduction in laxative use is advised (National Collaborating Centre for Mental Health, 2004).

6. Pancreas

Fasting and binge eating foods high in refined carbohydrates, especially if vomiting follows this, can lead to high levels of insulin release by the pancreas with large fluctuations in blood sugar levels. This may disrupt the appetite control mechanisms and the utilisation and deposition of energy. Serotonin is implicated in appetite regulation (there may be a particular role in carbohydrate balance); disruptions in serotonin levels may be affected by the impact of insulin on its precursor, tryptophan, and in turn acute tryptophan depletion may lead to an increase in calorie intake and irritability in bulimia nervosa and may be related to decreased mood, increased rating in body image concern and subjective loss of control of eating in people who have recovered from bulimia nervosa (National Collaborating Centre for Mental Health, 2004).

7. Conclusions

Bulimia nervosa is a common health problem in young people, has been reported worldwide both in developed regions and emerging economies, and its prevalence is arising. It can lead to serious medical complications. However, studies from the US and continental Europe suggest that only a fraction of people with bulimia receive specialised treatment for their eating disorder. The alimentary canal is the front line for the eating disorder patient. Therefore, the expression of the disease in the gastrointestinal tract may have a critical role in early diagnosis and management of the disease. New treatment strategies are now available, and evidence-based management of this disorder is possible. A specific form of cognitive behaviour therapy is the most effective treatment, although few patients seem to receive it in practice.

8. References

American Psychiatric Association. (1994). *Diagnostic and statistical manual of mental disorders (4th edn)*, ISBN 0-89042-062-9, Washington, USA.

Anderson L, Shaw JM, McCargar L. (1997). Physiological effects of bulimia nervosa on the gastrointestinal tract. *Can J Gastroenterol*, Vol.11, No.5, (July-August 1997), pp. 451-9, ISSN 0835-7900.

World Health Orgaganization. (1992). *International statistical classification of diseases and related health problems (ICD-10)*. ISBN 92-4-1546492, Geneva, Switzerland.

Treasure J, Claudino AM, Zucker N. (2010). Eating disorders. *Lancet*, Vol.375, (February 2010), pp. 583-93, ISSN 0140-6736.

Fairburn CG, Harrison PJ. (2003). Eating disorders. *Lancet*, Vol.361, (February 2003), pp. 407-16, ISSN 0140-6736.

National Collaborating Centre for Mental Health. (2004) National Clinical Practice Guideline: eating disorders: core interventions in the treatment and management of anorexia nervosa, bulimia nervosa, and related eating disorders. National Institute for Clinical Excellence. Available from 27.10.2009 at http://www.nice.org.uk/search/guidancesearchresults.

4

Treatment Strategies for Eating Disorders in Collegiate Athletics

Kendra Ogletree-Cusaac and Toni M. Torres-McGehee
University of South Carolina, Columbia, SC
United States

1. Introduction

Eating disorders such as Anorexia Nervosa, Bulimia Nervosa, not otherwise specified eating disorders, and binge eating disorder are on the rise in collegiate athletes and aesthetic dancers (Greenleaf, Petrie, Carter, & Reel, 2009; Johnson, Powers, & Dick, 1999; Torres-McGehee et al., 2009; Torres-McGehee, Monsma, Gay, Minton, & Mady, In Press). Due to the nature of specific sports and pressures of sport participation, eating disorder symptoms and etiology in athletes are slightly different than their non-athletic counterparts. Therefore, it is critical that treatment for eating disorders is unique to athletes. Preferably, the treatment of the athlete should be multi-dimensional (e.g., psychosocial interventions, nutritional management, and pharmacological interventions when necessary).

Treatment of Anorexia Nervosa in the early 1900s was considered a biologically based disease resulting from hormonal insufficiencies; therefore, treatment focused on correcting hormonal imbalances such as pituitary extract, insulin, estrogen, thyroid extract, and corticosteroids (Brumberg, 1998; Parry-Jones, 1985). Incorporation of psychotherapy was integrated as part of treatment in the 1930s. Bulimia on the other hand was not defined as a specific eating disorder until the late 1970s (Russel, 1979); and treatment then was primarily centered around eliminating patient's hungry appetites by imposing strict diets and prescribing medicines that were supposed to warm the stomach creating a sensation of being full. Additionally, individuals who have clinical eating disorders, like Bulimia, characteristically have low mood and higher-than-average levels of depressive symptoms, and are at greater risk of clinical depression (Fairburn et al., 1999; Fisher et al., 1995; Palmer, 1998; Muscat & Long, 2008). It was theorized by Koenig and Wasserman (1995) that the high rates of co-morbidity found between eating disorders and depression may, in part, be caused by common features such as negative self-evaluation and general dissatisfaction with one's physical appearance (Muscat & Long, 2008). It is plausible that precursors to binge-eating which is the disordered eating behavior that can lead to Bulimia appear to be depression symptoms and low self-esteem. Therefore, psychologists integrate strategies to alleviate depressed mood that is often plagued with Bulimia Nervosa (Gleaves., 2000).

Current treatments focus on both the underlying psychopathologies and the obvious behaviors using protocols including: individual, family, and group psychotherapy; nutritional counseling; medications; exercise therapy, and experiential therapies (e.g., art, music, movement). This chapter will examine current treatment and prognosis strategies for comorbid conditions among collegiate athletes. The goal of this chapter is to provide clinicians/professionals with a deeper understanding of current treatments strategies tailored to collegiate athletes. It should be emphasized that this approach is a team approach that integrates a multi-dimensional approach by the dietitian, physician, athletic trainer, psychologist, coach and other health professionals as needed.

2. Current treatments and prognosis

Eating disorders are serious mental health problems which require appropriate diagnosis and specialized treatment interventions. Eating disorders are essentially "cognitive disorders," in that they share a distinctive "core psychopathology," the over evaluation of shape and weight and their control that is cognitive in nature (Fairburn, 2008). The leading treatment for Bulimia Nervosa is cognitive-behavioral therapy in the general population. It is currently the most researched, best established treatment for Bulimia Nervosa (Wilson, Grilo, & Vitousek, 2007). Other treatments with promise are interpersonal therapy, dialectical behavioral therapy and behavioral weight loss therapy for treating bulimia. Interpersonal therapy is the only psychological treatment for Bulimia Nervosa that has demonstrated long-term outcomes that are comparable to those of cognitive-behavioral therapy (Wilson & Shafran, 2005).

Developmental stages and life transitions are important in determining timing for the onset of eating disorders (Mussell, Binford, & Fulkerson, 2000). Eating disorders are more likely to develop when individuals are having difficulty adjusting and adapting to developmental challenges (Smolak & Levine, 1996). Bulimia has a high relapse rate; it is also recognized as an unstable eating disorder that can acquire additional disordered eating behaviors over time. Additionally, Bulimia has a slightly later age of onset than anorexia, typically in late adolescence or early adulthood (Fairburn, 2008). The transition to college may be a particularly threatening time for some individuals and serve as a catalyst for eating pathology (Smith & Petrie, 2008). For instance, dieting at the beginning of the freshman year may be the best predictor of bulimic behavior at the end of the first year of college (Krahn, Kurth, Bohn, Olson, Gomberg, & Drewnowski, 1995). Age is considered as a factor in treatment effectiveness rather than just symptom duration. Current treatments have been utilized with populations in accordance with the identified affected groups; however they are being evaluated for use with special populations, such as ethnic minority groups, athletes, and males all which have been underrepresented in the prevalence data. Collegiate student athletes are a subset of the athlete population that possesses unique characteristics particularly related to Bulimia.

2.1 Treatment strategies with collegiate student athletes

With regard to the treatment of eating disorders, adolescents seem to benefit the most from cognitive-behavioral therapy, conjoint family therapy (specifically for anorexia), and interpersonal therapy. In treating Bulimia, it is important to consider the onset of disordered eating symptoms, the duration of the symptoms, and the age of the client. All of these factors are problematic for identifying disordered eating symptoms for collegiate student athletes. Moore and colleagues (2007) established that it is clear from the empirical literature that for Bulimia Nervosa, there are treatments that are efficacious and those that have no empirical foundation for their use with this disorder. Thus, the practitioner should be utilizing empirically supported interventions specifically useful with the athletic population. Considering the uniqueness of the sport environment, collegiate student athletes present with unique challenges regarding treatment for Bulimia Nervosa. In addition to the same sociological and psychological issues related to disordered eating in the general population, athletes experience issues such as evaluation criteria, sport-specific weight restrictions, peer comparison, peer and coach pressure, and athletic performance demands (Moore et al., 2007). Also due to sport pressures, athletes are probably less likely to personally seek treatment for Bulimia Nervosa. If athletes are slow to seek treatment, that extends the potential success of intervention applied for treatment.

The collegiate student athlete experiences life transitional issues similar to other college students, such as independence, responsibility, coping strategies, and building new relationships. In addition to these experiences, collegiate student athletes have transitional issues related to their sport, such as adjusting to a new team structure (i.e., coaches, teammates, trainers, etc.), balancing sport and academics, and the pressures of being a student-athlete (i.e., peers, expectations, media). The practitioner needs to be thoroughly knowledgeable about the complexities of eating disorders in athletes, for example, knowing the physical warning signs, general psychosocial functioning, emotion regulation, parental and coaching pressures, weight restrictions for competition, perceptions about body size and shape, perceived environmental control, self-worth, and any other factors that may place an athlete at risk for developing an eating disorder (Moore et al., 2007). Thus, interventions developed for athletes need to address general and sport-specific factors regarding the presence of Bulimia and disordered eating behaviors (Smith & Petrie, 2008).

2.2 Cognitive behavioral theory

The cognitive-behavioral theory for treatment of eating disorders such as Bulimia Nervosa, stresses that central to the maintenance of Bulimia is clients' dysfunctional scheme for self-evaluation. This self-evaluation is largely or even exclusively, in terms of their shape and weight and their ability to control them (Fairburn & Cooper, 2010). Cognitive behavioral theory can also be used to identify dysfunctional thought patterns (e.g., "I am a bad person") that trigger eating disordered behaviors (Stien et al., 2001), and reestablishing those thought patterns to reduce behaviors. This dysfunction is observed throughout all facets of their life, including dietary intake and restraint, perceived body image, and methods related to weight control. If the dysfunctional scheme is central to the maintenance of bulimic symptoms and is considered the core psychopathology, this criterion is especially problematic when working with collegiate student athletes. Collegiate student athletes with Bulimia Nervosa or disordered eating symptoms potentially experience the dysfunctional scheme for self-evaluation significantly differently from their nonathlete peers. They tend to internalize the pressures of their sport and physical appearance and it is not clear that their self-evaluation regarding their athletic potential as related to their physical appearance is always considered dysfunctional.

Another essential feature of Bulimia Nervosa is binge eating episodes. The cognitive-behavioral theory proposes that binge eating is largely a product of the clients' distinctive form of dietary restraint, which then maintains the core psychopathology by intensifying concerns about their ability to control their eating and weight (Cooper & Fairburn, 2010). Athletes are trained to pay attention to their dietary intake particularly as it relates to the interaction of their physique and athletic performance. It is inherently expected that athletes exhibit some form of dietary restraint which can inadvertently lead to the disordered eating cycle of dietary slips and binges. Purging and compensatory behaviors could be viewed as shortcuts to those slips and binges. However, they do not realize that vomiting, for example, only retrieves part of what has been eaten and that laxative misuse has little or no effect on energy absorption (Fairburn, 1995). Athletes often have the impression that their weight control and maintenance should have immediate effects. Binge eating could be especially problematic as the athlete may try to utilize extreme measures to control their weight when it is necessary to maintain appropriate caloric intake due to their level of energy expenditure. In addition, weight loss may interfere with athletes' ability to train and compete, decreasing their performances rather than producing the desired or expected effects of improvement (Smith & Petrie, 2008).

Cooper and Fairburn (2010) outline that cognitive-behavioral theory of the maintenance of Bulimia Nervosa has clear implications for treatment due to attempts to change binge eating and purging behaviors. Treatment must address dietary habits, self-evaluation of weight, and external events that may be influencing disordered eating behaviors. Athletes could benefit from the systematic nature of cognitive-behavioral treatment. Interventions for athletes, however, should consider the influence of the sport context when challenging the thoughts maintaining the disordered eating patterns.

2.3 Empirically supported treatments

2.3.1 Cognitive-behavioral therapy (CBT) and enhanced cognitive-behavioral therapy (CBT-E)

Cognitive-behavioral therapy was originally developed by Aaron T. Beck and colleagues and has become one of the most influential and well-validated models of psychotherapy available (Pike, Carter, & Olmsted, 2010). It has demonstrated efficacy for a broad range of psychiatric disorders, including depression, anxiety disorders, and substance abuse (Wilson, Grilo, & Vitousek, 2007). Cognitive behavioral therapy is also well-recognized as an empirically supported treatment for eating disorders. With regards to Bulimia, specifically it has shown effectiveness in reducing symptomatic behaviors, such as binge eating and purging episodes.

The foundation of cognitive-behavioral therapy maintains that symptoms of a psychiatric condition, such as an eating disorder are preserved by the interaction between cognitive and behavioral disturbances. In therapy, an individual is challenged about distorted beliefs, and subsequent behaviors that correspond to the maintenance of the beliefs. The goal is to modify the behaviors and ultimately change the beliefs to be more adaptive. Enhanced cognitive-behavioral therapy (CBT-E) is the latest version of the leading empirically supported treatment for eating disorders (Fairburn, 2008). It is treatment specifically for eating disorders, and it is equally suitable for males and females. It is individualized, and is generally time-limited. CBT-E focuses on working with the individual to the point where the primary maintaining mechanism, their "core psychopathology," has been disrupted and continued improvements are being experienced (Fairburn, 2008). It is understood that overcoming an eating problem is difficult but worthwhile and that treatment should be given priority (Fairburn, 2008). The core of CBT-E that differs from CBT is that the most powerful way of achieving cognitive change is by helping individuals change the way that they behave and then analyzing the effects and implications of those changes (Fairburn, 2008). Individuals are encouraged to observe themselves enacting their formulations live, and to become intrigued by the effects, and implications, of trying different ways of behaving (Fairburn, 2008).

2.3.2 Interpersonal psychotherapy (IPT)

Interpersonal psychotherapy is a brief and focused psychotherapy intervention that addresses the interpersonal issues in mental health disorders highlighting that one's psychological maladjustment is due to responses to the social environment. It has most widely been used for depression; however, IPT has garnered some empirical support as a treatment modality for Bulimia. IPT takes longer for symptom relief; however, it should be considered an alternative to cognitive-behavioral therapy. IPT is designed to improve interpersonal functioning and self-esteem, reduce negative affect, and in turn, decrease eating disorder symptoms (Tanofsky-Kraff & Wilfley, 2010).

With the bulimic client, interpersonal psychotherapy seeks to help them identify and modify current interpersonal problems that are hypothesized to be maintaining the eating disorder (Wilson, Grilo, & Vitousek, 2007). Interpersonal theory identifies relationships and social roles as critical components of psychological adjustment and well-being. In the case of Bulimia, interpersonal theory suggests that it occurs in the social and interpersonal context, and that the onset, response to treatment, and outcomes are influenced by the interpersonal relationship between the client and significant others (Tanofsky-Kraff & Wilfley, 2010).

Collegiate student-athletes have a unique context which inadvertently supports Bulimia symptomatology, body image issues, ideal vs. real sport weight, peer comparisons, and coach/judges' evaluations. Interactions with coaches, teammates, parents, and other athletic personnel (e.g., athletic trainers) could be the focus of the IPT in addressing the influence of the social environment on the bulimic symptoms.

2.3.3 Dialectical behavior therapy (DBT)

Dialectical behavior therapy was originally developed by Marsha Linehan to treat borderline personality disorder or the "difficult-to-treat clients". It is based on a dialectical worldview that stresses the fundamental interrelatedness or wholeness of reality and connects the immediate to the larger contexts of behavior (Safer, Telch, & Chen, 2009). It is based in cognitive-behavioral therapy with an emphasis on emotion regulation. The primary dialectical strategy is to focus on what is the balance between acceptance and change (Safer, Telch, & Chen, 2009). Implementing validation and problem-solving strategies allows the individual to be challenged and supported regarding their current situational context. DBT has shown promising results with eating disorders, particularly Bulimia and binge eating disorder. Learning to control one's emotions could directly impact the incidence of binges and the loss of control experienced during the binge episode.

Biosocial theory is the underlying theoretical construct for dialectical behavior therapy. It emphasizes affect regulation, highlighting that when applied to eating disorders, intense affect is a frequent precursor to binge eating, which may provide a means, albeit maladaptive, of regulating emotions (Chen & Safer, 2010). When considering the collegiate student athlete, it is conceivable that disordered eating behaviors may become negatively reinforced (i.e., as escape behaviors) or result in secondary emotions such as shame or guilt, which then may signal further disordered eating behaviors (Chen & Safer, 2010). Biosocial theory postulates that an invalidating environment and an emotionally vulnerable individual may inadvertently provide intermittent reinforcement of emotional escalation over time (Chen & Safer, 2010). For collegiate athletes an invalidating environment could include weight-related teasing or over concern with weight by peers, coaches, and family (Chen & Safer, 2010). DBT is useful with comorbid disorders such as, depression symptomatology, particularly suicidal ideation, and borderline personality disorder.

2.3.4 Medication management

Eating disorders at times should involve psychotropic medication (e.g., medications used to treat psychological disorders such as antidepressants) and monitoring by a psychiatrist or physician with specialized experience. It is critical to understand that these medications should be used to treat symptoms of eating disorders (e.g., depression or anxiety), rather than solely treating the eating disorder alone. Previous research supports that antidepressants promoted a decrease in bulimic patients' preoccupation with food and weight; and a decrease in a patients' binging and vomiting episodes (Hudson, Pope, & Carter, 1999).

With collegiate athletes, the psychiatrist would have to keep in mind the sport context and types of psychotropic medications and the associated side effects in addition to the constraints of the drug testing policies and procedures in athletics. It is important to be aware of the side effects of antidepressants. The most common may cause diaphoresis (i.e., excessive sweating), gastrointestinal distress, nausea, drowsiness, and dizziness (Lacy et al., 2002), all of which may decrease or limit an athlete's performance. If an athlete reports any of these symptoms, the medication dosage may have to be altered or daily routine depending on the symptoms. For example, if an athlete is becoming drowsy, the timing of the medication should be changed. It is recommended that the athlete takes two smaller doses per day or takes the medication at night before bed and then gradually increase dosage if necessary (Joy et al., 1997; Zetin & Tate 1999). Another recommendation would be to increase fluid intake if the athletes has increased sweating. Alternative medications should also be considered. Lithium carbonate (a mood stabilizer) and clonidine (an appetite stimulant) have also been used to treat patients with Bulimia Nervosa (Hudson, Pope, & Carter, 1999; Kaye, 1999).

3. Disordered eating and eating disorders and comorbidity

Disordered eating is often paired with other mental health disorders, some of the disorders that have comorbidity include mood disorders, anxiety disorders, substance use disorders and personality disorders. It is often believed that athletes do not experience psychological difficulties the same as the general population; however, more recent evidence is supporting a different prevalence in athletes. The sport context is pressure-filled with constant evaluation from those who can impact an athlete's opportunity to perform. In addition, lack of skills to effectively cope with the pressure make collegiate athletes at risk.

3.1 Mood disorders

Depression is a mental health disorder, in which the person experiences mood disturbance, appetite changes, sleep changes, anhedonia, and a lack of energy. Collegiate athletes experience depression at similar rates to the nonathlete population. They are particularly vulnerable for their experience of depression being overlooked or even misdiagnosed. Symptoms of depression may present differently, and inconsistently, and the athlete may or may not continue to perform well. The presence of depression may be subtle, if clear to others at all. An awareness of the possibility that an individual could be depressed is important for appropriately intervening. Depression is frequently comorbid with Bulimia Nervosa and can guide a student athlete down a spiraling and potentially destructive path. A collegiate athlete with Bulimia Nervosa and depression may also engage in excessive exercise as a form of weight control or to alter their shape, but some also use it to modulate their mood (Fairburn, 2008). Excessive exercising is a form of noncompensatory purging; however, for collegiate athletes, it increases the risk of injury and other physical ailments due to lack of consistent caloric intake and compensatory purging (e.g., self-induced vomiting, laxative misuse). Depression is also hallmarked by thoughts of hopelessness, worthlessness, and helplessness, and when paired with the obsessiveness and lack of control with Bulimia could be a deadly combination.

3.3.1 Suicide

One of the key symptoms of a major depressive episode is the presence of suicidal ideation. When one is considering suicide, it is the person's perception of a sense of helplessness and/or worthlessness. The decision to commit suicide is an act of desperation and highlights the individual's inability to see other options or less disastrous consequences. Collegiate athletes as a group are formulating their identity, self-image, and self-worth throughout their undergraduate career. They may be particularly susceptible to criticisms from numerous sources about their performance as well as their physical appearance. The loss of control during binge eating, the guilt and other emotions present, and concerns about image all suggest that suicidal ideation for athletes should be monitored more effectively. Hospitalization is clinically indicated if the eating disorder has comorbidity with depression and suicidal ideation. Close supervision is prudent upon discharge.

3.3.2 Anxiety disorders

Anxiety disorders are related to how a person perceives threat in their environment and the way in which they cope with their emotions. They are the class of disorders that are characterized by worry, apprehension, and fearfulness, and are exhibited by physical manifestations, such as muscle tremors, nausea, or heart palpitations (American Psychiatric Association, 2000). In athletes, the presence of an anxiety disorder could hurt performance, and if the anxiety disorder is comorbid with an eating disorder, a complicated diagnostic picture as well as intervention plan is the result. When comorbid with Bulimia Nervosa, anxiety disorders seem to magnify and intensify the experience of the disordered eating behaviors. Anxiety features tend to be more characteristic of individuals who have high levels of dietary restraint (Fairburn, 2008). People with eating disorders set multiple demanding, and highly specific, dietary rules designed to limit the amount that they eat, and as a result of these rules their eating becomes restricted in nature and inflexible (Fairburn, 2008). They adjust their lives around their preoccupation with food and the presence of an anxiety disorder further exacerbates the impairment that develops. Concentration is affected and socializing with friends and family are problematic, the individual worries about the pressure to eat in the presence of others.

The anxiety disorders frequently seen in the collegiate student athlete population include:

1. Generalized Anxiety Disorder (persistent and excessive anxiety and worry)
2. Obsessive-Compulsive Disorder (people have obsessions or compulsions that are severe enough to be time consuming or cause marked distress (American Psychiatric Association, 2000).
3. Panic Disorder (recurrent unexpected panic attacks)
4. Phobias (such as social phobia which can include performance anxiety)

As with mood disorders, anxiety disorders often implicate similar cognitive errors to those structuring eating disorders (Steiger & Israel, 2010). For example, a collegiate athlete with Bulimia Nervosa can experience general worry and anxiety regarding food intake and weight gain, obsessive preoccupations with body shape, compulsive reactions (such as the need to compensate after eating), or phobic elements (such as fear of weight gain; Steiger & Israel, 2010). Interventions need to categorize the symptoms of Bulimia Nervosa as well as the existence of an anxiety disorder, then applying strategies to control the persistence of cognitive errors.

3.3.3 Personality disorders

Personality disorders are difficult to identify in individuals with eating disorders because many features of personality disorders are directly affected by the presence of the eating disorder (Fairburn, 2008). Borderline personality disorder, for example, is a personality disorder that is marked by erratic or odd behaviors. Borderline personality disorder has a higher prevalence rate in females, and is considered to be marked by emotional difficulties, instability in relationships, fear of abandonment, and unpredictable emotional reactions. Specific psychopathological tendencies may accentuate specific components of eating disturbances - impulsivity driving high-frequency purging, compulsivity accentuating relentless dieting and pursuit of thinness, narcissism fueling overinvestments in achieving bodily (and other forms of) perfection (Steiger & Israel, 2010).

Personality disorder diagnoses are commonly given to individuals with eating disorders, thus when considering collegiate student athletes, two traits in particular—perfectionism and low self-esteem are evident, however, both are typically present before the eating disorder began (Fairburn, 2008). Additionally, it may be speculated that individuals who are perfectionist, independent, persistent, achievement oriented, and tolerant of pain and discomfort and who have high self-expectations yet low self-esteem are more susceptible to the development of disordered eating (Garfinkel, Garner, & Goldbloom, 1987). These personality traits have been shown to be the key to success in sports, which may help clarify the increased risk of eating disorders among athletes (Garner, Rosen, & Barry, 1998).

4. Future directions

There is increased interest in upgrading classic psychotherapeutic interventions with the fast-paced technological era. Interventions for eating disorders have been identified as a potential area that can be enhanced by utilizing technology as additional tools. Research is beginning to focus on studying the impact and effectiveness of using technology for adjuncts to treatment. Advances in treatment include the use of the internet, email, text messaging, and social networking sites.

5. Internet and treatment (e-mail, text messaging, social networking sites)

Technology has advanced and has allowed for therapeutic interventions to be monitored and tracked at increasing rates. The use of email, text and instant messaging, and social networking sites are changing the way that individuals can communicate with their psychologist, update progress on homework assignments, and receive helpful information between office visits. The internet is reportedly easy to use, readily accessible, convenient, and efficient (Bauer, Golkaramnay, & Kordy, 2005; Robinson & Serfaty, 2003); and is considered an alternative to face-to-face treatment with a therapist. Such use of technology has been shown to be effective particularly with weight loss strategies, self-esteem enhancement, and challenges to cognitive distortions (Nakagawa et al., 2010, Osgood-Hynes et al., 1998; Newman, Consoli, & Taylor, 1999). With CBT-E, for example, ongoing self-monitoring and the successful completion of homework tasks are of fundamental importance, thus use of technology can assist in the therapeutic process.

Using the internet as a component to treatment can offer additional support as well as encouragement for successfully completing treatment protocols. Previous research has investigated e-mail therapy in Bulimia Nervosa patients, and found that e-mail therapy helped to engage individuals in treatment who would otherwise have been unlikely to ask for help through more traditional therapy (Robinson & Serfaty, 2003). It is common that most cases of Bulimia Nervosa in the community are unknown to their general practitioners (van Hoeken, Lucas, & Hoek, 1998) and receive no treatment (Fairburn et al., 1996).

It is known that many ethical and practical questions have been asked in relation to the delivery of this therapy; however it is not recommended for all patients. This type of therapy may work for those that may not have access for a specialist in the eating disorder field or for patients who wish to receive individual therapy in a more anonymous setting. This new method of treatment delivery may have many advantages over the face-to-face methods; such advantages are related to increasing empowerment, accountability, affordability, convenience and privacy (Fingeld, 1999). Additionally, there are some benefits for the clinician as well. Robinson and Serfaty (2003) stated that E-therapy is a strategy that can be used to identify therapist competence by providing a method to monitor general competency and adherence to a specific therapeutic model.

Social networking sites (e.g., Facebook) are starting to be utilized for clients to interact with fellow treatment members, clinicians, and to access resources. These sites have tremendous potential to further aid the therapeutic process over time. As a best practice and to maintain appropriate ethical standards for clinicians, these new forms of therapeutic strategies (i.e., E-therapy, text messaging) are best utilized in conjunction with traditional therapeutic approaches. Specific strategies to ensure confidentiality are essential, such as encryption software on the clinician's computer, password protections on mobile devices, and address books privacy protected.

6. Clinical practice research

In conducting clinical practice research more work is needed to evaluate the effectiveness of interventions such as cognitive-behavioral therapy, interpersonal therapy, and dialectical behavior therapy with the athletic population. It is imperative that the research designs for studying effectiveness of interventions involve control groups, comparative trials, sequencing of treatment applications, randomization, and significant sample sizes to give sufficient statistical power. Clinical practice research needs to have clear, precise procedures for interventions being evaluated. The focus on clinical practice research should be on developing promising treatment approaches. The emphasis should be on symptom presentation and specific populations (ethnic minority groups, athletes, etc.). Other issues such as levels of care (e.g., inpatient, outpatient) also need to be evaluated in terms of effectiveness.

7. Summary

Collegiate student athletes who have Bulimia Nervosa are a specialized population who need particular consideration for treatment interventions. The sport environment is influential on the presence, development, and maintenance of disordered eating symptoms. Clinicians treating collegiate student athletes with Bulimia Nervosa should be knowledgeable about the sport culture and its overarching influence on their experience with the eating disorder. Empirically supported treatments for Bulimia Nervosa include cognitive-behavioral therapy specifically enhanced cognitive-behavioral therapy, interpersonal therapy, and dialectical behavior therapy. All of these treatments have promise for the collegiate student-athlete population; however, more rigorous clinical practice research needs to be done as well as investigating the impact of comorbid disorders on treatment outcomes. Medication management has been effective in treating Bulimia Nervosa as well as addressing any comorbid disorders. A multidisciplinary team approach is essential for intervening with collegiate student-athletes, including a psychologist, dietitian, athletic trainer, coach and physician. Lastly, technological advances, such as the Internet, emails, text messaging and social networking sites are being utilized to assist in the therapeutic process for people with Bulimia Nervosa, and holds potential as useful strategies for collegiate student athletes.

8. References

American Psychiatric Association. (2000). *Diagnostic and Statistical Manual of Mental Disorders* (4th ed.). Arlington, VA: American Psychiatric Association.

Armstrong, S. & Ooman-Early, J. (2009). Social Connectedness, Self-Esteem, and Depression Symptomatology Among Collegiate Athletes Versus Nonathletes. *Journal of American College Health (57) 5* , 521-528.

Bauer, S., Golkaramnay, V., & Kordy, H. (2005). E-mental health: Neue Medien in de psychosozialen Versorgung [E-mental health: The use of new technologies in psychosocial care]. *Psychotherapeutic.* 50, 7-15.

Brumberg, J.J. 1988. *Fasting girls: The history of anorexia nervosa.* New York: Plume.

Coelho, G.M.O., Soares, E.A., & Ribeiro, B.G. (2010). Are female athletes at increased risk for disordered eating and its complications. *Appetite, 55* , 379-387.

Cooper, Z. & Fairburn, C.G. (2010). Cognitive Behavior Therapy for Bulimia Nervosa. In C.M. Grilo & Mitchell, J.E., *The Treatment of Eating Disorders: A Clinical Handbook* (pp. 243-270). New York: Guilford.

Fairburn, C. G., & Cooper, Z. (1993). The eating disorder examination. In C. G. Fairburn, & G. T. Wilson, *Binge Eating: Nature, Assessment, and Treatment* (pp. 317-360). New York, NY: Guilford Press.

Fairburn, C. G. (1995). The prevention of eating disorders. In K. D. Brownell & C. G. Fairburn (Eds.), *Eating disorders and obesity: A comprehensive handbook* (pp. 289–293). New York: Guilford Press.

Fairburn, C.G., Welch, S.L., Norman, P.A., O'Connor, M.E., Doll, H.A. (1996). Bias and bulimia nervosa: How typical are clinic cases? *American Journal of Psychiatry,* 153, 386-391.

Fairburn, C. (2008). *Cognitive Behavior Therpay and Eating Disorders.* New York: Guilford.

Fingeld, D.L. (1999). Psychotherapy in cyberspace. *Journal of American Psychiatric Nursing Association,* 5, 105-110.

Fisher, M., Golden, N.H., Katzman, D.K., Keripe, R.E., Rees, J., Scebendach, J., Sigman, G., Ammerman, S., & Hoberman, H.M. (1995). Eating disorders in adolescents: A position paper of the society for adolescent medicine. *Journal of Adolescent Health, 16,* 420-437.

Garfinkel, P.E., Garner, D.M., & Goldbloom, D.S. (1987). Eating disorders: Implicationsfor the 1990's. *Canadian Journal of Psychiartry,* 32, 624-631.

Garner, D.M., Rosen, L.W., & Barry, D. (1988). Eating disorders among athltes: Research and recommendations. *Sport Psychiatry,* 7, 839-857.

Gleaves, D.H., Miller, K.J., Williams, T.L., & Summers, S.A. (2000). Eating disorders: An overview. In *Comparative treatments for eating disorders,* ed. Miller, K.J. and Mizes, J.S. New York. Springer.

Greenleaf, C., Petrie, T. A., Carter, J., & Reel, J. (2009). Female collegiate atheltes: Prevalence of eating disorders and disordered eating behaviors. *Journal of American College Health, 57,* 489-495.

Johnson, C., Powers, P. S., & Dick, R. (1999, 1). Athletes and Eating Disorders: The National Collegiate Athletic Association Study. *International Journal of Eating Disorders, 26,* 179-188.

Joy, E., Clark, N., Ireland, M.L., Martire, J., Nattiv, A., & Varechok, S. (1997). Team management of the female athlete triad. Rounttable. Part 1. What to look for? What to ask? *Physician and Sportsmedicine,* 25, 55-69.

Hausenblas, H. &. Carron, A. (1999). Eating disorder indicies and athletes: An integration. *Journal of Sport and Exercise Psychology, 21* , 230-258.

Holm-Denoma, J.M., Scaringi, V., Gordon, K.H., Van Orden, K.A., & Joiner Jr., T.E. (2009). Eating Disorder Symptojs among Undergraduate Varsity Athletes, Club Athletes, Independent Exercisers, and Nonexercisers. *International Journal of Eating Disorders, 42 (1),* 47-53.

Hudson, JI., Pope, Carter, W.P. (1999). Pharmacologic therapy of bulimia nervosa. In The management of eating disorders and obesity, ed. Goldstein, D.J. Totawa, NJ: Humana.

Kaye, W.H. (1999). Pharmacologic therapy for anorexia nervosa. In *The management of eating disorders and obesity,* ed. Goldstien, D.J. Totawa, NJ: Humana.

Keel, P. &. (2003). Are Eating Disorders Culture-Bound Syndromes? Implications for Conceptualizing Their Etiology. *Psychological Bulletin , 129* (5), 747-769.

Koenig, L.J., & Wasserman, E.L. (1995). Body image and dieting failure in college men and women: Examining links between depression and eating problems. *Sex Roles.* 32(3-4), 225-249.

Krahn, Kurth, Bohn, Olson, Gomberg, & Drewnowski. (1995). Predictors of at-risk and bulimic behaviors in college women. Paper presented at Seventh Internationsl Conference on Eating Disorders, New York.

Lacy, C.F., Armstrong, L.L., Goldman, M.P., Lance, L.L. (2002). *Drug information handbook.* Hudson, OH: Lexi-Comp.

Moore, Z.E., Ciampa, R. Wilsnack, J., & Wright, E. (2007). Evidence-Based Interventions for the Treatment of Eating Disorders. *Journal of Clinical Sport Psychology, 1* , 371-378.

Muscat, A. C., & Long, B. C. (2008). Critical comments about body shape and weight: Disordered eating of female athletes and sport participation. *Journal of Applied Sport Psychology, 20*(1), 97-115.

Mussell, M.P., Binford, R.B., & Fulkerson, J.A. (2000). Eating Disorders: Summary of risk factors, prevention programming, and prevention research. *Journal of Counseling Psychology, 46* , 42-50.

Nakagawa, A., Marks, I.M., Park, J.M., Bochofen, M., Baer, L., Dottl, S.L., & Greist, J.H. (2000). Self-treatment of obessive-compulsive disorder guided by manual and computer-conducted telephone interview. *Journal of Telemedicine & Telecare,* 6, 22-26.

Newman, M.G., Consoli, A.J., & Taylor, C.B. (1999). A palmtop computer program for the treament of generalsed anxiety disorder. *Behaviour Modification,* 23, 597-619.

Osgood-Hynes, D.J., Greist, J.H., Marks, I.M., Baer, L., Heneman, S.W., Wenzel, K.W., Manzo, P.A., Parkin, J.R., Spierings, C.J., Dottl, S.L., & Vitse, H.M. (1998). Self-administered psychotherapy for depression suing a telphone-accessed computer system plus booklets: An open US-UK study. *Journal of Clinical Psychiatry,* 59, 358-365.

Palmer, R. (1998). Etiology of bulimia nervosa. In J. T. H.W. Hoek, *Neurobiology in the treatment of eating disorders* (pp. 345-362). West Sussex: Wiley.

Parry-Jones, W.L. 1985. Archival exploration of anorexia nervosa. *Journal of Psychiatric Research,* 19 (2/3): 95-100.

Petrie, T.A., Greenleaf, C., Reel, J.J. & Carter, J.E. (2009). An Examination of Psychosocial Corelates of Eating Disorders Among Female Collegiate Athletes. *Research Quarterly for Exercise and Sport*, 621-632.

Pike, K.M., Carter, J.C., & Olmsted, M.P. (2010). Cognitive-Behavioral therapy for anorxia nervosa. In Grilo, C.M., & Mitchell, J.E., *The treatment of eating disorders: A clinical handbook*. E-book. 83-107.

Robinson, P., & Serfaty, M. (2003). Computers, e-mail, and therapy in eating disorders. *European Eating Disorder Review*, 11, 210-221.

Russel, G. 1979. Bulimia nervosa: An ominous variant of anorexia nervosa. *Psychological Medicine*, 9, 379-383.

Safer, D.L., Telch, C.F., & Chen, E.Y. (2009). Orientation for Therapists. In D. T. Safer, *Dialectial Behavior Therapy for Binge Eating and Bulimia* (pp. 16-29). New York: Guilford Press.

Smith, A. & Petrie, T. (2008). Reducing the Risk of Disordered Eating among Female Athletes: A Test of Alternative Interventions. *Journal of Applied Sport Psychology, 20 (4)* , 392-407.

Smolak, L., & Levine, M.P. (1996). Adolescent transitions and the development of eating problems. In M. B. Mussell, *Eating Disorders: Summary of risk factors, prevention programming, and prevention research* (pp. 764-796). The Counseling Psychologist, 28.

Smolak, L., Murnen, S., & Ruble, A. (2000). Female athletes and eating problems: A meta-analysis. *International Journal of Eating Disorders, 27*, 371-380.

Steiger, H. & Israel, M. (2010). Treatment of Psychiatric Comorbidities. In C.M. Grilo & Mitchell, J.E., *The Treatment of Eating Disorders: A Clinical Handbook* (pp. 447-457). New York: Guilford.

Stein, R.L., Saelens, B.E., Dounchis, J.Z., Lewczyk, C.M., Swenson, A.K., & Wilfley, D.E.. (2001). Treatment of eating disoreders in women. *Counseling Psychologist*, 29, 695-732.

Tanofsky-Kraff , M., Wilfley, D.E., Young, J.F., Mufson, L., Yanovski, S.Z, Glasofer, D. R., Salaita, C., & Schvey, N.A. (2010). A pilot study of interpersonal psychotherapy for preventing excess weight gain in adolescent girls at-risk for obesity. *International Journal of Eating Disorders*, 43, 701-706.

Torres-McGehee, T. M., Green, J. M., Leeper, J. D., Leaver-Dunn, D., Richardson, M., & Bishop, P. A. (2009). Body Image, anthropometric measures, and eating-disorder prevalance in auxiliary unit members. *Journal of Athletic Training, 44*, 418-426.

Torres-McGehee, T. M., Monsma, E. V., Gay, J. L., Minton, D. M., & Mady, A. N. (2011). Prevalence of eating disorder risk and body image distortion among National Collegiate Assocation Division I varsity equestrian athletes. *Journal of Athletic Training, 46*, 345-351.

Van Hoeken, D., Lucas, A.r., & Hoek, H.W. (1998). Epedemiology. In Hoek, H.W., Treasure, J.L., & Katzman, M.A. (Eds), *Neurobiology in the treatment of eaitng disorders.* Chichester: John Wiley & Sons.

Wilson, G.T., & Shafran, R. (2005). Eating Disorders guidelines from NICE. *Lancet*, 365, 79-81.

Wilson, G.T., Grilo, C.M., & Vitousek, K.M. (2007). Psychological treatment of eating disorders. *American Psychologist*, 62 (3), 199-216.

Ziten, M., & Tate, D. (1999). The psychopharmacology sourcebook. Los Angeles, CA: Lowell House.

Part 2

Early Identification and Intervention

5

Practical Screening Methods for Eating Disorders for Collegiate Athletics

Toni M. Torres-McGehee and Kendra Olgetree-Cusaac
University of South Carolina, Columbia, SC
United States

1. Introduction

Eating disorders are distinct severe disturbances in eating behavior (e.g., Anorexia Nervosa, Bulimia Nervosa, and Eating Disorders Not Otherwise Specified; American Psychiatric Association [APA], 2000, pg.583). Sociocultural, biological, and psychological factors are intricate in the development of eating disorders (Beals & Manore, 1999; Beals, 2004); though causation may be multifactoral. Extensive research has been conducted in eating disorders and body image disturbances, and many psychologists (e.g. Daniel & Bridges, 2010; Fredrickson & Roberts, 1997; Mazzeo & Espelage, 2002; Tylka & Subich, 2004) have presented model frameworks that eloquently combine variables to explain eating disorder and body image dissatisfaction symptomology in males and females. In the last decade, eating disorders and body image disturbances in the collegiate athletic population has received increasing attention (Black et al., 2003; Greenleaf et al., 2009; Johnson et al. 1999; Petrie et al., 2008; Sundgot-Borgen & Torstveit, 2004). Older research by Johnson, Powers, and Dick (1999) revealed in a hetergeneous sample of collegiate athletes that both females and males were at risk for eating disorders (males: 38% at risk for Bulimia Nervosa and 9.5% risk for Anorexia Nervosa; females: 38% at risk for Bulimia Nervosa and 34.75% at risk for Anorexia Nervosa). Whereas, more current research has estimated 20% for men (Petrie et al, 2008) and 25.5% for female collegiate athletes (Greenleaf et al., 2009). However, estimated prevalence in these studies have been conducted in an anonymous and controlled research environments; thus no data has been presented while examining eating disorder symptomology in a practical setting (pre-participation physical examinations [PPE]) screening for associated risk factors in collegiate athletes.

The sport context is influential on athletes in positive as well as negative ways, thus it is expected that the sport environment could have a considerable impact on the occurrence of eating disorders. Sports can be perceived as its own culture, with its own rules, customs and traditions, and expectations. A culture bound syndrome, as defined by Prince (1985), is "a collection of signs and symptoms (excluding notions of cause) which is restricted to a limited number of cultures primarily by reason of certain of their psychosocial features" (p.201). In a review, Keel and Klump (2003) suggested that Bulimia Nervosa may be a culture-bound syndrome, influenced by weight concerns, anonymous access to large quantities of food, and a motivation to prevent the effects of binge eating on weight through the use of inappropriate compensatory behavior (e.g. self-induced vomiting, excessive exercise, use of diet pills or laxatives, or fasting). Consequently, if the sport environment is conceptualized as its own culture, then the incidence of eating disorders, such as Bulimia in athletes would potentially have similar and dissimilar etiology from nonathletic populations. In addition, it is plausible that precursors to binge-eating, which is the disordered eating behavior that can lead to Bulimia, appear to be depression symptoms and low self-esteem.

It was theorized by Koenig and Wasserman (1995) that the high rates of co-morbidity found between eating disorders and depression may, in part, be caused by common features such as negative self-evaluation and general dissatisfaction with one's physical appearance (Muscat & Long, 2008). Therefore, to better understand the etiology of eating disorders, researchers have focused on the role of body image. Theorists agree that perceptions such as body image distortion and dissatisfaction play a crucial role in the development of disordered eating (Henriques et al., 1996; Ackard et al., 2002) and maladaptive weight control behaviors such as dietary restriction, excessive dieting, laxative use, over exercising and purging (Fredrickson & Roberts, 1997; Stice & Agras,1999; Sundgot-Borgen & Torstveit, 2004; Tylka & Subich, 2004). Some theorist (e.g., Fredrickson & Roberts, 1997; Maine, 2000; Pipher, 1994; Thompson et al., 1999) suggested that sociocultural pressures for thinness directly predict perceptions of poor social support and negative affect (e.g., low self-esteem). It is suggested that being pressured to obtain an unrealistic body image (e.g. thin) by others is more likely to lead into feeling unsupported (Pipher, 1994). Similarly, previous research examining athletes have revealed pressures from coaches (Beisecker & Martz, 1999; Griffin & Harris; 1996; Petrie et al., 2009), family members and peers (Field et al. 2001; Petrie et al. 2009; Vincent & McCabe, 1999) in the development of body image concerns and unhealthy weight-loss practices in athletes.

Body image disturbance, depression, and low self-esteem have been shown to have an association with eating disorders; however they are often not included in the screening process for athletes during PPEs. The National Athletic Trainers' Association and the American College of Sports Medicine have developed position statements for assisting clinicians by providing recommendations for screening and diagnosis of eating disorders and the female athlete triad in athletes (Bonci, et al., 2008; Nativi et al, 2007). Although both statements are very thorough, little attention is given to screening other psychological constructs (body image disturbance, depression, and low self-esteem) that are associated with eating disorders. Self-reported psychometric questionnaires such as the Eating Disorder Inventory (EDI; Garner, et al, 1983, pg.173-184), the Eating Disorders Examination (EDE-Q; Fairburn & Cooper, 1993) and the Eating Attitudes Test (EAT; Garner et al., 1982) are commonly used in the athletic population. Although these questionnaires have well established reliability and validity, it is recognized that most test administrators in the athletic setting for PPEs (e.g., athletic trainers) are either relatively unfamiliar with screening tests or have minimal knowledge or background in standardized test administration or psychometrics. Questionnaire can be fee-based or time consuming (e.g., EDI or EDE-Q), therefore with institutions with limited resources may utilize the EAT-26 because it's free, short in nature, and easy to score.

When it comes to examining body image dissatisfaction, both the EDI and the EDE-Q have subscales; however a more practical alternative used in the literature is the Stunkard Figural Stimuli Scale (Stunkard et al., 1983). A common version of the scale involves nine gender-specific BMI-based silhouettes (SILs). Bulik et al. (2001) examined 16,728 females and 11,366 males ranging in age from 18-100 and transformed the nine SILS and associated each pictorial image with a specific BMI increment. One way of understanding body image is through the use of gender-specific BMI-based SILs is to represent images of actual physique appearance compared to ideal appearance (Stunkard et al., 1983; Bulik et al., 2001). In addition, a recent strategy by Torres-McGehee et al. (2009), undercovered possible sources of negative body image (actual - ideal > 0) by associating SILs scales with reference questions pertaining to daily clothing verses uniform type in aesthetic (Torres-McGehee et al., 2009; Torres-McGehee et al., In Press) and perceptions by others (e.g., friends/peers, parents, cosches; Torres-McGehee & Monsma, n.d); however non-aesthetic sports were not represented in these samples. This strategy is useful for detecting differences from specific social agents.

Due to the large number of athletes at NCAA Division I institutions, screening athletes for potential eating disorder symptomology may be challenging during PPEs. Therefore, this study seeks to examine a retrospective data set compiled from two consecutive years of PPE screening for eating disorder risk and associated symptoms in Division I collegiate athletics. Practitioners utilized reliable and validated instruments commonly used for the general population were used (e.g., EAT-26, Center for Epidemiological Studies Depression Scale, Rosenberg's Self-Esteem Scale, BMI-based silhouette scale, Exercise Dependence Scale). Furthermore, this study will present preliminary findings associated with: (1) estimated prevalence of eating disorder risk, depression, low self-esteem and exercise dependence among female and male athletes; (2) weight pressures, (3) distribution of compensatory behaviors, and (3) body image disturbances associated with clothing type and perceptions of others. Due to the sensitivity of screening for eating disorder symptomology, it is expected that the estimated prevalences among eating disorders risk, associated symtomology, and compensatory behaviors will be lower than estimated prevalence among previous studies (Black & Burckes-Miller, 1988; Carter & Rudd, 2005; Johnson et al.,1999; Greenleaf et al., 2009, Petrie et al., 2008). It is proposed that negative body images thought to be held by others (i.e., actual - ideal), or perceived body ideals from others, are generated in reference to specific social agents (e.g., friends, parents, coaches), with the greatest influence from the coach.

2. Method

2.1 Design and procedure

This study was a retrospective, descriptive and cross-sectional study design. After acquiring appropriate institutional review board approval, two consecutive years of data were obtained from a secure online pre-participation physical examination for eating disorder and mental health screening database used by one NCAA Division I institution. For the protection of the athletes, specific dates of screening is not disclosed; however the two years of data obtained was within the last 5 years. Screening instruments included: (1) Eating Attitudes Test (EAT-26), (2) Center for Epidemiological Studies Depression Scale (CES-D), (3) Rosenberg's Self-Esteem Scale (RSES), (4) BMI-based silhouette scale, (5) Exercise Dependence Scale (EDS), (6) questions regarding weight and pressures in sport and (7) demographic information included athlete's age, gender, and sport, race/ethnicity.

2.2 Participants

One NCAA Division I institution's retrospective data from pre-participation eating disorder and mental health screening was used to examine athletes over a 2 year period (Year 1: n = 355, females: n = 243 and males: n = 112; Year 2: n = 340, females: n = 208, and males n: =

132). Academic background and self-reported physical measurements are represented in Table 1. Total sample of athletes for Years 1 and 2 classified themselves as: 81.8% vs. 82.6% Caucasian, 11.8% vs. 10.3% African American/Black, 1.5% vs. 3.5% Hispanic, 0.6% vs. 0.3% Native American/Indian, 0.3% vs. 0.9% Asian American, and 4.1% vs. 2.4% reported other. Distribution of males for Years 1 and 2 participated in the following sports: baseball, n = 23 vs. n = 23; swimming and diving, n = 27 vs. n = 21; basketball, n = 4 vs. n = 2; cheerleading, n = 8 vs. n = 14; football, n = 8 vs. n = 24; golf, n = 5 vs. n = 1; soccer, n = 12 vs. n = 20; track and field, n = 20 vs. n = 21; and tennis, n = 5 vs. n = 6 respectively. Distribution of females for Years 1 and 2 participated in the following sports: volleyball, n = 9 vs. n = 15; swimming and diving, n = 39 vs. n = 37; basketball, n = 7 vs. n = 5; cheerleading, n = 34 vs. n = 32; cross country, n = 21 vs. n = 11; golf, n = 6 vs. n = 5; soccer, n = 23 vs. n = 27; softball, n = 15 vs. n = 13; track and field, n = 41 vs. n = 25; equestrian, n = 27 vs. n = 34; dance, n = 17 vs. n = 0; and tennis, n = 5 vs. n = 4 respectively.

2.3 Measure

2.3.1 Eating Attitudes Test (EAT-26)

The EAT-26 was administered to screen for eating disorder characteristics and behaviors. Although not diagnostic, the EAT-26 is commonly used as a screening tool to identify early characteristics and behaviors indicating the potential presence of eating disorders (Garner et al.,1982). The EAT-26 is composed of three subscales: dieting, bulimia, and food preoccupation/oral control and followed by five supplemental questions: binge eating; vomiting to control weight or shape; use of laxatives, diet pills or diuretics to lose or to control weight; and exercise more than 60 minutes a day to lose or control weight. Supplemental questions were measured on a Likert-scale (e.g., never, once a month or less, 2-3 times a month, once a week, 2-6 times a week, or once a day or more). In addition, participants answered "Yes" or "No" to whether or not they had lost 20 pounds or more in the past 6 months. Individuals were identified as "at risk" if their total EAT-26 score was greater than 20 or if an individual met the "risk" criteria for one supplemental question. If the EAT-26 score is lower than 20 and individual does not meet the "risk" criteria for supplemental questions, then the individual is considered "not at risk." The EAT-26 has a reliability (internal consistency) of alpha = 0.90 (Garner et al.,1982). In a cross-validation sample, Mazzeo and Espelage (2002) reported coefficients alphas for subscales: dieting, α = .89; bulimia, α = .79; and oral control, α = .53. The alpha coefficients in the present study were as follows: total score, α = .91; dieting, α = .92; bulimia, α = .65 and oral control, α = .56 supporting subsequent analyses. Alpha coefficients across gender in this study were as follows: females, α = .91; dieting, α = .92; bulimia, α = .68 and oral control, α = .53 and males, α = .87; dieting, α = .89; bulimia, α = .60 and oral control, α = .60.

2.3.2 Center for Epidemiological Studies Depression Scale (CES-D)

Center for Epidemiological Studies Depression Scale (CES-D) was used to assess depression (Radloff, 1977). The CES-D is a 20-item self-report measure of depression. It consists of statements that may reflect persons' feelings throughout the week. These items are answered on a four-point scale from 1 = rarely to none of the time to 4 = most of the time. Total score of 16 or higher was considered depressed. The CES-D has 4 separate factors: Depressive affect, somatic symptoms, positive affect, and interpersonal relations. The CES-D has very good internal consistency with alphas of .85 for the general population (Radloff, 1977). The alpha coefficient for all athletes in this study was .89 (females: α = .90 and males: α = .88).

2.3.3 Rosenberg's Self-Esteem Scale (RSES)

The RSES was designed to provide a unidimensional measure of global self-esteem (Rosenberg, 1965). The instrument consists of 10 self-reported items related to overall feelings of self-worth or self-acceptance. These items are answered on a four-point Likert scale ranging from 1=strongly agree to 4=strongly disagree. Scores lower than 15 indicated low self-esteem. The scale is widely used and reported to have a high alpha reliabilities ranging from .72 to .85. The alpha coefficient for all athletes in this study was .90 (females: $\alpha = .90$ and males: $\alpha = .89$).

2.3.4 Gender-specific BMI figural Stimuli Silhouette (SIL)

The Figural Stimuli Survey examined body disturbance based on perceived and desired body images for both males and females (Stunkard et al., 1983). Stunkard's findings were extended by Bulik et al. (2001) by associating specific BMI anchors for each image. The Figural Stimuli is a scale links gender-specific BMI SILs associated with Likert-type ratings of oneself against one of nine SILs associated with a number which then represent a specific BMI ranging from 17.8 - 44.1 kg/m^2 and age range from 18-30 years (e.g., SIL 1 = 17.8, SIL 2 = 18.8, SIL 3 = 20.3, SIL 4 = 22.6, SIL 5 = 26.4. SIL 6 = 31.3, SIL 7 = 36.7, SIL 8 = 40.8, and SIL 9 = 44.1; Bulik et al. 2001). Previous research reported test-retest analyses for females' actual body image as $r = .85$ ($p < .0001$) and ideal body image, $r = .82$ ($p < .0001$; Peterson et al., 2003). Male BMI values for ages 18-30 years ranged from 18.8-49.4 kg/m^2 (e.g., SIL 1 = 18.8, SIL 2 = 20.2, SIL 3 = 21.4, SIL 4 = 22.9, SIL 5 = 25.4. SIL 6 = 28.2, SIL 7 = 33.1, SIL 8 = 35.8, and SIL 9 = 49.4; Bulik et al. 2001). The correlations between BMI and perceived actual SILs from others ranged from .42 to .55 ($p > .001$), and .11 ($p > .05$) to .28 ($p < .01$) for ideal SILs from others. This study's alpha coefficient for all body image SILs was .97 (females: $\alpha = .96$, males: $\alpha = .98$), and .98 for perceived SILs (females: $\alpha = .96$, males: $\alpha = .98$), and .96 for ideal SILs (females: $\alpha = .94$, males: $\alpha = .96$).

Consistent with previous research (Torres-McGehee et al. 2009; Torres-McGehee et al, In Press), SILs augmented by reference phrases were utilized to capture perceptions of actual and ideal body images in daily clothing and competitive uniform. Participants were provided with specific instructions to utilize the SILs (numbered 1-9) to identify which picture best represents: a) 'your appearance (now) in everyday clothing (e.g., what you wear to school)', b) 'the appearance you would like to be in normal daily clothing', c) 'your appearance (now) in your competitive uniform', and d) 'the appearance you would like to be in a competitive uniform'. Similar to Torres-McGehee & Monsma (n.d), additional questions were used to capture perceived body ideal from friends, parents and coaches: a) 'if your peers (friends) pick a picture that represents you now, what picture do you think they will pick,' and b) 'how do you think your peers (friends) would like your appearance to look like,' c) 'if your parents pick a picture that represents you now, what picture do you think they will pick,' d) 'how do you think your parents would like your appearance to look,' e) 'if your coach picks a picture that represents you now, what picture do you think they will pick,' and f) 'how do you think your coach would like your appearance to look.'

2.3.5 Exercise Dependence Scale-21

Exercise dependence was measured by the Exercise Dependence Scale (Hausenblas and Downs (2002)). The survey provides a mean overall score of exercise dependence symptoms; differentiates between at risk, nondependent-symptomatic, and dependent-symptomatic. In addition it specifies whether an individual has evidence of psychological dependence or no psychological dependence and whether individuals have evidence of physiological dependence (i.e., evidence of tolerance or withdrawal) or no physiological dependence (i.e., no evidence of tolerance or withdrawal). Exercise dependence is measured in the scale by the presence of 3 or more of the following: tolerance, withdrawal, intention effect, lack of control, time, reduction in other activities, and continuance. The 21-item questionnaire designed as a 6-point Likert scale. Scale has been validated for the general population (18 years or older; Hausenblas & Down, 2002); however the scales has not been used for the athletic population. For this reason, instructions for the scale were modified as "refer to current exercise beliefs and behaviors outside of regular scheduled practice with your team that have occurred in the past 3 months". The alpha coefficient for all athletes in this study was .93 (females: α = .94 and males: α = .93).

2.3.6 Weight and pressures in sports

Athletes were asked the following questions regarding pressures within their sport: (1) 'do you gain or lose weight regularly to meet the demands of your sport?'; (2) 'has anyone pressured you to change your weight or eating habits?'; and (3) do you feel pressured to look a certain way for your sport?'.

2.4 Data analysis

SPSS statistical software (version XVIII; SPSS Inc. Chicago, IL) was used for all analyses. For the privacy and protection of the athletes, all data was de-identified prior to release to the researchers. Due to the inability to determine whether an athlete repeated the screening two consecutive years the data was assessed within each individual year and across gender. Prevalence of eating disorder characteristics and behaviors, supplemental EAT-26 questions, depression, self-esteem, and exercise dependence was estimated using the number of "at risk" individuals at a 95% confidence level. Chi-square analyses were used to examine the significance and distribution of all at risk variables among males and females. In addition, Chi-square was used to determine the significance and distribution of variables which included: a) college education level, b) ethnicity, c) sport and d) pressures to lose weight.
An a priori α level set at $p = .05$.
Body image dissatisfaction was examined using the Likert SIL anchor data, four ANOVAs with a repeated measures on the last two factors were used to examine clothing type and perceptions of others' body image variation for both Year 1 and Year 2: (a) 2 (gender: females, males) x 2 (clothing type: SIL daily clothing, SIL competitive uniform) x 2 (actual body image, ideal body image) and (b) (a) 2 (gender: females, males) x 3 (perceptions of others: SIL friends, SIL parents, SIL coach) x 2 (actual body image, ideal body image). Mauchly's Test of Sphericity was examined to determine whether a correction factor should be applied. An a priori α level set at $p = 0.05$. BMI-based SIL means established by Bulik et al (2001) are provided for comparative purposes but were not used in statistical analyses examining body image variation across groups because the distance in BMI values associated with each incremental Likert anchor is uneven and would inherently inflate type I error rate (Torres-McGehee et al., n.d).

3. Results

Academic status and self-reported physical measurements (i.e., BMI, height, weight, ideal weight, etc.) of collegiate athletes are reported in Table 1. Distribution of athletes classified as "at risk" for eating disorders, depression, low self-esteem, and exercise dependence in athletes are reported in Table 2. Chi square values are represented for differences between females and males within each year. No significant differences were found among females and males for eating disorders (Year 2), depression, low self-esteem and exercise dependence; however, females in Year 1 reported significantly higher risk for eating disorders than males $\chi^2(1, n = 243) = 4.1, p = .04$. In addition, Year 2 females reported significantly higher pressure to look a certain way for their sport $\chi^2(1, n = 208) = 39.9, p < .01$ and pressured to change their weight or eating habits $\chi^2_1(1, n = 208) = 8.2, p < .01$ compared to males. Distribution of pathogenic behaviors (i.e., binging, vomiting to control or lose weight, use of diet pills/laxatives, excessive exercise) are reported in Table 3.

Repeated measures ANOVA results indicated a between subjects effect between clothing type and gender for both Years 1 and 2 respectively: $F(1,353)=52.3$, $p < .001$, $\eta^2 = .13$ and $F(1,338)=85.8$, $p < .001$, $\eta^2 = .20$. A main effect on perceptions was significant ($p < .001$) with a significant interaction by the clothing type by actual and ideal body image for Year 1: $F(1,353) = 30.2$, $p < .001$, $\eta^2 = .08$ and Year 2: $F(1,338) = 43.9$, $p < .001$, $\eta^2 = .12$. This indicated athletes desired to be smaller than their actual body image for each of the clothing types (Table 4). Repeated measures ANOVA results indicated a between subjects effect for perceptions from others and gender for both Years 1 and 2 respectively: $F(1,353)=49.7$, $p < .001$, $\eta^2 = .12$ and $F(1,338)=69.2$, $p < .001$, $\eta^2 = .17$. A main effect on perceptions was significant ($p < .001$) with a significant interaction by the all three variables (gender,

	Year 1						Year 2					
	All (n = 355)		Females (n = 243)		Males (n = 112)		All (n = 340)		Females (n = 208)		Males (n = 132)	
	M	*SD*	*M*	*SD*	*M*	*SD*	*M*	*SD*	*M*	*SD*	*M*	*SD*
Age	20.1	4.9	20.1	5.9	19.9	1.3	19.6	1.5	19.4	1.5	19.8	1.5
Weight (kg)												
Current	69.1	16.1	61.8	10.9	84.8	14.3	71.6	16.7	62.8	10.4	85.6	15.3
Ideal	68.0	16.3	59.8	9.3	85.4	13.8	71.0	17.5	60.8	9.6	87.1	14.7
High	72.3	16.5	65.0	11.1	88.1	15.3	74.6	17.7	65.7	11.2	88.7	16.9
Low	64.9	14.4	58.0	8.9	79.8	12.7	67.3	15.4	58.9	9.7	80.4	13.6
Current - Ideal	1.3	6.2	1.9	5.5	-1.0	7.1	.65	3.9	2.1	2.5	-1.6	4.6
Height (cm)	172.1	10.5	167.2	8.1	182.6	6.9	173.3	13.9	167.6	8.6	183.4	6.9
BMI (kg/m^2)	23.1	3.7	22.0	3.0	25.4	3.9	23.5	3.5	22.3	2.7	25.4	3.8
Academic Status	%	*n*	%	*n*	%	*n*	%	*n*	%	*n*	%	*n*
Freshman	28.8	98	19.1	65	9.7	33	30.3	103	19.4	66	10.9	37
Sophomore	24.4	83	15.6	53	8.8	30	25.6	87	14.7	50	10.9	37
Junior	24.4	83	13.5	46	10.9	37	21.2	72	14.1	48	7.1	24
Senior	22.4	76	12.9	44	9.4	32	22.9	78	12.9	44	10.0	34

Table 1. Academic status and self-reported physical measurements of collegiate athletes.

	Year 1							Year 2						
	All (n = 355)		Females (n = 243)		Males (n = 112)			All (n = 340)		Females (n = 208)		Males (n = 132)		
	%	*n*	%	*n*	%	*n*	χ^2	%	*n*	%	*n*	%	*n*	χ^2
EAT-26 At Risk	12.9	44	9.7	33	3.2	11	4.1*	14.1	48	8.8	30	5.3	18	.04
EAT Scales	1.5	5	1.5	5	0	0		0.6	2	0.3	1	0.3	1	
Behaviors	9.1	31	6.5	22	2.6	9		10.9	37	6.5	22	4.4	15	
Both	2.4	8	1.8	8	0.6	2		2.4	8	1.8	6	0.6	2	
Depression At Risk	19.8	67	8.3	28	11.5	39	.29	12.4	42	9.1	31	3.2	11	3.2
Self-Esteem At Risk	4.1	14	3.2	11	0.9	3	1.9	3.5	12	2.6	9	0.9	3	1.0
Exercise Dependence							2.6							.33
At Risk	3.2	11	2.4	8	0.9	3		4.4	15	2.6	9	1.8	6	
Nondependent - Symptomatic	45.9	156	29.7	101	16.2	55		39.1	133	23.2	79	15.9	54	
Nondependent - Asymptomatic	50.9	173	29.1	99	21.8	74		56.5	192	35.3	120	21.2	72	
Weight & Pressures														
Change weight to meet demands of sport	17.9	61	11.8	40	6.2	21	.61	17.1	58	10.9	37	6.2	21	.65
Pressure to change weight	31.5	107	20.3	69	11.2	38	.72	14.4	49	11.5	39	2.9	10	8.2*
Pressure to look a certain way	29.1	99	17.9	61	11.2	38	.01	25.6	87	22.9	78	2.6	9	39.9*

* p = <.05

Table 2. Proportion of participants classified as "at risk" for eating disorders, depression, low self-esteem, and exercise dependence in athletes. Chi square values are represented for differences between females and males within each year.

perceptions from others and by actual and ideal perceptions) for Year 1: $F(1,353) = 11.7$, $p < .001$, $\eta^2 = .03$ and Year 2: $F(1,338) = 17.8$, $p < .001$, $\eta^2 = .05$. This indicated differences between actual and ideal perceptions were dependent on perceptions from others (e.g., friends, parents, coaches) and across gender. In both Years 1 and 2, females perceived the largest discrepancy in body image from coaches, revealing a much smaller image compared to friends and parents (Table 5). Similarly, males perceived the highest body image discrepancy in perceptions from coaches; however Year 1 data represented a much smaller ideal image than to Year 2 with a larger body image compared to perceptions from friends and parents (Table 5).

Study	Population (n)	Binge Eating	Vomiting	Laxatives	Diet Pills or Dieting	Diuretics	Excessive Exercise	Lost > 20 pounds
Current Study Year 1	Males & Females (n = 355)	5.9	2.9	3.2†	--	--	1.8	2.1
Current Study Year 2 (n = 340)	Males & Females (n = 340)	6.5	1.8	1.8†	--	--	3.8	2.6
Black & Burckes-Miller, (1988)	Males & Females (n = 695)	--	5.6	3.7	10.6	3.2	55.8	--
Johnson et al., (1999)	Males (n = 883)	12.6	2.0	1.0	0.57	0.23	--	--
	Females (n = 562)	16.2	6.4	1.8	1.4	0.53	--	--
Carter & Rudd, (2005)	Males							
	Females							
Petrie et al., (2008)	Males (n = 203)	3.4*	3.0*	2.5	3.0	3.0	20.7	--
Greenleaf et al., (2009)	Females (n = 204)	15.2	2.9	0.98	15.7	1.5	25.5	--
Torres-McGehee et al. (n.d)	Cheerleaders (n = 136)	11.8	9.6	19.9†	--	--	1.5	2.2
Torres-McGehee et al. (2009)	Dancers (n = 101)	14.9	9.9	18.9†	--	--	--	--
Torres-McGehee et al. (2011)	Equestrian (n = 138)	24.6	11.6	15.2†	--	--	--	--

Note: --No reported measures for these variables
*Reported 1-2 times/per week
†Included laxatives, diet pills, and diuretics in one question.

Table 3. Comparison of prevalence rates (proportions) of pathogenic behaviors among athletes in the current study, cheerleaders, varsity equestrian athletes, auxiliary performers and other female and male athletes. (Torres-McGehee et al., In Press)

4. Discussion

4.1 Eating disorder risk

This is study is unique because we examined retrospective screening data for eating disorders and associated symptomology (e.g., depression, low self-esteem, excessive exercise, body image) in Division I collegiate female and male athletes' PPEs. Another unique feature is that the data retrieved was not obtained in a controlled research environment, but rather part of the athletes' medical record. Overall estimated prevalence

	BMI SILs Anchor Means (kg/m²)											
	Year 1						Year 2					
	All (n = 355)		Females (n = 243)		Males (n = 112)		All (n = 340)		Females (n = 208)		Males (n = 132)	
	M	*SD*	*M*	*SD*	*M*	*SD*	*M*	*SD*	*M*	*SD*	*M*	*SD*
Self-Reported BMI	23.1	3.7	22.0	3.0	25.4	3.9	23.5	3.5	22.3	2.7	25.4	3.8
SIL Daily Clothing												
Actual	22.2	2.8	21.7	2.7	23.4	2.5	22.6	2.6	21.9	2.5	23.6	2.6
Ideal	21.3	2.3	20.5	1.9	23.1	1.9	21.7	2.3	20.7	1.9	23.4	1.9
SIL Uniform												
Actual	22.1	2.8	21.6	2.7	23.2	2.5	22.7	3.2	22.0	2.8	23.9	3.4
Ideal	21.3	2.4	20.5	2.2	23.1	1.9	21.9	2.8	20.7	1.8	23.7	3.1

	Likert SIL Anchor Means											
	All		Females		Males		All		Females		Males	
	M	*SD*	*M*	*SD*	*M*	*SD*	*M*	*SD*	*M*	*SD*	*M*	*SD*
SIL Daily Clothing												
Actual	3.6	1.1	3.6	1.1	3.6	1.1	3.8	.97	3.6	.87	4.1	1.0
Ideal	3.3	1.0	3.2	1.0	3.3	1.0	3.5	.94	3.1	.76	4.1	.83
SIL Uniform												
Actual	3.6	1.1	3.6	1.1	3.5	1.1	3.8	1.0	3.6	.83	4.2	1.1
Ideal	3.3	1.0	3.2	1.1	3.3	1.0	3.5	1.0	3.0	.77	4.2	1.0

Table 4. Descriptive statistics for self-report-BMI and Likert SILs for clothing type body image variables (e.g., daily clothing and competitive uniform).

for eating disorder risk among all athletes was estimated at 12.9% for Year 1 and 14.1% for Year 2; which is significantly lower than previous research (Johnson et al., 1999; Greanleaf et al., 2009; Petrie et al., 2008). Due to the protection of athletes and the institution, sport context was not evaluated; therefore our study examined differences across gender. Interestingly, there was not a significant difference between males and females for Year 2; however results in Year 1 revealed that females portrayed higher risk symptoms for eating disorders than males (9.7% vs. 3.2%). Although, females reported to be higher risk, the estimated prevalence was still lower than previous studies examining female athletes (Black et al., 2003; Greenleaf et al., 2009; Sundgot-Borgen & Torstveit, 2004; Torres-McGehee et al., 2009; Torres-McGehee et al., In Press). Our study had representation of female athletes across 12 different sports. Similarly, in a sample of 204 female athletes, Greenleaf et al. (2009) estimated eating disorders risk across 17 female sports (e.g., gymnastics, rowing, softball, basketball, cross country, etc.), and classified athletes with eating disorders (2.0%; n=4), as symptomatic (25.5%; n=52) and asymptomatic (72.5%; n=148). In addition, no significant differences were found between sport team classification and eating disorder classification.

	BMI SILs Anchor Means (kg/m²)											
	Year 1						Year 2					
	All (n = 355)		Females (n = 243)		Males (n = 112)		All (n = 340)		Females (n = 208)		Males (n = 132)	
	M	*SD*	*M*	*SD*	*M*	*SD*	*M*	*SD*	*M*	*SD*	*M*	*SD*
Self-Reported BMI	23.1	3.7	22.0	3.0	25.4	3.9	23.5	3.5	22.3	2.7	25.4	3.8
SIL Friends												
Actual	22.0	2.6	21.4	2.5	23.4	2.5	22.4	2.8	21.7	2.6	23.6	2.7
Ideal	21.7	2.3	21.0	1.9	23.3	2.1	22.1	2.2	21.3	1.9	23.4	1.9
SIL Parents												
Actual	22.1	2.7	21.5	2.6	23.3	2.7	22.3	2.6	21.7	2.6	23.3	2.2
Ideal	21.7	2.2	20.9	1.9	23.2	2.1	22.1	2.3	21.1	1.7	23.5	2.2
SIL Coach												
Actual	22.3	2.8	21.7	2.7	23.5	2.7	22.6	3.1	22.0	2.7	23.7	3.3
Ideal	31.3	21.4	20.5	2.0	23.2	2.0	21.8	2.8	20.7	1.7	23.8	3.0
	Likert SIL Anchor Means											
	All		Females		Males		All		Females		Males	
	M	*SD*	*M*	*SD*	*M*	*SD*	*M*	*SD*	*M*	*SD*	*M*	*SD*
SIL Friends												
Actual	3.5	1.1	3.5	1.1	3.5	1.1	3.7	1.1	3.4	.96	4.1	1.1
Ideal	3.4	1.0	3.4	1.0	3.4	1.0	3.6	.87	3.4	.75	4.1	.84
SIL Parents												
Actual	3.5	1.1	3.6	1.1	3.5	1.1	3.6	.97	3.5	.91	4.0	.98
Ideal	3.4	.99	3.4	.98	3.4	1.0	3.6	.92	3.2	.74	4.1	.93
SIL Coach												
Actual	3.6	1.1	3.6	1.1	3.6	1.2	3.8	1.0	3.6	.96	4.1	1.1
Ideal	3.3	1.1	3.2	1.1	3.3	1.1	3.5	1.0	3.0	.82	4.2	.95

Table 5. Descriptive statistics for self-report-BMI and Likert SILs for perceptions by others (e.g., friends, parents, and coaches).

Other studies, have examined eating disorder risk across categorized sport groups or specific individual team sports (Black et al., 2003; Sundgot-Borgen & Torstveit, 2004; Torres-McGehee et al., 2009; Torres-McGehee et al., In Press; Torres-McGehee et al., n.d). More specifically, Black and et al., (2003) estimated their highest eating disorder prevalence to be among cheerleaders (33%), while also finding disordered eating occurring frequently among gymnasts (50%), modern dancers (45%), and cross country athletes (45%). Similarly to Black et al. (2003), Torres-McGehee and colleagues (2009, In Press, n.d) estimated high risk among collegiate dancers (29%), cheerleaders (33%) and equestrian athletes (42%). Whereas, Sundgot-Borgen & Torstveit (2004) revealed eating disorder prevalence among categorized athletic sport groups vs. individual sports and revealed eating disorder risk in the following: technical sports (17%; e.g., bowling, golf), ball game sports (16%; e.g., team handball, soccer, tennis, volleyball); aesthetic sports (42%; e.g., gymnastics, dancing, figure skating, diving) and endurance sports (24%; e.g., aerobics, long-distance running).

This study revealed males to have a lower eating disorder risk (Year 1 = 3.2% vs. Year 1 = 5.3%) than male athletes in a studies conducted by Johnson et al. (1999) and Petrie et al., (2008). More specifically, Johnson et al. (1999) found males to be 9.5% for Anorexia Nervosa and 38% risk for Bulimia Nervosa; whereas Petrie et al. (2008) reported symptomatic eating disorders in male athletes across categorized sports (e.g., 13% for endurance sports, 20% for ball game sports, and 22% for power sports). However, our results were slightly higher than those reported among Australia elite male athletes (n = 108; Bryne & McLean, 2002). Byrne & McLean (2002) reported prevalence in the thin-build category (e.g., long distance running, swimming, gymnastics, diving) to be 4% at risk for Anorexia Nervosa, 2% Bulimia Nervosa, and 2% EDNOS. No eating disorders were identified among male normal-build athletes.

4.2 Compensatory/pathogenic behaviors

Clinical and subclinical eating disorders involve the use of specific disordered eating and compensatory weight-control behaviors to manage emotions, weight and body size (APA, 2000). In our study, ~17% of male and female athletes reported they gained or lost weight to regularly meet the demands of their sport. More specifically they reported highest prevalence with compensatory behaviors in: binging in Year 2 (6.5%), vomiting to control or lose weight in Year 1 (2.9%), use of diet pills and diuretic to control or lose weight in Year 1 (3.2%), and excessive exercise in Year 2 (3.8). Our findings were aligned with several studies examining compensatory behaviors in athletes (e.g., Table 3, Carter & Rudd, 2005; Johnson et al., 1999) but lower than Black and Burckes-Miller (1988), Greenleaf et al. (2009), Petrie et al., 2008; and studies that focused solely on aesthetic sports (e.g., Table 3, Torres-McGhee et al, 2009; Torres-McGehee et al., In Press; Torres-McGehee et al, n.d). However, these numbers may be lower due to the timing of PPEs. Previous research has found that athletes who engage in chronic dieting, fasting, laxative use, and/or self-induced vomiting do so during certain times of the year (e.g., in-season athletes attempting to maintain a certain weight (Sundgot-Borgen, 1994).

4.3 Depression, low self-esteem and weight pressures

Eating disorders have high rates of comorbidity with other psychological illnesses, such as depression and low self-esteem (Mischoulon et.al., 2010). Individuals, who have clinical eating disorders, characteristically have low mood and higher-than-average levels of depressive symptoms, and are at greater risk for clinical depression (Muscat & Long, 2008). It is often that athletes will be at higher risk for depression because of the commitment to competitive athletics. Although, we did not compare non-athletes in our study, our estimated prevalence for depression was similar to Armstrong et al. (2009). Armstrong et al. (2009) revealed collegiate athletes had significantly lower levels of depression and significantly greater levels of self-esteem than non-athletes (33.5% non-athletes vs. Year 1: 19.8% and Year 2: 12.4% in our study). In addition, Armstrong et al. (2009) reported that being an athlete was not a predictor of depression when compared with other variables such as gender and self-esteem. Similarly, our results revealed no significant difference between gender for both years; however our data was inconsistent for males for Years 1 and 2 (11.5% vs. 3.2%). On the other hand, Yang et al. (2007) took the analysis a little further and revealed that males were at 19.2% and females at 25.6% reported symptoms of depression, which were both significantly higher than males in females in both years of reported data.

One of the important psychological factors that have been studied in association with eating disorders is self-esteem. Petrie and colleagues (2009) identified self-esteem as a potential moderator between eating disorders and body dissatisfaction in that positive self-esteem affects the likelihood of female athletes internalizing sport-specific pressures about appearance or weight. Our results reflected higher levels of self-esteem in collegiate athletes. Although these are only estimates, it may be speculated that athletes may be protected from depression because of their regular exercise regime associated with sports, increased self-esteem (Armstrong et al., 2009; Dishman et al., 2006), and being more socially connected (Baumeister et al., 1995; Armstrong et al., 2009). Whereas, non-athletes reported higher levels of depression, and lower levels of self-esteem and social connectedness predicted higher levels of depression (Armstrong et al., 2009). Interestingly, in Year 1, 31.5% of athletes reported they had felt pressure to change their weight or eating habits; ~17% of athletes for both years revealed they gained or lost weight to regularly meet the demands of their sport; and on average ~27% felt pressured to look a certain way for their sport. Due to nature of sports, it may be speculated that athletes may have higher levels of social connectedness; however, the these pressures to maintain a certain weight or appearance may increase concerns regarding body image thus decreasing self-esteem and possibly triggering depression and/or low self-esteem. Another possibility of increased depression in athletes may arise when athletes have a severe athletic injury. The inability to continue participation with the team or individual sport or a decrease in athletic performance often leads to difficulty with coping with the injury cognitively, emotionally and behaviorally (Wiese-Bjornstal et al., 1998).

4.4 Body image disturbance

Aligned with the tenets from researchers (Fredrickson & Roberts, 1997), this study considered body related perceptions from others and in competitive uniform verses daily clothing, which was similar to previous research (Torres-McGehee et al., 2009; Torres-McGehee et al., In Press; Torres-McGehee & Monsma, n.p). Body image has links to both socio-culturally driven pressures to achieve a certain body shape and contextual demands for thinness to enhance performance (Bonci et al., 2008). The role of body image disturbance was examined from the perspective of clothing type (e.g., daily clothing, competitive uniforms) and perceptions from others (e.g, friends, parents, coach). Our study revealed significant differences in body image disturbances between males and females for both daily uniform and competitive uniform; however, there were no significant differences between actual and ideal discrepancies between daily clothing and competitive uniform within male and female athletes. Therefore, regardless of clothing type, all athletes wanted to be smaller for their ideal image. Our findings were consistent with recent studies on collegiate dancers, cheerleaders and equestrian athletes (Torres-McGehee et al., 2009; Torres-McGehee et al., In Press; Torres-McGehee & Monsma, n.d); however, males were not used in these studies. Therefore, this is the first study to examine collegiate male athletes and their associated actual and ideal discrepancies in daily clothing and uniform.

Previous research has examined external pressures and the delelopment of body image concerns from social agents (e.g., coaches, family members, and friends, Beisecker & Martz, 1999; Field et al. 2001; Griffin & Harris; 1996; Petrie et al., 2009; Vincent & McCabe, 1999). A unique part of the study was that actual and ideal discrepancies from social agents were examined. Data revealed a significant difference between gender, actual –ideal discrepancy, and between perceptions from others; therefore the differences between actual and ideal discrepancies were dependent on perceptions from others (e.g., friends, parents, coaches) and across gender. Similar to Torres-McGehee & Monsma (n.d), females perceived the largest discrepancy in body image from coaches, revealing a much smaller image compared to friends and parents (Table 5). Similarly, males perceived the highest body image discrepancy in perceptions from coaches; however Year 1 data represented a much smaller ideal image than to Year 2 with a larger body image compared to perceptions from friends and parents (Table 5). It was also interesting to note that in Year 2, males reported coaches' ideal perceptions to be slightly larger than Year 1. This may be due the larger number of football athletes who completed the screening.

4.5 Limitations

There were several limitations to this study. First, the data set was retrieved from only one institution; therefore, the outcomes cannot be generalizable to the entire athletic population. However results can be used as a guideline to integrating eating disorder screening into PPEs. Although the EAT-26 is commonly used and a psychometrically sound instrument; it is a screening rather than diagnostic tool. In this study, the EAT-26 was used to identify individuals at risk or displayed risk eating behaviors pathology. Because we screened for, rather than diagnosed, eating disorder characteristics and behaviors, we cannot absolutely conclude that athletes classified as "at risk" actually had an eating disorder. Possible causes of false-positive, high EAT-26 scores may include subjects with eating disorders not otherwise specified (EDNOS) or generally disturbed individuals who respond positively on surveys without having significant eating concerns could have also inflated the EAT-26 scores in the absence of a diagnosable eating disorder (Fairburn & Cooper, 1993; Wilfley et al., 2000). Due to the scoring of the EAT-26, it is likely to have similar EAT-26 total score mean values for those athletes classified as "at risk" and "not at risk" (e.g., an "at risk" with a total EAT-26 score < 20, but reported "at risk" due to values on the Likert scale for the behavioral questions). Finally, due to the nature of the screening (not being anonymous), athletes could have under reported their responses. Many factors could lead to under reporting: 1) athletes are in denial of possible eating disorder or associated symptomology, 2) athletes may be afraid it will affect their playing time, 3) athletes may be scared to lose their athletic scholarship, or 4) being medically disqualified. Although there are some limitations to scoring the EAT-26, it is important to note the purpose of the instrument is to "screen" athletes. If suspicions of eating disorders or associated symptomology arise from interpretation of questionnaire results, an in-depth personal interview by a member of the health care team should follow for a more accurate interpretation of circumstances (Black et al., 2003; Bonci et al., 2008; Sundgot-Borgen & Torstveit, 2004). It is suggested that future research examines the association of eating disorders risk, associated symptomology and specific clinical outcomes throughout an athletes' career.

5. Conclusion

It is important to note that athletes with disordered eating symptomology; will rarely self-identify due to the secrecy, shame, denial, and fear of reprisal (Currie & Morse, 2005; Johnson et al., 1999; Ryan, 1992). Therefore, integrating eating disorder screening in conjunction with PPE may help identify those athletes presented with elevated risk. Previous research has examined the influence of sport on the occurrence and prevalence of psychological variables, and psychological well-being in athletes (Petrie et al., 2009). It was suggested future research should identify psychosocial factors associated with eating disorders such as body image concerns, general and sport-specific weight pressures (e.g., coaches, teammates, parents, etc.), internalization of the ideal, restrained eating, negative affect, and modeled behaviors (e.g., family, friends, teammates, etc.). While this study didn't capture all of those variables, the instruments used for screening during PPEs were instrumental in identifying those athletes that presented elevated symptomology for potential eating disorder risk. However, specific questions items designed to assess disordered eating behaviors and attitudes should not only be incorporated into the medical history portion of the PPE; but also followed up with appropriate medical personal for more in-depth screening (Bonci et al., 2008). Moreover, a benefit for screening all athletes during PPEs is that individual institutions will be able to acquire an overall glance at the health and well-being of their student athletes. It is suggested that overall screening data is utilized to identify target areas of concern for all student athletes; and then followed up with solutions to integrate prevention programing for both the student athletes and coaches. Finally, our study also confirmed an understanding of how males and female athletes perceive their bodies. Evidence from this study exposed external pressures (e.g., clothing type and perceptions of others) for actual -ideal discrepancy which is indicative of possible risk for developing eating disordered thoughts and behaviors. These actual -ideal discrepancies may have practical implications for weight loss behaviors and mental status (e.g., depression and low self-esteem) in collegiate athletes. Therefore, it is suggested to examine mental health and compensatory behaviors to control or lose weight independent of eating-disorder risk status.

6. References

Ackard, D. M., Croll, J. K., & Kearnedy-Cooke, A. (2002). A deiting frequency among college females: association with disordered eating, body image, and related psycholgoical problems. *Journal of Psychosomatic Research, 52*, 129-136.

American Psychiatric Association. (2000). *Diagnostic and Statistical Manual of Mental Disorders* (4th ed.). Arlington, VA: American Psychiatric Association.

Armstrong, S., & Oomen-Early, J. (2009). Social connectedness, self-esteem, and depression symptomatology among collegiate athletes verses nonathletes. *Journal of American College Health, 57*, 521-526.

Baumeister , R. F., & Leary, M. R. (1995). The need to belong: desire for interpersonal attachments as a fundamental human emotion. *Psychological Bulletin, 112*, 461-484.

Beals, K. A. (2004). Etiology of eating disorders in athletes. In *Disordered eating among athletes: A comprehesive guide for health professionals* (pp. 41-52). Champaign, IL: Human Kinetics.

Beals, K. A., & Manore, M. M. (1999). Subclinical eatng disorders in physically active women. *Topics in Clinical Nutrition, 14*, 14-29.

Biesecker, A. C., & Martz, D. M. (1999). Impact of coaching style on vulnerability for eating disorders: An analog study. *Eating Disorder Journal of Treatment and Prevention*, 235-244.

Black, D. R., & Burckes-Miller, M. E. (1988). Male and female college athletes: Use of anorexia nervosa and bulimia nervosa weight loss methods. *Research Quarterly for Exercise and Sport, 59*, 252-256.

Black, D. R., Larkin, L. J., Coster, D. C., Leverenz, L. J., & Abood, D. A. (2003). Physiological screening test for eating disorders/disordered eating among female collegiate athletes. *Journal of Athletic Training, 38*, 268-297.

Bonci, C. M., Bonci, L. J., Granger, L. R., Johnson, C. L., Malina, R. M., Milne, L. W., et al. (2008). National Athletic Trainers' Association Position Statement: Preventing, Detecting, and Managing Disordered Eating in Athletes. *Journal of Athletic Training, 43*, 80-108.

Bulik, C. M., Wade, T. D., Heath, A. C., Martin, N. G., Stunkard, A. J., & Eaves, L. J. (2001). Relating body mass index to figural stimuli population-based normative data for Caucasians. *International Journal of Obesity, 25*, 1517-1524.

Byrne, S., & McLean, N. (2002). Elite athletes: Effects of the pressure to be thin. *Journal of Science and Medicine in Sport, 5*, 80-94.

Carter, J., & Rudd, N. (2005). Disordered eating assessment for college student-athletes. . *Women in Sport and Physical Activity Journal, 14*, 62-75.

Currie, A., & Morse, E. D. (2005). Eating disorders in athletes: managing the risks. *Clinicals in Sports Medicine, 24*, 871-883.

Daniel, S., & Bridges, S. K. (2010). The drive for muscularity in men: Media influences and objectification theory. *Body Image, 7*, 32-38.

Dishman, R. K., Hale, D. P., Pfeiffer , K. A., Felton, G. A., Saunders, R., Ward, D. S., et al. (2006). Physical self-concept and self-esteem mediate cross-sectional relations of phsyical activity and sport participation with depression symptoms among adolescent girls. *Health Psychology, 25*, 396-407.

Fairburn, C. G., & Cooper, Z. (1993). The eating disorder examination. In C. G. Fairburn, & G. T. Wilson, *Binge Eating: Nature, Assessment, and Treatment* (pp. 317-360). New York, NY: Guilford Press.

Field, A. E., Camargo, C. A., Taylor, C. B., Berkely, C. S., Roberts, S. B., & Colditz, G. A. (2001). Peer, parent, and media influences on the development of weight concerns and frequent dieting among preadolescents and adolescents girls and boys. *Pediatrics, 107*, 54-60.

Fredrickson, B., & Roberts, T. (1997). Objectification theory. *Psychology of Women Quarterly, 21*, 173-206.

Garner, D. M., Olmstead, M. P., Bohr, Y., & Garfinkel, P. E. (1982). The eating attitdues test: Psychometric features and clinical correlates. . *Psychological Medicine, 12*, 871-878.

Garner, D. M., Olmsted, M. P., & Polivy, J. (1983). *The Eating Disorder Inventory: A measure of cognitive-behavioral dimensions of Anorexia Nervosa and Bulimia. Anorexia: Recent developments in research.* New York, NY: Alan R. Liss.

Greenleaf, C., Petrie, T. A., Carter, J., & Reel, J. (2009). Female collegiate atheltes: Prevalence of eating disorders and disordered eating behaviors. *Journal of American College Health, 57*, 489-495.

Griffin, J., & Harris, M. B. (1996). Coaches' attitudes, knowledge, experiences, and recommendations regarding weight control. *The Sports Psychologist, 10*, 180-194.

Hausenblas, H. A., & Downs, D. S. (2002). *Exercise Dependence Scale-21 Manual.* Copyright.

Henriques, G. R., Calhoun, L. G., & Cann, A. (1996). Ethnic differences in women's body satisfaction: An experimental investigation. *Journal of Social Psychology, 136*, 689-697.

Johnson, C., Powers, P. S., & Dick, R. (1999, 1). Athletes and Eating Disorders: The National Collegiate Athletic Association Study. *International Journal of Eating Disorders, 26*, 179-188.

Keel, P. K., & Klump, K. L. (2003). Are eatingdisorders culture-bound syndromes? Implications for conceptualizing their etiology . *Psycholgoical Bulletin, 129*, 747-769.

Koenig, L. J., & Wasserman, E. L. (1995). Body image and dieting failure in college men and women: Examining links between depression and eating problems. *Sex Roles, 32*, 225-249.

Maine, M. (2000). *Body wars: Making peace with women's bodies.* Carlsbad, CA: Gurze Books.

Mazzeo, S. E., & Espelage, D. L. (2002). Associatoin between childhood physical and emotional abuse and disordered eating behaviors in female undergraduates: an investigation of the mediating role of alexithymia and depression. *Journal of Counseling Psychology, 49*, 86-100.

Mischoulon, D., Eddy, K. T., Keshaviah, A., Dinescu, D., Ross, S. L., Kass, A. E., et al. (2010). Depression and eating disorders: Treatment course. *Journal of Affective Disorders*, doi:10:1016/j.jad.2010.10.043.

Muscat, A. C., & Long, B. C. (2008). Critical comments about body shape and weight: Disordered eating of female athletes and sport participation. *Journal of Applied Sport Psychology, 20*(1), 97-115.

Nativi, A., Loucks, A. B., Manore, M. M., Sanborn, C. F., Sundgot-Borgen, J., & Warren, M. P. (2007). American College of Sports Medicine Position Stand: The female athlete triad. *Medicine and Science in Sports and Exercise , 39*, 1867-1882.

Peterson, M., Ellenberg, D., & Crossan, S. (2003). Body-image perceptions: Reliability of a BMI-based silhouette matching test. *American Journal of Health Behavior, 27*, 355-363.

Petrie, T. A., Greenleaf, C., Reel, J., & Carter, J. (2008). Prevalence of eating disorders and disordered eating behaviors among male collegiate athletes. *Psychology of Men and Masculinity, 9*, 267-277.

Petrie, T. A., Greenleaf, C., Reel, J., & Carter, J. (2009). Personality and psychological factors as predictors of disordered eating among female collegiate athletes. *Eating Disorders, 17*, 302-321.

Phipher, M. (1994). *Reviving Ophelia: Saving the selves of adolescent girls.* Carlsbad, CA: Gurze Books.

Prince, R. (1985). The concept of culture-bound syndromes: Anorexia nervosa and brain-fag. *Social Science and Medicine, 21*, 197-203.

Radloff, L. S. (1977). The CES-D scale: A self-report depression scale for research in the general population. *Applied Psychological Measurement, 1*, 385-401.

Rosenberg, M. (1965). *Society and the adolscent self-image.* Princeton, NJ: Princeton University Press.

Ryan, R. (1992). Management of eating problems in athletic settings. In K. D. Brownell, & J. H. Wilmore, *Eating, Body Weight, and Performance in AThletics: Disorders of Modern Society* (pp. 344-362). Philadelphia, PA: Lea & Febiger.

Stice, E., & Agras, W. S. (1999). Subtyping bulimic women along dietary restraint and negative affect dimensions. *Journal of Consulting and Clinical Psychology, 67*, 460-469.

Stunkard, A., Sorensen, T., & Schulsinger, F. (1983). Use of the Danish Adoption Register for the study of obesity and thinness. In S. S. Ketty, L. P. Roland, R. L. Sidman, & S. W.

Matthysse, *The genetics of neurological and psychiatric disorders* (pp. 115-120). New York: Raven Press.

Sundgot-Borgen, J. (1994). Risk and trigger factors for the development of eating disorders in female elite athletes. *Medicine Science for Sports and Exercise, 26*, 414-419.

Sundgot-Borgen, J., & Torstveit, M. (2004). Prevalence of eating disorders in elite athletes is higher than in the general population. *Clinical Journal of Sports Medicine, 14*, 25-32.

Thompson , J. K., & Heinberg , L. J. (1999). The media's influence on body image distrubance and eating disorders: We've reviled them, now can we rehabilitate them? *Journal of Social Issues, 55*, 339-353.

Torres-McGehee , T. M., & Monsma, E. V. (n.d). Eating disorder risk and the role of context specific body images among collegiate cheerleaders. *Manuscript submitted for publication.*

Torres-McGehee, T. M., Monsma, E. V., Dompier, T. P., & Washburn, S. A. (n.d.). Eating Disorder Risk and the Role of Clothing on Body Image in Collegiate Cheerleaders. *Manuscript submitted for publication.*

Torres-McGehee, T. M., Green, J. M., Leeper, J. D., Leaver-Dunn, D., Richardson, M., & Bishop, P. A. (2009). Body Image, anthropometric measures, and eating-disorder prevalance in auxiliary unit members. *Journal of Athletic Training, 44*, 418-426.

Torres-McGehee, T. M., Monsma, E. V., Gay, J. L., Minton, D. M., & Mady, A. N. (In Press). Prevalence of eating disorder risk and body image distortion among National Collegiate Assocation Division I varsity equestrian athletes. *Journal of Athletic Training, 46*, 345-351.

Tylka, T. L., & Subich, L. M. (2004). Examining a multidimensional model of eating disorder symptomatology among college women. *Journal of Counseling Psychology, 51*(3), 314-328.

Vincent, A., & McCabe, M. P. (2000). Gender differences among adolescents in family and peer influences on body dissatisfaction, weight loss, and binge eating behaviors. *Journal of Youth and Adolescence, 29*, 206-221.

Weise-Bjornstal, D. M., Smith, A. M., Shaffer, S. M., & et al. (1998). An integrated model of the response to sport injury: Psychological ad sociological dynamics. *Journal of Applied Sports Psychology, 10*, 46-69.

Wilfley, D. E., Schwartz, M. B., Spurrell, E. B., & Fairburn, C. G. (2000). Using the eating disorder examinatino to identify the specific psychopathology of binge eating disorder. *International Journal of Eating Disorders, 27*, 259-269.

Yang, J., Peek-Asa, C., Corlette, J. D., Cheng, G., Foster, D. T., & Albright, J. (2007). Prevalence of and risk factors associated with symptoms ofdepression in competitive athletes. *Clinical Journal of Sports Medicine, 17*, 481-487.

6

Targeted Prevention in Bulimic Eating Disorders: Randomized Controlled Trials of a Mental Health Literacy and Self-Help Intervention

Phillipa Hay[1,6], Jonathan Mond[2], Petra Buttner[3], Susan Paxton[4], Bryan Rodgers[5], Frances Quirk[6] and Diane Kancijanic[1]

[1]*School of Medicine, University of Western Sydney,*
[2]*School of Health Sciences, University of Western Sydney,*
[3]*School of Public Health, Tropical Medicine, and Rehabilitation Sciences, James Cook University, Townsville, Australia University of Western Sydney,*
[4]*School of Psychological Sciences, La Trobe University,*
[5]*Australian Demographic and Social Research Insittute, The Australian National University,*
[6]*School of Medicine and Dentistry, James Cook University, 7 School of Medicine, University of Western Sydney,*
Australia

1. Introduction

Eating disorders (EDs) in the community are associated with high burden and poor quality of life (Mathers et al., 2000, Hay & Mond, 2005). It is also known that people with EDs have frequent chronic medical complications (Mehler, 2003), increased risk of obesity especially for the more common bulimic EDs such as binge eating disorder (Neumark-Sztainer et al., 2006; Hudson et al., 2007)) and high levels of co-morbidity with both depression and anxiety (Hudson et al., 2007). However, there is a wide gap between the presence of a disorder and its identification and treatment. It is well-documented that the overwhelming majority of people in the community with an ED do not seek help for their eating behaviours (Hart et al., in press; Welch & Fairburn 1994), and that even fewer access appropriate or evidence-based treatments (Cachelin & Striegel-Moore,2006; Mond et al., 2009). This is problematic as many randomised controlled trials support the efficacy of treatments, such as cognitive-behaviour therapy for bulimic EDs (Hay et al., 2004) and unmet treatment needs likely add to the general community burden from psychiatric disorders (Andrews et al., 2000). In addition, these disorders often become chronic with longitudinal studies indicating persistence of symptoms over many years (Fairburn et al., 2000, Evans et al., 2011).

It has been argued that factors contributing to the low rates of help-seeking amongst people with EDs include poor knowledge about treatments amongst sufferers (Cachelin & Striegel-Moore, 2006; Hepworth & Paxton, 2007; Mond & Hay, 2008), feelings of shame (Cachelin & Striegel-Moore, 2006; Hepworth & Paxton, 2007), perceived stigmatisation of EDs (Stewart et al., 2006), ambivalence towards change (Hepworth & Paxton, 2007), cost (Cachelin &

Striegel-Moore, 2006; Hepworth & Paxton, 2007), and a belief that one could or should handle the problem alone (Becker et al., 2004; Cachelin & Striegel-Moore, 2006).

Many of these reasons for the under-utilisation of health care in eating disorders are features of 'mental health literacy', a term introduced and defined by Jorm as "knowledge and beliefs about mental disorders that may aid in their recognition, management and treatment" (Jorm et al, 1997). Jorm and colleagues, and others, have argued that poor mental health literacy is a major factor in the individual, social and economic burden of mental health problems (Andrews et al., 2000; Jorm et al., 2000). There have been attempts to evaluate the efficacy of mental health literacy interventions in improving outcomes for patients with problems such as depression. In one study Jorm and colleagues (2003) reported a large community-based RCT (n=1094) for an evidenced based guide to treatments versus a general brochure for people with depressive symptoms. They found more positive outcomes in the former group but the effects were not large.

In the area of eating disorders we have conducted a small randomized controlled study of a brief postal mental health literacy intervention in community women with bulimic eating disorders. At the end of a year symptomatic improvement, less pessimism about how difficult eating disorders are to treat, improved recognition and knowledge, as well as increased help-seeking were observed in both groups (Hay et al., 2007a). Those randomized to receive the mental health literacy intervention also had improved mental health related quality of life. The study supported further investigations of the role of targeted health literacy interventions in eating disorders described in this chapter.

2. Randomised controlled trial of an eating disorder (bulimia nervosa) mental health literacy intervention (BN-MHL)

2.1 Aims of BN-MHL trial

The study aims were to test the efficacy of a mental health literacy intervention for eating disorders in a non-clinical sample of adult women. Outcomes included mental health literacy regarding treatments for a common eating disorder, bulimia, perceived health related quality of life and general and specific eating disorder psychological symptoms.

2.2 Methods of BN-MHL trial

The sample was derived from a longitudinal survey of women with disordered eating recruited through advertisements in four universities and colleges of higher education in two Australian States (Queensland and Victoria). Details of the total sample at baseline have been reported in Mond et al. (2010). Recruitment strategies varied and included approaches via central University email/web mail, printed advertisements in student bulletins and halls of residence and direct approach to students in University common areas. For individuals approached via email, participants were given the option of completing an on-line questionnaire. For other participants, questionnaires were provided in hard copy with reply-paid envelopes. The questionnaire included measures of eating disorder psychopathology and health-related quality of life (as completed by the first sample, see below).

The sample for the trial comprised 217 symptomatic young women (all $\geq$ 18 years, mean age 24.5 years SD 7.6) who agreed to follow-up. They were included if they had current extreme weight/shape concerns and/or current regular (e.g. occurring weekly over the past three months) binge eating and/or any extreme weight control behaviours such as self-induced vomiting and/or laxative/diuretic use and/or fasting or severe food restriction and/or 'driven' exercise and/or who self-identified on the BN-MHL survey as currently having a problem like that of 'Naomi' (see below - only one was included on this criteria alone). The majority of students (179, 84%) were Australian born and 150 (72%) were never married.

At the start of the first year (baseline) the participants who agreed to follow-up were randomised to receive either a bulimia nervosa mental health literacy (BN-MHL) intervention (n=97) or information about their symptom scores and local mental health services only, with the comparison group (as required by ethical consideration) receiving the intervention at the end of the first year. The intervention comprised a single posted package of information about treatment of BN and related disorders, purchasing information on the book "Binge eating and Bulimia nervosa: A guide to recovery" (Cooper, 1995). The recommended book included a detailed psycho-educational section and a self-directed cognitive-behaviour therapy. The package also provided recommended websites for further information on treatments, lists and contact details of local eating disorder specialist treatment facilities, and contact details for the (local) eating disorders support group and consumer organisation. At baseline the control group (n=120) received information about local mental health services only.

Randomisation was by means of SPSS RV.BINOM (1,0.5) function and allocation was concealed from the research officer who communicated with the participants. In the covering letter informed consent was obtained, along with permission for follow-up in order to "find out how health issues and general health and well-being impacts on people's quality of life over time". Participants were not told they were part of a randomised controlled trial. Three respective institutional ethics committees approved the research (namely James Cook, La Trobe and Western Sydney universities), with the proviso that control participants were provided with the intervention at one year.

ED symptoms were assessed with the Eating Disorder Examination Questionnaire (EDE-Q). The EDE-Q has been validated in community and clinic samples of people with EDs (Fairburn & Beglin, 1994; Mond et al., 2004). It yields a global score of ED attitudes and restraint, and four sub-scales (i.e. shape, weight and eating concern and dietary restraint) and also frequency of ED behaviours such as binge-eating over the preceding four weeks.

BN-MHL was assessed with a questionnaire designed for this research (Mond et al., 2010). A vignette describing a (fictional) 19-year-old female suffering from BN called Naomi (N) was presented. Care was taken to ensure that the core features of the disorder were present while avoiding the use of medical terminology. The text of the vignette was: *N is a 19-year-old second year arts student. Although mildly overweight as an adolescent, N's current weight is within the normal range for her age and height. However, she thinks she is overweight. Upon starting university, N joined a fitness program at the gym and also started running regularly. Through this effort she gradually began to lose weight. N then started to "diet," avoiding all fatty foods, not eating between meals, and trying to eat set portions of "healthy foods," mainly fruit and vegetables and bread or rice, each day. N also continued with the exercise program, losing several more kilograms. However, she has found it difficult to maintain the weight loss and for the past 18 months her weight has been continually fluctuating, sometimes by as much as 5 kilograms within a few weeks. N has also found it difficult to control her eating. While able to restrict her dietary intake during the day, at night she is often unable to stop eating, bingeing on, for example, a block of chocolate and several pieces of fruit. To counteract the effects of this bingeing, N takes water tablets. On other occasions, she vomits after overeating. Because of her strict routines of eating and exercising, N has become isolated from her friends.*

Following presentation of the vignette, participants were asked: "What would you say is N's *main* problem?" They were required to choose one answer only from a list of options provided. Options, listed in a pre-determined, random order, were: "bulimia nervosa"; "anorexia nervosa"; "an eating disorder, but not anorexia or bulimia"; "yo-yo dieting"; "poor diet"; "low self-esteem/lack of self-confidence"; "depression"; "an anxiety disorder or problem"; "stress"; "a nervous breakdown"; "a mental health problem"; and "no real problem, just a phase." Participants were asked to indicate which of a number of possible interventions within each of three categories—people (15 options), treatments/activities (12 options), and medicines/pills (4 options)—they believed would be most helpful for N as well as the person that they would first approach for advice or help were they to have a problem such as the one described. At 6 and 12 months the name and age of the person in the vignette was changed but gender remained female and the symptom profile remained that of purging type BN.

Mental health related quality of life was assessed with the well-validated 12-item Short Form-12 Health Status Questionnaire (SF-12; Ware et al., 1996). This provides a mental health related component score presented in this chapter. A score below 50 indicates impairment and below 40 moderate to severe impairment. General psychiatric symptoms were assessed with the Kessler-10 item distress scale (K-10). It is designed to detect cases of anxiety and affective disorders in the general population (Andrews & Slade, 2001) and it has been used in our previous research (e.g. Mond et al., 2004b). Scores range from 10 to 50 as there are ten items scored from 1 to 5. Scores of 19 or above indicate likely psychiatric disorder such as major depression or an anxiety disorder. Body Mass Index (BMI; kg/m^2) was calculated from self-reported height and weight.

Differences between groups were tested statistically using SPSS v 18 and with independent t-test and chi square or independent sample Mann-Whitney U tests respectively. Due to multiple testing significance was set at alpha ≤ 0.01.

2.3 Results of BN-MHL trial

At baseline the participants' BN-MHL and ED symptoms did not differ between groups. Eighteen percent correctly identified the problem in the vignette as BN and the most common response (27%) response was that the person's problem was low self-esteem (Table 1). Regard for evidence based treatments or specialists was modest. Only one person at baseline, two at 6-months and five at 12-months thought a self-help treatment manual would be helpful.

ED symptoms were high with mean (SD) scores on the EDE-Q subscales of eating concern 2.4 (1.4), shape concern 4.2 (1.2), weight concern 3.8 (1.2), and restraint 3.0 (1.5). The majority (80%) were binge eating (objective and /or subjective type), 32 (15%) were vomiting for weight control, 30 (14%) were using laxatives and three (1.4%) had used diuretics in the past four weeks. Follow-up responses at 6 months were 66% and 62% at 12 months. There were no significant differences at baseline on outcome variables between those who were and were not followed to 12-months.

Further results and comparative findings of the groups randomised or not to the BN-MHL intervention over the 12-months are shown in Table 1 below. At follow-up there were no significant differences between the intervention and information-only groups in BN-MHL or in symptomatic outcomes or in mental health related quality of life (see Table 2). A sensitivity analysis (to test for completer only analysis bias) was therefore not done. (Whilst on inspection it appeared that those in the intervention group were more likely to identify the problem as BN or another eating disorder ED at 6 and 12 months these differences were did not reach significance. There was a significant trend for those in the information only group to have fewer subjective binges at 6-months.)

	Baseline	**6-months**		**12-months**	
		BN-MHL	**I-only**	**BN-MHL**	**I-only**
N	217	65	78	62	72
Main problem					
Bulimia nervosa	39 (18%)	18 (28%)	26 (33%)	10 (16%)	8 (6.7%)
Other ED	35 (16%)	15 (23%)	8 (6.7%)	16 (26%)	19 (16%)
Low self-esteem	58 (27%)	14 (22%)	16 (13%)	13 (21%)	19 (16%)
Other	82 (38%)	18 (28%)	28 (36%)	22 (36%)	25 (35%)
Not answered	3 (1.4%)	0	0	1 (1.6%)	1 (1.3%)
Most helpful therapy					
Getting information	42 (20%)	23 (36%)	24 (31%)	20 (32%)	27 (38%)
Cognitive-behaviour	39 (19%)	10 (15%)	12 (15%)	12 (19%)	11 (16%)
Other psychotherapy	33 (15%)	7 (11%)	6 (8%)	5 (8%)	4 (6%)
Other	92 (42%)	24 (37%)	36 (46%)	34 (55%)	29 (40%)
Not answered	11 (5%)	1	0	1 (1.6%)	1 (1.3%)
Most helpful medication					
Vitamins/minerals	116 (54%)	36 (55%)	43 (55%)	40 (65%)	30 (42%)
Anti-depressant	37 (17%)	14 (22%)	22 (28%)	12 (19%)	19 (26%)
Herbal	29 (14%)	4 (6%)	4 (5%)	4 (7%)	12 (17%)
Other	1 (0.4%)	0	2 (3%)	1 (1.6%)	0
Unsure/none	19 (9%)	7 (11%)	4 (5%)	2 (3%)	6 (8%)
Not answered	14 (7%)	4 (6%)	3 (4%)	3 (5%)	5 (7%)
Most helpful professional					
Dietitian	51 (24%)	4 (6%)	14 (18%)	14 (23%)	22 (31%)
Specialist	48 (22%)	13 (20%)	18 (23%)	12 (19%)	17 (24%)
Non-specialist	30 (14%)	17 (26%)	13 (17%)	13 (21%)	12 (17%)
Family doctor	32 (15%)	12 (19%)	7 (9%)	7 (11%)	7 (10%)
Other	46 (21%)	16 (25%)	23 (30%)	15 (24%)	13 (18%)
Not answered	10 (5%)	3 (5%)	3 (4%)	1 (1.6%)	1 (1.3%)

Table 1. **Bulimia nervosa mental health literacy (BN-MHL) outcomes following a BN-MHL intervention.** All data is in the form of n (%), I=information, ED=eating disorder, specialist refers to psychiatrist or psychologist, non-specialist refers to a counsellor or social worker, all between group differences not significant.

	Baseline6-months			12-months	
		BN-MHL	I-only	BN-MHL	I-only
N	217	65	78	62	72
			Mean (SD)		
Global EDE-Q	3.3 (1.1)	2.9 (1.2)	2.6 (1.3)	2.7 (1.3)	2.4 (1.2)
EDE-Q Eating concern	2.4 (1.4)	1.9 (1.4)	1.7 (1.4)	1.9 (1.5)	1.6 (1.3)
EDE-Q Shape concern	4.2 (1.2)	3.6 (1.4)	3.4 (1.6)	3.0 (1.5)	3.4 (1.5)
EDE-Q Weight concern	3.9 (1.2)	3.4 (1.3)	3.1 (1.5)	3.1 (1.4)	2.9 (1.5)
EDE-Q Restraint	3.0 (1.5)	2.6 (1.5)	2.2 (1.5)	2.4 (1.4)	2.0 (1.4)
SF-12 MH	39 (12)	41 (11)	42 (11)	43 (12)	46 (12)
K-10	23 (8)	22 (8)	21 (9)	22 (8)	21 (8)
BMI kg/m^2	26 (6)	25 (6)	26 (6)	26 (6)	26 (5)
			Median (IQ range)		
Objective binge eating	1 (0-8)	0 (0-5)	0 (0-5)	0 (0-4)	0 (0-3)
Subjective binge eating	4 (0-10)	2 (0-6)	0 (0-2)*	0 (0-4)	0 (0-4)

Table 2. **Health outcomes following a mental health literacy intervention in women with disordered eating.** SF-12 MH (mental health component score) measures mental health related quality of life, the K-10 measures psychological distress, BMI=body mass index, mean and SD, all p not significant excepting *p=0.01

2.4 Summary and introduction to trial of self-help approaches

In the trial of BN-MHL intervention we found the participants' BN-MHL at baseline to be similar to that in our previous surveys (Mond et al., 2010). Participants were most likely to identify the problem for the women with BN as one of low self-esteem and had modest or low regard for evidence based or specialist therapies compared to non-specialists. As we found previously (Hay et al., 2007a) a BN-MHL intervention had no significant impact on changing attitudes or improving symptoms and in this study it also had no significant impact on improving mental health related quality of life.

The findings indicated that merely providing people with information about treatments for bulimic EDs and also advising them to seek help did not result in notable changes in behaviour or beliefs. Our question then was - what interventions might help people with EDs improve recognition and understanding of treatments for their problem and thereby prompt effective help-seeking? We thus planned a second feasibility trial to investigate the impact of enhancing the MHL intervention by adding an evidence-based self-help treatment manual to the MHL intervention.

3. Self-help as a targeted intervention for bulimic EDs in primary care

3.1 Introduction to feasibility trial of self-help

Self-help therapies have been introduced to help fill the gap between the high prevalence of bulimic-type EDs in the general population, and the lack of specialised professionals. Self-help can be appropriate for partial or less severe conditions, with guidance from trained non-specialised professionals in primary care services (GSH), or utilised in specialised services as a first step of a more comprehensive treatment, i.e. in a "stepped-care" approach.

Manuals studied have included: *"Overcoming Binge Eating"* (Fairburn, 1995) or translations/adaptations of it; the manual: *"Bulimia Nervosa: a guide to recovery"* (Cooper, 1995) since updated; and the manual: *"Getting Better Bit(e) by Bit(e)"* (Schmidt & Treasure 1993).

Hay et al. (2004) and Stefano et al. (2006) examined abstinence rates from ED behaviours such as binge eating in meta-analyses of trials pure self-help (PSH) vs waitlist in bulimic disorders such as BN or binge eating disorder. Rates ranged from 30% to 36% for PSH - and were better for GSH which ranged from 33% to 43%, the latter of which can be comparable to full CBT in its outcomes. In all meta-analyses PSH was however favoured over waitlist where abstinence rates were, for example, between 5% and 11%. Despite promising if modest findings, there have been a number of problems with these studies including variable levels of therapist training and variation in evaluation tools and outcome measurements. Whilst it has been argued that self-help can be a first step in management for selected people seeking help for EDs its role in assisting people with EDs not accessing services or treatments is thus less clear.

In addition, as weight concern and seeking help to lose weight is a common feature of women who do not seek help for their ED (Hay et al., 1998; Mond et al., 2007) we thought it important to add nutrition and lifestyle intervention strategies to self-help to assist women who are overweight or obese to reduce further weight gain and/or maintain weight in the healthy range. This included specific advice on healthy exercise. We also chose a vignette of someone with binge eating disorder as that is a common bulimic eating disorder and is more frequently associated with weight disorder (Hudson et al., 2007, Darby et al., 2009). We thus developed the intervention to be for both eating and weight disorder health literacy (EWD-HL).

We based this second trial in general practice as unrecognised bulimic eating disorders are common in women attending their family doctors (King, 1989; Whitehouse et al. 1992; Hay et al., 1998; Mond et al., 2009). The family doctor is also the point of access for psychological treatments for people in Australia. To inform the present study we conducted an investigation into the dissemination of an EWD-HL intervention into primary care at two general practices in late 2005 (Hay et al., 2006). One hundred and fifty-five women (aged 18-45 years) attending the two practices (over 3 months) in North Queensland (Australia) were screened through the distribution of an ED symptom and an ED-MHL survey by reception staff. Fourteen (9%) had a bulimic ED, and a further 12 (7.7%) had clinically significant symptoms. Attractive booklets containing information about ED and their treatments, a brief assessment screening questionnaire for Eating Disorders (the SCOFF (Morgan et al., 1999)) and information on local services and consumer groups were left in the waiting rooms, and a poster containing the SCOFF questions was displayed inviting patients to take a copy of the 'guide' booklet.

This survey confirmed a high level of untreated bulimic EDs in primary care settings as of the 23% women who self-identified an ED problem only one had sought professional help, in this instance from a counselor. In addition, patients reported they were prompted to discuss their ED symptoms with their GP as a result of reading the booklet. However, screening utilising reception staff was problematic and very inefficient compared to our previous method of embedding a research assistant (RA) in the practices (e.g. Hay et al., 1998). We also found the booklets needed to be provided to participants directly as, while many participants (54%) were interested in receiving a copy of the booklet when their attention was drawn to it, very few (14%) had picked it up in the waiting rooms. This occurred despite the waiting room poster drawing their attention to the booklet. Thus our intent in the randomized controlled trial was to ensure dissemination of the EWD-HL intervention to all women who were symptomatic.

The aims of the present feasibility trial were to test the ease of screening women in general practice for untreated EDs and the acceptance of an unsolicited self-help and EWD-HL intervention. Secondary aims were to inspect symptomatic and MHL outcomes compared to a non-specific self-help intervention.

3.2 Methods of self-help trial

Participants were identified by an author (DK) from sequential surveys of consecutive women attendees in two family doctor waiting rooms over a series of morning, afternoon, evening and weekend clinics. They first completed a survey including informed consent, EDE-Q (see above section 2.2) screening questions, and reported weight and height. Respondents who were symptomatic were asked to complete the remaining survey questionnaires and were subsequently posted or not posted the relevant intervention packages. Assessments were conducted at baseline and a 3-month postal follow-up.

Assessments were the same as in the first trial described in section 2.2 above with the vignette being of that of a women with binge eating disorder (BED) and BMI 26 (i.e. above the normal range but not overweight or obese) and addition of a self-esteem questionnaire (Robson 1998, 1989). The background to the development of the questionnaire is described in the 1988 paper where self-esteem was defined as: "The sense of contentment and self-acceptance that stems from a person's appraisal of his own worth, significance, attractiveness, competence, and ability to satisfy his aspirations" (Robson, 1988). The Robson questionnaire aims to quantify this sense of self-esteem or the individual elements of self-appraisal. Seven components of self-esteem are evaluated: subjective sense of significance; worthiness; appearance and social acceptability; competence; resilience and determination; control over personal destiny; and the value of existence. The items are scored on an 8-point Likert scale from "completely disagree" (zero score) to "completely agree" (score of seven). The total score is a summation of the scores on each item. The reliability and validity of the questionnaire has been assessed in one non-patient group and two patient groups (Robson, 1989). In the non-patient group the split-half reliability score was 0.96 and the Cronbach alpha coefficient was 0.89. The test-retest correlation was 0.88 ($p<0.0001$).

The text used in the BED-MHL vignette was: *Emily (E) is a 25 year-old student who has been "chubby" since she was 13. Over the years she has tried several diets, but she has never been able to stick with the recommendations for very long. E has just started a new job and is finding it hard to adjust. To make herself feel better, E "treats" herself with her favourite foods. When E gets home from work she often goes to the kitchen for a snack and then finds that she is unable to stop eating, for example, a sandwich, a chocolate bar, a slice of cheesecake, some ice cream and some fruit. Later in the evening she will eat dinner and sometimes she loses control with this as well and eats the leftovers, along with that another slice of cake, some cereal, and some more ice cream. These episodes of overeating occur, on average, two to three times per week. The next day she will try to eat less to "make up" for overeating. E feels ashamed of herself when she loses control of her eating like this and she despises the shape of her body, although she has never talked to anyone about it. She has often thought about more extreme methods of controlling her weight, such as fasting, vomiting after eating, or using laxatives, but she has never tried any of these things. She has been told by her doctor that she is just over the 'normal' weight for her height.*

Participants were included if they were over 18 years, had current extreme weight and/or shape concerns and current regular clinically significant ED behaviours (as in the first trial). Women who at baseline were receiving treatment for an ED and women who were at high risk if left untreated, specifically those who were pregnant, and of very low weight (BMI$\leq$ 17.5) were excluded.

Participants were blind to their group and outcome assessments were blind to the group allocation. A second author (PH) was responsible for randomization (using a sequence generated using SPSS RV.BINOM (1,0.5) function), allocation concealment and posting out of the intervention packages. This trial was approved by the University of Western Sydney Human Research Ethics Committee.

The EWD-HL intervention was presented in booklet format which included (i) information on different types of eating disorders and associated mental health and weight problems, (ii) available evidence based treatments for EDs and what they involve, (iii) information on eating and lifestyle for maintaining a healthy weight, or for weight loss or gain in those who are overweight or underweight, designed specifically for those with eating disorders, (in accordance with National Health and Medical Research Council Australian guidelines for levels of exercise and nutrition (NHMRC, 2003) and a reference to a self-help book (Kausman, 1998: "If not dieting, then what?"), (iv) information regarding attitudes and beliefs likely to sustain symptoms and/or hinder treatment-seeking, (v) lists and contacts of local community and specialist treatment facilities and the (local) EDs support group or consumer organisation, (vi) the cognitive-behavioural self-help manual and book by Cooper (1995) "Bulimia nervosa and Binge Eating: A guide to recovery" that has specific guidance through the stages of therapy, checklists of progress, encouragement when treatment goals are obtained and advice on 'lapses' and when and where to go for more help if needed, and (vii) an ED screening questionnaire the "SCOFF" (Morgan et al., 1999) to assist participants self-identify an ED. In addition participants received a full copy of the book by Cooper (1995).

The control group received the self-help book "Overcoming Low Self-esteem" (Fennell, 1999). This utilises cognitive and behavioural techniques in a self-help guide format for readers. It is comparable in length and context to the Cooper manual for EDs. Low self-esteem is common in people with EDs and has been the target of primary prevention programs and general strategies to improve self-esteem have been included in other self-help manuals for BN (e.g. Schmidt & Treasure (1993)). In addition (and as described above) we have found community women and symptomatic women most frequently identify the main problem for a women with BED or similar ED as one of 'low self-esteem' (e.g. Mond & Hay, 2008). However, findings in RCTs targeting self-esteem in universal programs aimed to reduce ED risk factors have been inconsistent (Wade et al., 2003).

3.3 Results of self-help trial

Three hundred and twenty six women were approached over 6-months in two general practices. One hundred and sixty-three women were screened of whom 44 (13.5%) women met criteria and 36 (80%) agreed to do the full assessments and to have a follow-up assessment. Most were in full or part-time employment (57%) or employed in home duties (20%). Sixty per cent were married or living as married, 15% were separated or divorced, 74% had children, 43% had at least completed high school and 47% had completed a tertiary level qualification or degree. Mean age was 40.1 years (SD 11.9) and mean BMI was 30 (SD 7.5). The majority 40 (90%) were binge eating (7 subjective bingeing only) and 9 (20%) were using laxatives, diuretics or self-induced vomiting.

Twenty-three (52%) participants completed 3-month follow-up. There were no statistically significant differences in level of ED symptoms on the EDE-Q or other outcome variables between those who did and did not complete follow-up. Because of the small absolute numbers per group who completed follow-up descriptive data only are reported, no between group statistical tests were performed and sensitivity analyses were not performed. At baseline the MHL responses found most identified the problem as one of low self-esteem (see Table 3), vitamins and minerals were more favorably regarded than evidence based

	Baseline	**3-month follow-up**	
		EWD-HL & ED SH	Self-esteem SH
N	36	12	11
Main problem			
Bulimia nervosa	2 (5%)	0	0
Binge eating disorder	6 (17%)	4	1
Other ED	2 (5%)	0	0
Low self-esteem	18 (50%)	0	5
Other	7 (19%)	5	4
Not answered	1 (3%)	3	1
Most helpful therapy			
Getting information	8 (22%)	4	5
Cognitive-behaviour	4 (11%)	2	1
Other psychotherapy	4 (11%)	0	0
Self-help manual	0 (0%)	0	1
Other	16 (44%)	5	3
Not answered	4 (11%)	1	1
Most helpful medication			
Vitamins/minerals	21 (58%)	9	5
Anti-depressant	8 (22%)	2	2
Herbal	5 (14%)	0	4
Other	0	0	0
Not answered	2 (5%)	1	0
Most helpful professional			
Dietitian	8 (22%)	4	2
Specialist	5 (14%)	1	2
Non-specialist	5 (14%)	0	0
Family doctor	11 (31%)	3	3
Other	5 (14%)	4	4
Not answered	2 (5%)	0	0

Table 3. **Binge eating disorder mental health literacy (BED-MHL) outcomes following a EWD-HL/Self-Help (SH) intervention.** Specialist refers to psychiatrist or psychologist, non-specialist refers to a counsellor or social worker. Because of low numbers % are not presented for follow-up data.

medication (antidepressants), and primary care or other non-specialists were more often regarded as helpful than specialist care. BED was identified as the main problem by 17%, and increased at follow-up in those who had the EWD-HL intervention and ED self-help book, indicating some effect on recognition at least with this. Perceived helpfulness of evidence base treatments such as cognitive-behaviour therapy or anti-depressants did not seem to change and regard for specialists as the most helpful professionals did not increase. There was improvement overall but few differences in symptoms, mental health related quality of life or self-esteem between randomized groups at follow-up (as shown on Table 4). There were reduced numbers with objective but not subjective binge eating in those who received the self-esteem book.

No-one listed a self-help manual as most helpful at baseline but one person who received the self-esteem self-help book did list a self-help manual as most helpful treatment at follow-up. At follow-up 8/12 reported reading the ED self-help book (and most read about 50% of it), all found it not difficult to understand, 6/12 thought it informative (notably the first psycho-educative section of the book) but only 1 described it as personally helpful. Seven of 11 reported reading the self-esteem self-help book (and most read around 40% of it), all found it not difficult to understand, 7/11 thought it informative and 4/11 described it as personally helpful with again most finding the psycho-education sections more helpful than the self-help treatment section.

	Baseline	**3-month follow-up**	
		BED-MHL & ED SH	**Self-esteem SH**
N	44	12	11
		Median (IQ range)	
Objective binge eating	4 (0-8)	2 (0-4)	0 (0-5)
Subjective binge eating	5 (0-10)	2 (0-4)	2 (0-10)
		Mean (SD)	
EDE-Q Global score	3.3 (0.9)	2.7 (1.2)	3.1 (1.0)
EDE-Q Restraint	2.9 (1.4)	2.9 (1.6)	2.5 (1.3)
EDE-Q Eating concern	2.0 (1.4)	1.4 (1.4)	2.5 (1.3)
EDE-Q Weight concern	3.9 (0.9)	3.4 (1.6)	3.7 (0.9)
EDE-Q Shape concern	4.4 (1.0)	4.1 (1.6)	4.1 (1.2)
N	36	12	11
SF-12 mental health	42.2 (11.1)	44.0 (11.0)	42.6 (9.5)
K-10	19.2 (7.4)	18.1 (7.4)	16.5 (4.2)
BMI kg/m^2	30 (7.5)	31.8 (8.9)	31.8 (9.0)
Self-esteem	48.6 (7.7)	52.4 (4.7)	51.3 (7.9)

Table 4. **Health outcomes following a EWD-HL/Self-Help (SH) intervention.** SF-12 measures mental health component score of health related quality of life, the K-10 measures psychological distress, BMI=body mass index

Although more than half of the respondents reported reading and understanding a significant proportion of the self help material, this appears to have had no impact on curbing attempts to lose weight. At assessment, 29 (85%) women reported trying to lose weight in the previous six months whilst in the three month period between assessment and follow up 21 (91%) reported they had been trying to lose weight.

4. Conclusions

In this chapter we describe two attempts to identify and assist women with EDs in the community, one a sample of younger women from tertiary education institutions and one a sample of older women attending their family doctors. In the first trial we did not replicate the positive findings of an earlier study which found a brief BN-MHL intervention improved mental health related quality of life when compared to a control condition of information about ED services only. The MHL intervention had little impact on changing attitudes and beliefs about EDs, their identification or their treatment. However, the present studies were possibly underpowered to show differences. The second study was with an enhanced intervention that included provision of an evidence-based self-help book. There may have been a small impact on identification of the ED but overwhelmingly participants still had a comparatively low regard for specialist treatments and rated getting more information as the most helpful approach for a fictitious person with a bulimic ED.

Given that identifying the main problem for the woman with a bulimic ED in the vignette as low self-esteem it was of interest that the self-esteem self-help book appeared better received and more found it personally helpful than the ED self-help book. Anecdotal comments were that the title of the ED book was disconcerting and some women were puzzled as to why they had received it. Although not overt we suspected that it may have been perceived as stigmatising by some participants. Many community women perceive significant stigma and discrimination for those who have a known ED (Hepworth & Paxton, 2007) and particularly for those with binge eating and (over) weight (Darby et al., manuscript in preparation). We think it is likely that self-help books for binge eating and BN such as that used in the present study are thus best provided in the context of a consultation where their role and relevance can be explained.

An additional factor (the 'elephant in the room') is the ambivalence people have towards the ED behaviours. We have found that despite distress from ED symptoms, people with EDs have a favourable regard for ED weight losing strategies (Mond et al., 2010) and are much more likely to seek help to lose weight than to modify disordered eating (Hay et al., 1998; Mond et al., 2007; Evans et al., 2011). This apparent paradox is perhaps understandable in the context of widespread public and community concerns about obesity and negative community attitudes towards weight disorders with widespread cultural positive regard for being thin. If a woman's main concern is to receive help for a perceived or actual over-weight problem, then she may be less likely to want to engage in treatments that are not known to reduce weight. In addition, we have found many women and up to a third of general practitioners and other key health professionals consider weight gain to be likely with treatment for bulimia nervosa (Hay et al., 2007b).

The question of how best to improve ED-MHL for people with disordered eating, and if an improvement subsequently leads to an increase in accessing evidence-based treatments from appropriately trained professionals thereby reducing community and individual burden from EDs is still unanswered. Large scale universal public health campaigns and /or programs that target health care professionals are alternatives to the targeted programs described here. One focussing on depression and its treatment has likely had an effect in improving community attitudes in Australia (Jorm et al., 2006). However their impact for reducing impact from depression for individuals is hard to evaluate. New approaches in developing strategies to help people with EDs understand their problems and how to effectively seek treatment may need to more directly target weight concern and deliver community interventions in mental health stigma-free contexts such as 'lifestyle' or 'well being' centres.

5. Acknowledgement

The first trial was funded by a grant from the Australian Rotary Health Research Fund. The second trial was funded by an internal UWS research grant to PH. We thank Amber Sajjad for assistance with data management.

6. References

Andrews., G., Slade, T. (2001) Interpreting scores on the Kessler Psychological Distress Scale (K10). *Aaustralian and NewZealand Journal of Public Health* Vol 25, pp. 494-497.

Andrews, G., Sanderson, K., Slade, T. & Issakidis,C. (2000). Why does the burden of disease persist? Relating the burden of anxiety and depression to effectiveness of treatment. *Bulletin of the World Health Organization*, Vol 78, pp. 446-454.

Becker, A. E., Franko, D. L., Nussbaum, K., & Herzog, D. B. (2004). Secondary Prevention for Eating Disorders: The Impact of Education, Screening, and Referral in a College-Based Screening Program. *International Journal of Eating Disorders,* Vol 36, pp. 157–162.

Cachelin, F. M., & Striegel-Moore, R. H. (2006). Help seeking and barriers to treatment in a community sample of Mexican American and European American women with eating disorders. *International Journal of Eating Disorders,* Vol 39,pp. 1544-1561.

Cooper P. (1995) *Bulimia Nervosa and Binge Eating. A guide to recovery*. London: Robinson Press.

Darby, A., Hay, P., Mond, J., Quirk, F., Buettner, P., & Kennedy, L. (2009). The rising prevalence of co-morbid obesity and eating disorder behaviours from 1995 to 2005 *International Journal of Eating Disorders,* Vol 42, pp. 104-108.

Darby, A., Hay, P., Mond, J., Quirk, F. (in preparation). Societal reaction toward eating disorder sufferers: A paradox of positive regard and discrimination.

Evans, E. J., Hay, P. J., Mond, J. M, Paxton, S. J., Quirk, F., Rodgers, B., Jhajj, A. K., Sawoniewska, M. A. (in press 2011). Barriers to help-seeking in young women with eating disorders: A qualitative exploration in a longitudinal community survey. *Eating Disorders: The Journal of Treatment and Prevention,* Vol 19, pp 270-285.

Fairburn, C. G. (1995). *Overcoming binge eating*. New York: Guilford.

Fairburn, C.G., & Beglin, S.J. (1994). Assessment of eating disorders: Interview or self-report questionnaire? *International Journal of Eating Disorders,* Vol 16, pp. 363-370.

Fairburn, C., Cooper, Z., Doll, H., Norman, P.,& O'Connor, M. (2000) The natural course of bulimia nervosa and binge eating disorder in young women. *Arch Gen Psychiatry* Vol 57, pp. 659–665.

Fennall, M. (1999) *Overcoming low self-esteem.*. London: Constable Robinson.

Hart, L. M., Granillo, M. T., Jorm, A. F., Paxton, S.J. (in press). Unmet need for treatment in the eating disorders: A systematic review of eating disorder specific treatment seeking among community cases. *Clinical Psychology Review.*

Hay, P. J., & Mond, J. (2005). How to 'count the cost' and measure burden?: a review of health related quality of life in people with eating disorders. *Journal of Mental Health* Vol 14, pp. 539-552.

Hay, P., Darby, A., & Hogg, A. (2006) A targeted intervention for Eating Disorders in primary care: A pilot study. Presentation to State-wide Eating Disorder Reference group, QLD, 02/2006.

Hay, P., Claudino, A. (2010) Evidence-Based Treatment for the Eating Disorders. *In* Oxford Handbook of Eating Disorders. Ed Stewart Agras. New York: Oxford University Press. pp 452-279.

Hay, P. J., Marley, J., & Lemarn S. (1998) Covert eating disorders: The prevalence, characteristics and help-seeking of those with bulimic eating disorders in general practice. *Primary Care Psychiatry*, Vol 4, pp 95-99.

Hay, P. J., Bacaltchuk, J., & Stefano, S. (2004). Psychotherapy for bulimia nervosa and binge eating. *Cochrane Database of Systematic Reviews*, 3, CD000562.

Hay, P.J., Mond, J.M., Darby, A., Rodgers, B., & Owen, C. (2007a). What are the effects of providing evidence-based information on eating disorders and their treatments? A randomised controlled trial in a symptomatic community sample. *Early Intervention in Psychiatry,* Vol 1, pp. 316-324.

Hay, P. J., Darby, A., Mond, J. (2007b) Knowledge and Beliefs about Bulimia Nervosa and its Treatment: A Comparative Study of Three Disciplines. *Journal of Clininical Psychology in Medical Settings* Vol 14, pp. 59-68.

Hepworth, N. S., & Paxton, S. J. (2007). Pathways to help-seeking in bulimia nervosa and binge eating problems: A concept mapping approach. *International Journal of Eating Disorders Vol* 40, pp. 493-504.

Hudson, J. I., Hiripi, E., Pope, H. G. Jr., & Kessler, R. C. (2007). The Prevalence and Correlates of Eating Disorders in the National Comorbidity Survey Replication *Biological Psychiatry* Vol 61, pp. 348–358.

Jorm, A.F., Korten, A.E., Jacomb, P.A., Christensen, H., Rodgers, B., & Pollitt, P. (1997). Mental health literacy: A survey of the public's ability to recognise mental disorders and their beliefs about the effectiveness of treatment. *Medical Journal of Australia,* Vol 166, pp. 182-186.

Jorm, A.F., Angermeyer, M. & Katschnig, H. (2000), Public knowledge of and attitudes to mental disorders: A limiting factor in the optimal use of treatment services. In G. Andrews & S. Henderson (Eds.), Unmet need in psychiatry (pp.399-413). Cambridge: Cambridge University Press.

Jorm, A. F., Griffiths, K. M., Christensen, H., Korten, A. E., Parslow, R. A, & Rodgers, B. (2003) Providing information about the effectiveness of treatment options to depressed people in the community. *Psychological Medicine* Vol 33, pp. 1071-1079.

Jorm, A. F., Christensen, H., & Griffiths, K. M. (2006). Changes in depression awareness and attitudes in Australia: the impact of Beyond Blue: The National Depression Initiative. *Australian and New Zealand Journal of Psychiatry* Vol 40, pp. 42-46.

Kausman R. (1998) *If not dieting then what?* Allen & Unwin.

King, M. B. (1989). Eating Disorders in a general practice population. [Monograph] *Psychological Medicine,* Vol 14, pp. 1-34.

Mathers, C., Vos, T., & Stevenson, C. (1999). The burden of disease and injury in Australia. Canberra: Australian Institute of Health and Welfare.

Mehler, P. S. (2003) Clinical practice. Bulimia nervosa. *New England Journal of Medicine* Vol 28, pp875-81.

Mond, J. M., & Hay, P. J. (2008) Public perceptions of binge eating and its treatment. *International Journal of Eating Disorders* Vol 41, pp.419-426.

Mond, J.M., Hay, P.J., Rodgers, B., Owen, C., & Beumont, P.J.V. (2004). Validity of the Eating Disorder Examination Questionnaire (EDE-Q) in screening for eating disorders in community samples. *Behaviour Research and Therapy,* Vol 42, pp. 551-567.

Mond, J. M., Robertson-Smith, G., & Vitere A. (2006). Stigma and eating disorders: is there evidence of negative attitudes towards individuals suffering from anorexia nervosa? *Journal of Mental Health,* Vol 15,pp. 519-532.

Mond, J.M., Hay, P.J., Rodgers, B., & Owen C. (2007). Health service utilization for eating disorders: Findings from a community-based study. *International Journal of Eating Disorders,* Vol 40, pp.399-409.

Mond, J. M., Myers, T. C., Crosby, R. D., Hay, P. J., & Mitchell, J. E.(2009) Bulimic eating disorders in primary care: Hidden morbidity still? *Journal of Clinical Psychology in Medical Settings,* Dec 29, pp. 56-63.

Mond JM, Hay PJ, Paxton SJ, Rodgers B, Darby A, Nillson J, Quirk F, Owen C. (2010) Eating Disorders "Mental Health Literacy" in Low Risk, High Risk and Symptomatic Women: Implications for Health Promotion Programs. *Eating Disorders: The Journal of Treatment and Prevention* Vol 18, pp. 267-285.

Morgan, J. F., Reid, F., & Lacey, J. H. (1999) The SCOFF questionnaire. *British Medical Journal* Vol 319, pp. 1467-1468.

Neumark-Sztainer, D., Wall, M., Guo, J, et al. (2006) Obesity, disordered eating, and eating disorders in a longitudinal study of adolescents? *Journal of the American Dietetic Association* Vol 106, pp.559-568.

NHMRC. (2003) Dietary Guidelines for Australian Adults. Commonwealth of Australia: Canberra.

Robson PJ. Self-Esteem - A psychiatric view. British Journal of Psychiatry 153:6-15, 1988.

Robson PJ. Development of a new self-report questionnaire to measure self-esteem. Psychological Medicine 19:513-518, 1989.

Stefano, S. C, Bacaltchuk, J., Blay, S. L., & Hay, P. (2006). Self-help treatments for disorders of recurrent binge eating: a systematic review. *Acta Psychiatrica Scandinavica* Vol 113, pp. 1-8.

Stewart, M-C, Keel, P. K., & Schiavo, R. S. (2006). Stigmatization of Anorexia Nervosa. *International Journal of Eating Disorders,* Vol 39, pp. 320-325.

Schmidt, U. H., & Treasure, J. L. (1993). *Getting better bit(e) by bit(e): A survival kit for sufferers of bulimia nervosa and binge eating disorders.* Hove, UK: Psychology Press.

Wade, T. D., Davidson, J,& O'Dea J. A. (2003) A preliminary controlled evaluation of a school-based media literacy program and self-esteem program for reducing eating disorder risk factors. *International Journal of Eating Disorders* Vol 33, pp. 371-83.

Ware, J. E., Kosinski, M., Keller, S. D. (1996) A 12-item short-form health survey. *Medical Care* Vol 34, pp. 220-233.

Whitehouse, A. M., Cooper, P. J., Vize, C. V., Hill, C., & Vogel, L. (1992). Prevalence of eating disorders in three Cambridge general practices: Hidden and conspicuous morbidity. *British Journal of General Practice,* Vol 42, pp. 57-60.

7

Bulimia Nervosa and Dissatisfaction of Adolescent's Body Shape

Alice Maria de Souza-Kaneshima and Edilson Nobuyoshi Kaneshima
State University of Maringá. Maringá PR, Brazil

1. Introduction

Bulimia nervosa is an eating disorder that affects young people and causes serious damage to life quality and death in extreme cases (Affenito & Kerstetter, 1999; Cordás, 2004; Costa et al., 2008; Gucciardi et al., 2004). Since most people with the disorder have normal weight, the diagnosis of bulimia nervosa becomes a highly complex issue (Kaufman, 2000).

The etiology of bulimia nervosa has yet to be understood. However, low self-esteem, depression, social pressure on keeping oneself slim and a dissatisfaction with the body shape are factors that may be associated with the bulimia nervosa event, especially in the case of adolescents and female young adults (Affenito & Kerstetter, 1999; Alvarez-Rayon et al., 2009; Costa et al., 2008; Crosby et al., 2009; Gucciardi et al., 2004; Jauregui-Lobera et al., 2008; Thompson & Chad, 2000).

Excessive concern with weight gaining is not the only criterion for a diagnosis of bulimia nervosa. Nevertheless, adolescents with such concern have a seven-fold chance in developing some type of eating disorder (Grillo & Silva, 2004).

The fact that many young people are not satisfied with their own body shape may be an effect of pre-conceived ideas on idealized body images taken from aesthetic values transmitted by society or by the social media (Andrade & Bosi, 2003; Reato et al., 2000; Reato, 2002). The female adolescent finds herself in conflict between a fantasy-created image and her real body shape. From her perspective, there is a great difference between what is observed and what is desired. This event may lead towards dissatisfaction and low self-esteem which induces the development of eating disorders such as bulimia nervosa (Andrade & Bosi, 2003; Mond et al., 2004; Reato, 2002; Silva et al., 2003).

Many authors agree that the most prevalent aspect of female dissatisfaction occurs in issues referring to weight and appearance. Many women, including those with normal weight or even slim ones, have the impression that they are overweight or even obese. This is the reason why their body image distortion mainly affects female adolescent and young adult females (Alvarez-Rayon et al., 2009; Cordas, 2004; Costa et al., 2008; Mond et al., 2004; Nunes et al., 2001).

Studies related to adolescent's psychological and eating behaviour alterations are important for the determination of factors involved in the development of eating disorders in young populations. The use of self-evaluation scales is an asset in the detection of possible eating disorders or of sub-clinic individuals (Kjelsas et al., 2004; Wichstrom, 1995).

Bulimia nervosa affects males and females, although the latter are more prone to the disease. This is due to the fact that women have more conflicts related to meals, weight and body shape. Conflicts indeed change the female adolescents' emotional state; in their turn, they present a distorted body image and low self-esteem (Affenito & Kerstetter, 1999; Gucciardi et al., 2004; Mond et al., 2004). Although many bulimic syndrome cases have been reported in young women under 18 years, the occurrence of such eating disorder is also on the increase in males (Affenito & Kerstetter, 1999; Alvarez-Rayon et al., 2009; Appolinário & Claudino, 2000; Costa et al., 2008; Gucciardi et al., 2004; Jauregui-Lobera et al., 2008; Kaufman, 2000).

Several authors report that patients with bulimic events are also highly concerned with weight gain. The patient is prone to use non-appropriate compensatory methods even twice a week. Self-evaluation of body image in these patients is greatly affected by society-idealized images of body shape and weight (Alvarez-Rayon et al., 2009; Cordás, 2004; Costa et al., 2008; Gucciardi et al., 2004; Jauregui-Lobera et al., 2008; Miranda, 2000; Pedrinola, 2002; Thompson & Chad, 2000).

2. The evolution of beauty standards

The idea of a healthy and beautiful body underwent several changes throughout the ages. By the end of the Middle Ages the ideal feminine body emphasized its reproductive role with an underscoring of motherhood, as Botticelli's artistic representation of the *Birth of Venus* (1485) warrants. The beautiful and the desired female always featured a lady with a round body due to fat deposits in the waist, thighs, belly and breasts, round and full breasts (Castilho, 2001). Famines and lack of food were not infrequent during the period and a round-bodied female symbolized the strong woman with sufficient energy to face the vicissitudes of the time and protect her family (Almeida et al., 2005; Andrade & Bosi, 2003).

At the start of the 16th century any artifice to seek or enhance beauty was liable to punishment. Beauty was God's gift and the face should reveal the soul's innocence. Hands should be long, white and dainty, and tight corsets were mandatory so that the female bosom could be graceful and her body elegant. In the 17th century etiquette and body posing were highly appreciated. Moreover, beauty was the female's asset although male aesthetics distanced itself from the signs of power in which it was enmeshed. More radical changes of concepts occurred in the 18th century. Mirrors became popular and with them the possibility of observing the entire body, or rather, the body's profile, balance and movements, with a consequent increase in sensitiveness and awareness of one's own body. Walking was recommended by physicians so that one's posture could be strengthened and legs and arms mobilized (Vigarello, 2006).

In the 19th century other parts of the body began to be focused and notions of beauty lime-lighted shape and profile. Sales and use of cosmetics and make-ups increased throughout the century and the physical model of the female profile now comprised a tight waist and a puffed up bosom. The discovery of oxygen may have shown that large breasts symbolized life. By the end of the century while special emphasis was bequeathed to the legs, the beach was the site of leisure and rest (Vigarello, 2006).

The idealized female image of the beginning of the 20th century was represented by two opposite standards: the first one comprised an erotic profile which could be found in the fin-de-siècle cafés full of females exhibiting rounded contours and pronounced tights; the second revealed a slim and thin profile. The latter definitely supplanted the former and

advertisements featuring slim females became abundant. In fact, several massage methods were introduced to delete excesses in rounded profiles. It was during this period that a relationship between age, weight and height was established even though hard and fast rules were inexistent (Vigarello, 2006).
The end of the First World War brought about the female's plain and free shapes which displaced the erstwhile curve ideals. Women's wear of the 1920s abandoned the curvy outlines and corsets. Bodices were set aside. Since women started to support their breasts with vests that flattened their profile, during this period beauty was almost characterized by the absence of secondary female sexual traits. The female profile had an extended shape, legs were up for view and hairdressings were high (Castilho, 2001).
Fashion magazines of the 1920s demonstrated an association between professional life style and beauty care. Swimming became more frequent and dynamic moving half-naked bodies were exposed for anyone to look at and appreciate. Such a condition had an important influence on the concept of beauty since beauty became synonymous to a slim and muscular body with elegant and graceful movements. As a consequence, women started to maintain strict diets and extenuating physical exercises to decrease their body mass (Castilho, 2001; Vigarello, 2006).
In the wake of such a deep concern for weight loss the 1926 *New York Times* advertised that the New York Science Academy was calling a two-day conference to study "the explosion of food disturbances". Table 1 shows a 10-year historical series in which the ideal weight of women, height 1.60m, was suggested. The table below reveals the loss of weight trend according to the magazine *Votre Beauté*.

PERIOD	BODY MASS
January 1929	60.0 kg
April 1932	54.0 kg
August 1932	52.0 -53.0 kg
May 1939	51.5 kg

Table 1. Description of the ideal weight for women, height 1.60 m, at the beginning of the 20th century

Table 2 shows some measurements that the female figure, height 1.60 m, was expected to have in the 1930s, as described in the magazines *Votre Beauté* and *Marie Claire*. A trend had been introduced so that rates became smaller and smaller, corroborating the suggestion of progressive slimness (Vigarello, 2006). Progressive slimness of the female body throughout the ages may also be deduced from requirements on the agenda of Miss America Contest. In 1921 the Body Mass Index (BMI) of most of the candidates was 21.2 whereas in 1940 it decreased to 19.5. Specialized magazines exhibited the perfect body profile of film stars, and female editors were vying in giving counsels to the readers that all women may possess a

	1933 (*Votre Beauté*)	1938 (*Marie Claire*)	1939 (*Votre Beauté*)
Bosom	83 cm	85 cm	81 cm
Hips	87 cm	85 cm	75 cm
Waist	65 cm	60 cm	58 cm

Table 2. Measurements of the female figure, height 1.60 m

beautiful body if discipline, physical culture and adequate diets were practiced. Their motto was that "there are no ugly women but women who do not take care of their body" (Vigarello, 2006). Make-up had a basic role during the first half of the 20th century. In fact, the female face was considered uncared for in its absence. Concern with cellulite and creases was followed by repairing and aesthetic surgeries (Vigarello, 2006).

Body cult from the 1950s onward became a rage and won an unprecedented social dimension. Democratization of the beauty stance was rife. The social media exerted a great influence on people, spread the craze for fashion, expanded the consumption of beauty products, broadcasted the changes that occurred in the bodies of famous people who underwent plastic surgery and idealized physical appearance as a basic factor in female and male identity (Castilho, 2001).

In 1960 publicity on beauty products and the like made up 60 to 70% of women's fashion magazines, or rather, the double of the number in the 1930s. Further, as from the 1960s, the male body underwent a slimming process and men started to be concerned more and more with their aesthetics. Simultaneously the start of the feminization of body building could be observed. Consequently, beauty was not a criterion restricted to define the female or the male gender since both sought to model their bodies on slimness and by athletic and defined shapes (Almeida et al., 2005; Andrade & Bosi, 2003; Ferriani et al., 2005; Oliveira & Bosi, 2003). Linear shapes became a warrant of efficiency, agility, elegance and flexibility.

Cosmetics, make-up, aesthetic surgery and physical exercises triggered men and women to have an attractive body profile. Excuses for such complaints as being "not according to the figure" were severely rejected. An ugly person is a person who wants to be ugly and only those who want to age will get old. The body figure is shown to be a personal success since "fat and unsightly subjects do not exist; only lazy ones do" (Castilho, 2001).

The above shows that people may adopt any strategy to have the body they desire, including extremely restrictive diets and abuse in anorexigenous drugs, laxatives and diuretics. The use of anabolic hormones, excessive physical activities and numberless surgeries for the correction of small body defects may be the subjects' strategies to have an adequate muscular mass.

A study undertaken in the state of São Paulo, Brazil, with men and women featuring normal weight showed that 50% were unsatisfied with their bodies and 67% of the females would undergo plastic surgery to have the body they desire. This information corroborates the fact that Brazil is second (after the USA) in the number of cosmetic plastic surgeries (Finger, 2003). Such dissatisfaction reveals that the feminine body's ideal is gradually distancing itself from current female profiles (Hesse-Biber et al., 1987).

The fact that the number of obese people has tremendously increased in Western countries, including Brazil, exemplifies the situation previously described. The main causes are mainly an increase in the intake of hypercaloric food with high saturated fat rates and a sedentary life style that triggered an increase in leisure and a decrease in physical activities (Schwartz & Brownell, 2004; Stettler, 2004). Whereas in general people have increased their body mass, the social media insists in broadcasting the progressively slim person. Thus, current beauty standards require slimmer anthropometric measurements (Morrison et al., 2004; Schwartz & Brownell, 2004).

Although the physical consequences of obesity have been adequately described, the psychological and social consequences require further investigation even though they have already been established in the literature (Fonseca & Matos, 2005). Body cult is directly associated with power, beauty and social mobility and thus an increase in body mass may amplify dissatisfaction with one's body, especially among children and young people (Striegel-Moore et al., 2000, Striegel-Moore, 2001).

3. Aetiology and the establishment of body dissatisfaction

Since the two-year-old child is already self-aware of its identity and recognizes its body image reflected in the mirror, the body image may be developed concomitantly to the development of the human body (Castilho, 2001). As a rule, body images are dynamic, changeable and directly related to the outside world (Tavares, 2003). The distortion of body perception may occur when the subjects overestimate or underestimate their body size and form. Social and cultural influences, pressures by the social media and the continuous search for an ideal body standard associated with achievements and happiness are the main causes of changes in body image and cause deep dissatisfaction in individuals, especially in women (Conti et al., 2005a,b).

Young people undergo constant psychological, emotional, somatic and cognitive changes which contribute towards deep concern with physical appearance and a craze for the ideal body (Tavares, 2003). The body dissatisfaction developed by adolescents may be related to changes in their self-image and self-esteem, coupled to excessive preoccupations with weight, body form and fat. The above alterations and concerns show that there is a discrepancy between the perception and the desire for a specific body size and shape which may predispose young people to develop psychological disorders (Almeida et al., 2005; Conti et al., 2010; Neumark-Sztainer et al., 2006; Smolak et al., 1999). Food intake, self-esteem and physical and cognitive performance depend on the intensity of this dissatisfaction and may be the cause of altering several aspects in the subjects' life (Smolak & Levine, 2001).

It should be underscored, however, that disturbances in body perception are not merely a trait proper to young people who develop some type of eating disorder (Branco et al., 2006). In fact, body dissatisfaction, excessive concern with weight and a history of restrictive diets during adolescence are predisposing factors for the development of eating disorder behaviour such as bulimia nervosa, anorexia nervosa and binge eating disorder (Stein, et al., 1998). The social media, parents and friends are accountable for social comparisons on the physical aspects and idealizing concepts of slimness. They are thus related with the development of body dissatisfaction and, consequently, with low self-esteem, limitations in psychological and social performance and depression conditions (Robinson et al., 2001; Sands & Wardle, 2003; Stice, et al., 2000).

The social media is accountable for food behaviour disorders or the body image. In fact, it not merely broadcasts images of perfect body forms but stimulates the intake of non-healthy food. Since magazines, films and advertisements publish images of young people with slim, muscular bodies, they induce individuals to establish an idea of beauty which is totally personal, characterized by unreachable aesthetic standards, in spite of all the diversity and singularity presented (Saikali et al., 2004).

Whereas by the end of the 20th century, human manikins weighed 8% less than the average women at that time, currently they weigh 23% less. The difference may be associated with a decrease in the models' weight but also with women's weight gain in general. Body dissatisfaction, taken to be a standardized item in Western women, may be attributed to an increasing social and cultural pressure imposed by the social media in its portrayal of the ideal physical profile such as an unreal slimness for females and a muscular body for males (Becker et al., 2002; Rodin, et al., 1985; Stice et al., 2002). Such body image corresponds to that to which young people are constantly exposed to in advertisements, musical videos and films (Morrison et al., 2004; Stice & Shaw, 2002; Stice & Whitenton, 2002).

Feminine body dissatisfaction may be related to the social concepts advertised by the media which valorises and defines the slim body as physically more attractive and compensating; as a contrast, fat people's profiles are considered non-attractive and non-appealing. This situation reveals the female trend to acquire a body which will be an object of desire (Stormer & Thompson, 1996). Most TV film stars are slim and only 5% may be classified as fat (Silverstein et al., 1986).

Since human manikins advertised in women's magazines are represented statically, they reinforce the idea that the body is just an ornament (Duquin, 1989). Fashion magazines are important sources of information on beauty and excellence in form. Young women, who are their most frequent readers, demonstrate high dissatisfaction levels with regard to body form and most probably are prone to alter their social behaviour and food habits, such as practicing exhausting physical exercises or shunning meals, to decrease their body weight (Ferriani et al., 2005; Vilela et al., 2004). Women's constant contact with ideal body images advertised by the social media increases the occurrence of attitudes and behaviours which characterize eating disorders such as bulimia nervosa (Stice et al., 1994).

The social media also advertises the ideal male body as essentially muscular. It is actually a situation very similar to that among women where the male body is also an object of desire (Sommers-Flanagan et al., 1993). Several studies showed that most interviewed people had a hard conviction that the male body should be muscular while few replied that slimness is the true characteristic of the ideal male body (Murray et al., 1996). Consequently, very slim or very fat males represent a negative body image and, as a rule, are not in the media's limelight (Silverstein et al., 1986; Morrison et al., 2004). Concerns on the proper physical male profile have been intensified since the 1960s, with special emphasis on strength and body building so that the muscular body could be constructed (Petrie et al., 1996).

Since children aged between 8 and 11 years were aware of the slim body as the ideal to be attained, it may be surmised that their perception has been under the influence of the social media which is accountable for the broadcasting of body images of film stars and models as highly attractive and imitable (Cusumano & Thompson, 2001). A study on young females, aged between 12 and 29, from the southern region of Brazil, was undertaken. Most of the women desired to have size and body mass less than their present condition even though only one third of this group was classified with a BMI equivalent to overweight or obesity (Nunes et al., 2003).

Parents and friends, along with the social media, construct body dissatisfaction in people (Sands & Wardle, 2003). Eating habits and a body image may be built during the pre-adolescence period, although it is not an exclusive adolescence problem (Robinson, 2001). Concern with body weight afflicts 6- and 7-year-old girls due to concepts transmitted by society on what is attractive and graceful. These ideas foregrounding the girls' awareness on physical attractiveness, may very well be a reproduction of their mothers' opinions and attitudes (Castilho, 2001, Davison et al., 2000; Lowes & Tiggemann, 2003)

In fact, the desire to be slim is manifest at the very onset of puberty. There is, however, much evidence that even pre-puberty children are worried about their body's shape and loss of weight is a great concern (Carvalho et al., 2005). Dissatisfaction and concern with the body and their repercussions were reported in a population-based investigation in the southern region of Brazil, comprising students within the 8-11 years bracket. In fact, 82% of the children desired a different body form since they manifested low self-esteem and revealed perception levels with regard to their parents' and friends' expectations on their featuring a slim body (Pinheiro, 2003). Dissatisfaction with body shape already affects a great number of pre-adolescents, even in those with adequate weight. Regardless of nutrition state and sex, excessive concern with weight shows that many pre-adolescents are under pressure to adopt beauty stereotypes (Triches & Giugliani, 2007). Research reveals that during the first years of adolescence parents exert a great influence on their children's physical appearance and lifestyle (Robinson, 2001; Smolak at al., 1999).

Obese children are unhappy and dissatisfied with weight excess and reveal psychic sufferings, low self-esteem and insecurity due to jokes and pranks practiced on them by their school mates (Braet, et al., 1997). Parents of 5-year-old overweight girls reported very high levels of concern with regard to the body mass of their daughters when compared with those whose daughters' weight was "normal". Very early in life these girls are concerned with their body: whereas they normally reveal low body esteem, their knowledge on nutrition and diets is considerable (Abramovitz & Birch, 2000; Davison & Birch, 2001).

Further studies are required to have an in-depth evaluation on the origin and consequences of children's dissatisfaction with regard to their body, taking into account the degree of dissatisfaction and family, social and cultural influences. However, the above information is enough to make parents, educators and health professionals on the look out for such a high prevalence in body dissatisfaction among pre-adolescent children so that the necessary strategies for a better body satisfaction could be taken. The literature has abundant studies on the theme of the body in adolescence and on its influence in the subjects' health. In fact, several investigations report that 25 to 80% are not satisfied with their body (Stice & Whitenton, 2002). Western society highly values the slim and graceful body and fashion clothes are manufactured small size to this end. This condition causes a lack of body satisfaction in overweight subjects or in people with excessive weight, which is also associated with health concerns. In fact, the increasing number of obese people within a population, especially among children and adolescents, is a case of public health since they are in danger of developing diseases such as hypertension and Type 2 diabetes, coupled to problems in the spine, in bone articulations and in the lower members (Carvalho et al., 2005).

Overweight children and adolescents reveal a high rate of body dissatisfaction and a negative impact on the development of their self-image (Carvalho et al., 2005; Conti, 2005a,b; Davison & Birch 2001; Erling & Hwang, 2004). However, lack of satisfaction is not exclusive to this group since it has also been reported in over 15-year-old adolescents. Except those who are very slim, practically all desire to lose weight (Wardle & Cooke, 2005). Children and adolescents within the 9-16 years bracket have low self-esteem due to their physical characteristics, and their happiness and intelligence levels are lower when compared with slim or eutrophic types (Paxton et al., 1991). The above situation demonstrates that self-perception with regard to the body type may cause serious interference on the body.

Most girls develop an awareness of their body form in the wake of their observations of their parents' habits and attitudes. The family is actually the primary socializing agent and may influence the perceptive self-evaluation of the children and the development of their habits (Hill & Franklin, 1998). Parents may have an influence on their offspring's body dissatisfaction when they show concern with regard to their children's weight. This concern may occur implicitly when access to certain food is monitored or restricted, or explicitly when the weight and body form of other children are criticized or compared (Birch & Fisher, 1998).

Several non-overweight adolescents have reported their feeling on finding themselves fat. The feeling is associated with the body perception acquired during childhood and is related to parents' expectations with regard to children's ideal weight. Actually parents have a direct influence on their children's look up till the first year of adolescence. Moreover, the mother's excessive worry on the daughters' weight may decrease the body form perception regardless of their weight (Davison & Birch, 2001; Pinheiro & Giugliani , 2006a).

Since the role of the female model is proper to mothers and it is a well-known fact that they influence their children's food habits since childhood, it may be remarked that the highest rates of body dissatisfaction in children and young people may be related to the mothers' opinion with regard to their children's weight (Hill & Franklin, 1998; Keel et al., 1997; Mukai, 1996). Body satisfaction level in adolescents and the adoption and the frequency of diets reflect the mothers' attitudes and concepts. This fact reveals that adolescents' body dissatisfaction is not exclusively affected by their body self-awareness but also by the behaviour of their mothers (Hill & Franklin, 1998).

The mother's schooling level has been employed to assess economic social level. Daughters whose mothers have had less than eight years of schooling revealed an increased predisposition with regard to body dissatisfaction level. Such predisposition may be related to the need of acceptance by the social milieu since complying with the fashionable beauty standard may increase their possibility of social elevation due to their insertion within the artistic or fashion status (Cusumano & Thompson, 2001). However, several authors remark that female adolescents of the higher social classes also have greater concerns with the body shape and size (Ogden & Thomas, 1999). The above divergent results may be due to the employment of different research tools and different population samples. No significant difference in the proportion of subjects with or without body dissatisfaction was perceived in a study undertaken with several people with different ethnic and social-economical class backgrounds (Wang et al., 2005). Although parents may have an impact on boys so that they may gain weight and develop their muscles, further studies are required to evaluate the parents' influence in the boys' body image (Ricciardelli & McCabe, 2001).

Friends have a great impact on socialization during the period of adolescence and social comparison is a highly employed mechanism among them (Lattimore & Butterworth, 1999). Concerns in body weight among adolescents in the upper high school and a great probability of taking up restrictive diets may reflect the impact exerted by female friends. Several authors discuss that female friends' influence in late adolescence is higher than that provided by mothers with regard to diet attitudes and behaviour (Mukai, 1996; Taylor et al., 1998). Lack of body satisfaction among male adolescents is also related to the influence of friends and of the social media. Parents' impact is low during this period (O'Koon, 1997; Ricciardelli, et al., 2000).

As a rule, social comparison is proper to adolescents due to exhibited similar traits. Such a comparison may be related to the bearing for more or for less, and also to the characteristics of the target. When subjects with characteristics below their interest levels are compared, there is an automatic increase in subjective well-being; however, if social comparisons are directed towards subjects with better physical traits, the former subjects' well-being levels and their self-evaluation in attractiveness decrease considerably (Wheeler & Miyake, 1992). When target characteristics are taken into account, the general target consists of information provided by the media which is a powerful means to influence idealized standards presented by the specific target provided by friends and family (Irving, 1990).

Attractiveness self-evaluation decreases in subjects constantly exposed to the professional models in advertisements or fashion (Martin & Kennedy, 1993; Thornton & Moore, 1993). However, females who have taken up famous people (a general target) as a reference for their physical beauty standard also exhibited a decrease in their self-evaluation of attractiveness. As a consequence, they are prone to take up abnormal weight control practices such as vomit induction (Heinberg & Thompson, 1992).

A Canadian study on adolescents within the 15-19 age bracket showed that male and female groups had an inverse relationship with regard to their evaluation of body image, self-esteem and body satisfaction. Several male adolescents considered themselves very slim, or rather, with less musculature than male actors and models, with the consequent need to increase their muscle mass. On the other hand, female adolescents had a body perception of obese people. Such changes in body perception may be related to their exposition to the media through which ambiguous concepts on body form are acquired. They thus underwent an intense general social comparison which, as a rule, brings about low levels of self-esteem (Morrison et al., 2004).

4. Methodological aspects in the study of dissatisfaction with body image

People who are extremely worried with their physical appearance are also susceptible to a negative or distorted body image (Castilho, 2001). Recent studies show that dissatisfaction with the body has reached alarming levels and has affected people in several age brackets (Conti, 2008; Coqueiro et al., 2008; Tribess et al., 2010; Triches & Giugliani, 2007).

Leonhard and Barry (1998) remark that the very first studies on body image were restricted to and underscored body measurements, or rather, they focused on subjects classified as obese according to the BMI. The ideal current standard of feminine beauty corresponds to extreme slimness, whereas obesity is a negative factor in people's life. A high BMI is also related to discontent with one's body (Robinson et al., 2001).

Several analyses have shown that overweight school children and adolescents manifest low self-esteem and dissatisfaction with their body image when they compare themselves to eutrophic schoolmates (Gleaves et al., 1995; Pinheiro & Giugliani, 2006a; Stice et al., 1996; Tiggemann, 1994). An investigation among students in the USA showed that body dissatisfaction featuring weight concern is highly prevalent among both sexes, in different ethnic groups and in social and economical classes. In fact, high BMI rates were always related to body dissatisfaction (Robinson et al., 2001).

It has been verified in current study that most eutrophic girls desire to be slimmer in contrast to boys' ideal for a bigger body or a bigger body form (Robinson et al., 2001) From the feminine point of view the ideal beauty stereotype is basically a lean and slim body, similar to the Barbie® doll which represents the ideal feminine slimness (Norton et al., 1996), whereas the male's point of view focuses on the robust and muscular body shape as the ideal of beauty, very similar to the super-heroes dolls male children play with (Pope et al., 1999).

A study among Brazilian adolescents in the state of Paraná, aged 15 - 19 years, verified that 48.6% of female adolescents with negative body image were eutrophic; only 2.6% of adolescents classified with malnutrition or on the malnutrition border had such disturbances; 14.5% of adolescents who had body image disturbance were actually overweight or obese. In the case of male adolescents, only 10% of the eutrophic group had body image disturbances and 8.6% were overweight or obese (Souza-Kaneshima et al., 2006; Souza-Kaneshima et al., 2008).

When body weight awareness is higher than the body mass, the introduction of important changes in eating behaviour is enhanced. In fact, the discussion of the theme in different population segments is mandatory so that the significance of the phenomenon could be acknowledged and strategies to tackle the problem planned (Nunes et al., 2001). The development of tools to detect possible body image distortions in different population groups and the choice of such instruments are essential for the validity of the results.

Gender and ethnic groups manifest different types and degrees of body dissatisfaction. For instance, females have a higher propensity to develop body image discontent. This is due to the fact that they are constantly evaluated by society, especially with regard to their physical appearance. Even males may demonstrate body image distortions for the same reasons (Alvarez-Rayon et al., 2009; Costa et al., 2008; Cordas, 2004; Mond et al., 2004; Nunes et al., 2001).

Ethnicity-related physical characteristics also affect the adolescents' body satisfaction. A study in the state of Minnesota, USA, showed that Afro-American and mixed-race adolescents had a high body image satisfaction amounting to almost three times that in whites. On the other hand, Hispanics and Asians had the least satisfaction degree within the analyzed group (Kelly et al., 2005).

The age bracket also affects the evaluation of the body image. Young women show a higher rate of dissatisfaction as from their 13th or 15th year, while the male has a high degree of body image satisfaction at the same age. This is due to the fact that an increase in height and muscular mass occurs in male adolescents at this age, which brings them close to the ideal social and cultural image of the male body (Kelly et al., 2005; Raudenbush & Zellner, 1997). Male adolescents may later have difficulties in the maintenance of their physical profile and consequently a lowering of body satisfaction levels occurs (McCabe & Ricciardelli, 2004a).

The very first studies on this issue underscored body measurements even though social and behavioural aspects which may affect body image distortion were not taken into account. This occurred in spite of the fact that authors related gender, ethnic background and age bracket as factors that could affect body dissatisfaction.

The Body Cathexis Scale (Secord & Jourard, 1953) was one of the first self-evaluation ratings. In 1973, Berscheid et al. developed the Body Image Questionnaire and in 1984, Winstead & Cash introduced the Body-Self Relations Questionnaire (BSRQ). This questionnaire contains 140 items which the patients answer on a 5-point scale. Items deal with patients' attitudes and activities in three body areas: physical appearance, physical form and physical health.

The Body Attitudes Questionnaire (BAQ) (Ben-Tovim & Walker, 1994) is a self-report questionnaire with 44 items, developed for those with concerns for body appearance, and deals with the measurement of several attitudes related to the body. Answers may be grouped into six sub-scales which describe (1) overall fatness ("Feeling fat"); (2) self-disparagement ("Depreciation"); strength ("Strength and Physical Fitness"); (4) salience of weight ("Salience"); (5) feelings of attractiveness especially with people of the opposite sex ("Physical attraction"); (6) consciousness of lower body ("Lower limbs fatness"). High scores in the subscales "Feeling fat", "Depreciation", "Salience" and "Lower limbs fatness" produce negative attitudes with regard to the body. High scores in "Strength and Physical Fitness" and "Physical Attraction" cause positive attitudes with regard to the body.

Candy & Fee (1998) developed the Eating Behaviours and Body Image Test (EBBIT) to identify feeding behaviour and body image in pre-adolescent girls. It is a 42-item self-report questionnaire with four answer alternatives in which eating behaviour for each reply receives different marks. Answers range from "Most of the time" to "Never", while each alternative receives marks from 0 to 3, namely, 3 = most of the time; 2 = frequently; 1 = rarely; 0 = never. The test is subdivided into 3 sub-scales: (1) dissatisfaction with body image and food restriction, with 22 items; (2) compulsive eating behaviour, with 15 items; (3) 4 items for compensation behaviour associated to feeding disorders indicated by the Diagnostic and Statistical Manual of Mental Disorders (DSM IV). First and second scales are grouped for a total score and the items of the third scale are individually evaluated.

Due to their practical application and correction, the Body Shape Questionnaire (BSQ) and the Body Silhouette Figure method are currently the most quoted in the literature dealing with the evaluation of body image distortion in population studies (Mendelson et al., 2002).

The Body Shape Questionnaire (BSQ) has been developed by Cooper et al. (1987) and incorporates the influence of the social milieu. It also provides an underlying evaluation of body image disorders in clinical and non-clinical populations and may be employed to evaluate the influence of body image disorders in the development, maintenance and in treatment response to feeding disturbances (Branco et al., 2006; Lemes et al., 2001; Oliveira et al., 2003). The questionnaire is composed of 34 points, each with six alternative answers, varying between "always" and "never". Marks from 1 to 6 (always = 6; very frequent = 5; frequent = 4; sometimes = 3; rarely = 2; never = 1) are given to each answer. Test result is the sum of the 34 items in the questionnaire. Result classification features levels of concern with body image, or rather, less than 70 marks means normal standard and no concern with body image distortion; marks between 70 and 90 demonstrate a mild concern on body image distortion; marks between 91 and 110 mean a moderate concern with distortion; above 110 marks means a marked concern with body image distortion (Assunção et al., 2002).

Therefore, BSQ measures concerns with body form, with self-disparaging due to physical appearance and with the feeling of being 'fat'. Since it evaluates the body image's affective aspect, it is a very promising and helpful tool for the clinical follow-up of patients with eating disorders, such a bulimia nervosa (Conti, 2008; Kakeshita, 2004). Although BSQ initially evaluated the body image distortion in women with eating disorders, some studies show that it may also be used to measure concern on body form, weight and, in particular, the frequency people of both sexes, with or without eating disorder, feel that they are "fat" (Cooper et al., 1987; Freitas et al., 2002).

Other investigations evaluated BSQ in different populations without any eating disorders. Good discriminating indexes in the test's validity and reliability and its repetition, coupled to internal consistency, have been reported (Rosen et al., 1996) Although different studies may highly diverge in their dissatisfaction index with the body image, most authors agree on a high body dissatisfaction index during adolescence, mainly with the female sex, which influences the emotional (dissatisfaction) and the perceptive (high estimation) dimensions (Ferrando et al., 2002).

Almost 75% of adolescent high school students in the state of Paraná, Brazil, aged 15 - 19, reveal a normal BMI and therefore are eutrophic subjects. Nevertheless, the BSQ questionnaire revealed that half of them had body image disorders. Moreover, a comparative analysis between the sexes verified that only 34.2% of female adolescents failed to manifest any body image disturbances. The other interviewed adolescents manifested the following degrees in image: 23.9% with mild disorders; 31.6% with moderate disorders; 10.3% with marked disorders. On the other hand, body image disorders in male adolescents were lower, featuring 11.4 and 7.2% with mild and moderate disorders respectively (Souza-Kaneshima et al., 2006; Souza-Kaneshima et al., 2008).

Predominance of body image dissatisfaction reached 15.3% among university students in Brazil (Luz, 2003). In some countries, such as Spain, body image dissatisfaction amounted to 22.1% among female adolescents (Ferrando et al., 2002), whereas an Australian study identified body frustration in most female adolescents, aged 14 - 16 years. Further, 57% of Australian young women practiced unhealthy diets and 36% ingested anorexigenous pills, diuretics and laxatives, smoked and practiced extremely restrictive diets. The above attitudes clearly show the relationship between body dissatisfaction and abnormal behaviour, suggestive of eating disorders (Grigg et al., 1996). Moreover, a longitudinal investigation among Norwegian young women showed that body image disturbances predispose towards restrictive diets (Friestad & Rise, 2004). Frequent diet practice may be a risk factor favouring the development of eating behaviour disorders, such as bulimia nervosa (Morgan et al., 2002).

Weight dissatisfaction in a group of female university students of the Nutrition Course in Rio de Janeiro, Brazil, was also investigated by BSQ. The slim body ideal imposed by society also prevailed in the group since 58.7% desired a decrease of two or more kilos even though their weight was adequate. A similar desire was shown by almost all the female university students with moderate and marked body image disturbances. The above result is highly relevant since body image distortion may be a risk factor for the development of eating behaviour disorders, such as bulimia nervosa. It should be emphasized that future professionals should take a different view of the patient especially in situations featuring eating disorders. Therefore, awareness of one's own body is part and parcel of the multidimensional character of eating behaviour disorders and should be discussed with future nutritionists so that society's influence in the construction process of ideas of beauty might be assessed. Consequently, their clinical attitudes would include the limits in which weight loss brings a positive impact on people's health (Bosi et al., 2006).

Silhouette Figure Body Images were introduced by Stunkard et al. (1983) with 15 silhouettes for each gender, later developed by Thompson & Gray (1995) with a new 9-silhouette figures (Fig. 1) in individual cards containing a male and a female figure with several silhouettes. Card 1 shows a very slim person (BMI = 12.5 kg/m^2) and Card 9 a very obese one (IMC = 47.5 kg/m^2). The subjects choose a card with a silhouette that is closest to their body's image, identified as I; another card representing a healthy person is then chosen, identified as HEALTHY; finally, a card is chosen which represents the desired silhouette, identified as IDEAL.

Rating has five variables: 1) the number which corresponds to the current figure; 2) the number which corresponds to the healthy figure; 3) the number that corresponds to the ideal figure; 4) discrepancy scores between the healthy and current figures; and 5) discrepancy scores between the ideal and current figures. Scores range between - 8 and + 8, or rather, the higher the difference, the higher the body discrepancy and, consequently, a greater dissatisfaction rate. Discrepancy scores between the healthy and current figures is a more objective rating for body dissatisfaction, whilst the discrepancy score between the ideal and current figures represents a more emotional stance (Scagliusi et al., 2006).

The Figure Body Images is a fast, easy and simple method, highly efficient in evaluating body distortion and dissatisfaction with weight and body dimensions rate. In fact, it is widely accepted and used by several researchers since it is a valid tool for quantitative studies for body image perception in both sexes (Coqueiro et al., 2008; Damasceno et al., 2005; Gardner et al., 1998; Gardner et al., 1999; Kakeshita, 2004; Madrigal et al., 2000; Tribess

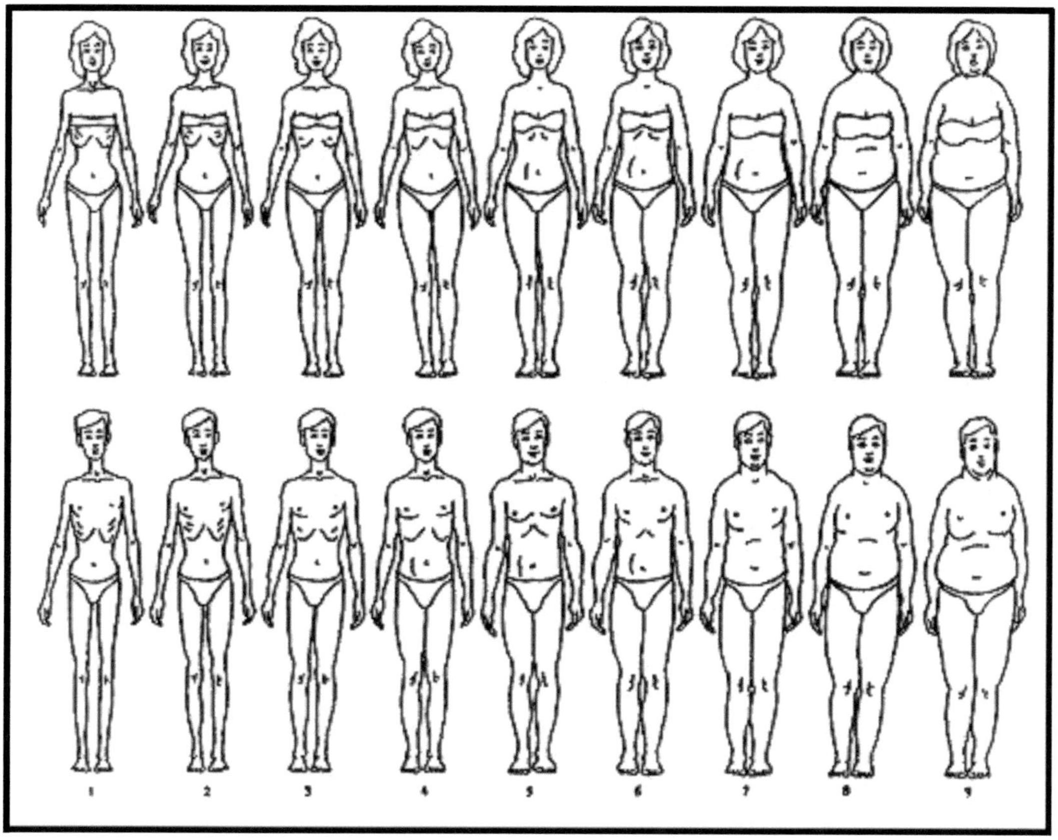

Fig. 1. Silhouette Figure Body Images developed by Stunkard et al. (1983) and modified by Thompson & Gray (1995).

et al., 2010). However, its main limitations are the contour figures designed in a linear bi-dimensional form which may reproduce shortcomings in body entireness and in fat distribution (O'Brien, et al., 2007). Further, the figures may be foregrounded on biotypes which do not correspond to the characteristics of the population under analysis.

Studies employing the Figure Body Images with children aged 6 – 12 years showed that in the case of girls the ideal body is substantially smaller that their own, whereas no difference in choice occurred in the case of boys (Williamson & Delin, 2001; McCabe & Ricciardelli, 2004a,b). Owing to a more critical stance by girls with regard to their body image, they manifest a high esteem for their body image which causes a self-awareness related to overweight and obesity. Thus, girls, albeit eutrophic, choose figures with the above-mentioned contours. Boys show an inverse distortion of reality, or rather, overweight boys choose figures with contours in eutrophic conditions (Branco et al., 2006)

The Figure Rating method (Stunkard et al., 1983), applied in several Brazilian studies, showed a prevalent 82% of school children dissatisfied with their body image (Erling & Hwang, 2004; Pinheiro & Giugliani, 2006b; Triches & Giugliane, 2007), coupled to 78.8% of university students and physically active adults (Coqueiro et al., 2008; O'Brien et al., 2007). All these analyses report that women desire a decrease in their body contour size, whereas men desire a stronger, more muscular body. Difference in the male's and female's preference of body

contours is due to the fact that women overestimate the body image and men underestimate it (Almeida et al., 2006; Atalah et al., 2004; Coqueiro et al., 2008; Damasceno et al., 2005; Kakeshita & Almeida., 2006; Madrigal et al., 2000; Tanaka et al., 2002).
Although percentages of the body image dissatisfaction prevalence may be different in Australia, Croatia, UK, Mexico, Switzerland and the USA, it is very high in all countries and this lack of satisfaction is not merely found in overweight or obese subjects but also in eutrophic ones (Ricciardelli & McCabe, 2001).
Due to incidence increase in eating disorders, such as anorexia nervosa and bulimia, several researches are relating them to body image disorders (Almeida et al., 2005; Conti et al., 2010; Killen et al., 1994; Neumark-Sztainer et al., 2006; Smolak & Levine, 2001, Stein et al., 1998; Souza-Kaneshima et al., 2006; Souza-Kaneshima et al., 2008). It should also be underscored that during the last years body image disorders have been found in still younger eutrophic populations too (Souza-Kaneshima et al., 2006; Souza-Kaneshima et al., 2008).

5. Consequences of body dissatisfaction

Since body image formation involves the subjects' relationship with their own body, positive and gratifying experiences are required with regard to the body so that a satisfactory development of the body image may occur. The subjects who refuse their own physical appearance undergo an interpersonal anxiety experience and have difficulties in their social interactions (Castilho, 2001).
Overweight and obesity in any age bracket are high stigmatizing conditions in society and negatively affect the subjects' vocational, professional and relationship opportunities. Fear of being obese, body dissatisfaction and the preoccupation in being thin may establish body image distortions in children and adolescents, produce health damaging behaviour such as the inadequate ingestion of food, risking cognitive development and the development of eating behaviour disorders, such as bulimia nervosa (Cooley & Toray, 2001; Crocker et al., 2003; Johnson & Wardle, 2005; Nunes et al., 2003; Pinheiro & Giugliane, 2006a; Stice et al., 2002; Vilela et al., 2004).
Girls who go on restrictive eating diets gain weight in the long run and thus a vicious circle ensues (Field et al., 2003; Stice et al., 1999; Stice et al., 2002). These situations are a source of concern to health professionals because of the high prevalence of adolescents with low body satisfaction levels (Smolak, 2004). Several studies have emphasized that body dissatisfaction is associated with eating disorders, such as anorexia nervosa and bulimia in adolescent and adult females (Cattarin & Thompson, 1994; Thompson & Smolack, 2001) and also in children (Gardner et al., 2002).
Several research works have associated body dissatisfaction and a wide variety of negative implication in health and behaviour, such as an increase in depression, low self-esteem, and anxiety, and an increase in dangerous habits such as smoking, alcoholism and drug-taking (Ackard et al., 2002; Granner et al., 2002; Ohring et al., 2002; Pesa et al., 2000; Rierdan & Koff, 1997; Stice & Shaw, 2002; Stice et al., 2000).
A five-year longitudinal study revealed that body-dissatisfied males and females frequently acquire eating compulsion, acquire bad eating behaviour, live a sedentary life and adopt unhealthy habits for weight control. The above study proved that low body dissatisfaction fails to be a motivation to get a healthy weight behaviour. On the contrary, it predisposes to types of behaviour that may put to risk adolescents' health and it increases chances in weight gaining (Neumark-Sztainer et al., 2006).

Since most adolescents are greatly affected by social pressures, the media, parents and friends, it is recommended that their convivial milieu be focused on healthy and physical activities rather than on body weight control. This will minimize the effects of enhancements of the slim body ideal in Western society and increase the probability that they will be satisfied with their body (Kelly et al., 2005).

Several authors report that the practice of physical activity by adolescents is related to body satisfaction (Savage et al., 2009; Damasceno et al., 2005; Neumark-Sztainer et al., 2006). Parents, educators and health professionals should stimulate adolescents to adopt programs for the promotion of the healthy body and for a positive body image. This will inhibit potential damaging behaviour, such as unhealthy control in body weight and eating binges.

6. Conclusion

While the social media and social culture associate a beautiful body with slimness, they transmit a beauty standard unattainable by most people. The body image's distortion may be related to the thin body as the ideal body type. Since the distortion is normally linked to diseases such as depression, it may also be associated with eating disorders such as anorexia and bulimia nervosa. In fact, such diseases are difficult to deal with and perhaps the best type of prevention is an improvement of satisfaction with the body image, especially during childhood and adolescence which are the periods in which subjects are building their body image.

Educational campaigns focused on healthy social milieus which make possible an emotional well-being are highly recommended. Campaigns, physical activities and the intake of healthy food should be adopted by the community and broadcasted by all the social media. Results in the subjects' health will be visible in a short space of time. Therefore, parents, educational personnel and health agents should not merely increase their knowledge on the potential risks of overweight during childhood and its consequences in adulthood but provide practical and concrete alternatives, such as linking leisure with physical activities. It will surely improve children and adolescents' body image. The family may also provide a wide variety of healthy food for children and the latter may choose their preferences.

Children and young people will have healthy feelings with regard to themselves coupled to a solid self-esteem. They will never have their physical value tainted by the social impositions on beauty. Avoidance of eating disorders, such as bulimia nervosa, and an improvement in their body's image will be achieved when there is a change in current ideal of beauty, which is already being sustained by many experts in the field.

7. References

Abramovitz, B.A. & Birch, L.L. (2000). Five-year-old girls ideas about dieting are predicted by mothers dieting. *Journal of the American Dietetic Association,* Vol.100, N°10, (October 2000), pp.(1157-1163), ISSN 0002-8223.

Ackard, D.M.; Crol, L, J.K. & Kearney-Cooke, A. (2002). Dieting frequency among college female: association with disordered eating, body image, and related psychological problems. *Journal of Psychosomatic Research.* Vol.52, N°3, (March 2002), pp.(129-136), ISSN 0022-3999.

Affenito, S.G. & Kerstetter, J. (1999). Position of the American Dietetic Association and Dietitians of Canada: women's health and nutrition. *Journal of the American Dietetic Association,* Vol.99, N°6, (June 1999), pp.738-751, ISSN 0002-8223.

Almeida G.A.N.; Santos, J.E.; Passian, S.R. & Loureiro, S.R. (2005). Percepção de tamanho e forma corporal de mulheres: estudo exploratório. *Psicologia em Estudo,* Vol.10, N°1, (Janeiro/Abril 2005), pp.(27-35), ISSN 1413-7372.

Alvarez-Rayon, G.; Franco-Paredes, K.; López-Aguilar, X.; Mancilla-Díaz, J.M. & Vázquez-Arévalo, J. (2009). Imagen corporal y trastornos de la conducta alimentaria. *Revista de Salud Pública,* Vol.11, N°4, (July/August 2009), pp.(568-578), ISSN 0124-0064.

Andrade, A. & Bosi, M.L.M. (2003). Mídia e subjetividade: impacto no comportamento alimentar feminino. *Revista de Nutrição,* Vol.16, N°1, (Janeiro/Março 2003), pp.(117-25), ISSN 1415-5273.

Appolinário, J.C. & Claudino, A.M. (2000). Transtornos alimentares. *Revista Brasileira de Psiquiatria,* Vol.22, supl.2, (Dezembro 2000), pp.(28-31), ISSN 1516-4446.

Assunção, S.S.M.; Cordas, T.A. & Araújo, L.F.S.B. (2002). Atividade física e transtornos alimentares. *Revista de Psiquiatria Clínica,* Vol.29, N°1, (Janeiro/Fevereiro 2002), pp.(4-13), ISSN 0101-6083.

Atalah, E. Urteaga, C. & Rebolledo, A. (2004). Autopercepción del estado nutricional en adultos de Santiago. *Revista Médica de Chile,* Vol. 132, N°11, (Novembro 2004), pp.(1383-1388), ISSN 0034-9887.

Becker, A.E.; Burwel, R.A.; Gilman, S.E.; Herzog, D.B. & Hamburg, P. (2002). Eating Behaviours and Attitudes Following Prolonged Exposure to Television among Ethnic Fijian Adolescent Girls. *The British Journal of Psychiatry,* Vol.180, N°6, (June 2002), pp.(509-514), ISSN 0960-5371.

Ben-Tovim, D.I. & Walker, M.K. (1994). The influence of age and weight on women's body attitudes as measured by the Body Attitudes Questionnaire (BAQ). *Journal of psychosomatic research,* Vol.38, N°5, (July 1994), pp.(477-481), ISSN 0022-3999.

Berscheid, E.; Walster, E. & Bohrnstedt, G. (1973). The happy American body: A survey report. *Psychology Today,* Vol.7, (November 1973), pp.(119-131), ISSN 0033-3107.

Birch, L.L. & Fisher, J.O. (1998). Development of eating behaviors among children and adolescent. *Pediatric,* Vol.101, N°3, (March 1998), pp.(539-549), ISSN 0031-4005.

Bosi, M.L.M.; Luiz, R.R.; Morgado, C.M.C.; Costa, M.L.S. & Carvalho, R.J. (2006). Auto-percepção da imagem corporal entre estudantes de nutrição. *Jornal Brasileiro de Psiquiatria,* Vol.55, N°2, (Abril/Junho 2006), pp.(108-113), ISSN 0047-2085.

Braet, C., Mervielde, I. & Vandereycken, W. (1997). Psychological aspects of childhood obesity: a controlled study in a clinical and nonclinical sample. *Journal of Pediatric Psychology,* Vol.22, N°1, (June 1996), pp.(59-710), ISSN 0146-8693.

Branco, L.M.; Hilário, M.O.E. & Cintra, I.P. (2006). Percepção e satisfação corporal em adolescentes e a relação com seu estado nutricional. *Revista de Psiquiatria Clínica,* Vol.33, N°6, (Novembro/Dezembro 2006), pp.(292-296), ISSN 0101-6083.

Candy, C.M. & Fee, V.E. (1998). Underlying Dimensions and Psychometric Properties of the Eating Behaviors and Body Image Test for Preadolescent Girls. *Journal of Clinical Child Psychology,* Vol.27, N°1, (March 1998), pp.(117-127). ISSN 0047-228X.

Carvalho, A.M.P.; Cataneo, C.; Galindo, E.M.C. & Malfara, C.T. (2005). Autoconceito e imagem corporal em crianças obesas. *Paidéia,* Vol.15, N°30, (Janeiro/Abril 2005), pp.(131-139), ISSN 0103-863X.

Castilho, S.M. (Ed.). (2001). *A imagem corporal*, ESETec Editores Associados, ISBN 978-85-88303-13-2, Santo André, SP.

Cattarin, J. & Thompson, J.K. (1994). A three year longitudinal study of body image and eating disturbance in adolescent female. *Eating Disorders: The Journal of Treatment & Prevention*, Vol.2, N°2, (Sum, 1994), pp.(114-125), ISSN 1064-0266.

Conti, M.A. (2008). Os aspectos que compõem o conceito de imagem corporal pela ótica do adolescente. *Revista Brasileira de Crescimento e Desenvolvimento Humano*, Vol.18, N°3, (Dezembro 2008), pp.(240-253), ISSN 0104-1282.

Conti, M.A.; Frutuoso, M.F.P. & Gambardella, A.M.D. (2005a). Excesso de peso e insatisfação corporal em adolescentes. *Revista de Nutrição*, Vol.18, N°4, (Julho/Agosto 2005), pp.(491-497), ISSN 1415-5273.

Conti, M.A; Gambardella, A.M.D. & Frutuoso, M.F. P. (2005b). Insatisfação com a imagem corporal em adolescentes e sua relação com a maturação sexual. *Revista brasileira de crescimento e desenvolvolvimento humano*, Vol.15, N°2, (Agosto 2005), pp.(36-44), ISSN 0104-1282.

Conti, M.A.; Scagliusi, F.; Queiroz, G.K.O., Hearst, N. & Cordás, T.A. (2010). Adaptação transcultural: tradução e validação de conteúdo para o idioma português do modelo da Tripartite Influence Scale de insatisfação corporal. *Cadernos de Saúde Pública*, Vol.26, N°3, (March, 2010), pp.(503-513), ISSN 0104-1282.

Cooley, E. & Toray, T. (2001). Body image and personality predictors of eating disorders symptoms during the college years. *The International journal of eating disorders*, Vol.30, N° 1, (July 2001), pp.(28-36), ISSN 0276-3478.

Cooper, P.J.; Taylor, M.; Cooper, Z. & Fairburn, C.G. (1987). The development and validation of the Body Shape Questionnaire. *The International journal of eating disorders*, Vol.6, N°4, (July 1987), pp.(485-494), ISSN 0276-3478.

Coqueiro, R.S.; Petroski, E.L., Pelegrini, A., & Barbosa, A.R. (2008). Insatisfação com a imagem corporal: avaliação comparativa da associação com estado nutricional em universitários. *Revista de Psiquiatria do Rio Grande do Sul*, Vol.30, N°1, (Janeiro/Abril 2008), pp.(31-38), ISSN 0101-8108.

Cordás, T.A. (2004). Transtornos alimentares: classificação e diagnóstico. *Revista de Psiquiatria Clínica*, Vol.31, N°4, (Julho/Agosto 2004) pp.(154-157), ISSN 0101-6083.

Costa, C.; Ramos, E.; Severo, M.; Barros, H.;Lopes, C. (2008). Determinants of eating disorders symptomatology in Portuguese adolescents. *Archives of pediatrics & adolescent medicine*, Vol.162, N°12, (December 2008), pp.(1126-1132), ISSN 1072-4710.

Crocker, P.; Sabiston, C.; Forrestor, S.; Kowalski, N.; Kowalski, K. & McDonoug, M. (2003). Predicting change in physical activity, dietary restraint, and physique anxiety in adolescent girls: examining covariance in physical self-perceptions. *Canadian journal of public health. Revue canadienne de santé publique*, Vol.94, N°5, (September/October 2003), pp.(332-327), ISSN 0008-4263.

Crosby, R.D.; Wonderlich, S.A.; Engel, S.G.; Simonich, H.; Smyth, J. Mitchell, J.E. (2009). Daily mood patterns and bulimic behaviors in the natural environment. *Behaviour Research and Therapy*, Vol.47, N°3, (March 2009) pp.(181-188), ISSN 0005-7967.

Cusumano, D.L. & Thompson, J.K. (2001). Media influence and body image in 8-11-year-old boys and girls: a preliminary report on the multidimensional media influence scale. *The International journal of eating disorders*, Vol. 29, N°1, (January 2001); pp.(37-44), ISSN 0276-3478.

Damasceno, V.O.; Lima, J.R.P.; Vianna, J.M.V.; Vianna, V.R.A. & Novaes, J.S. (2005). Tipo físico ideal e satisfação com a imagem corporal de praticantes de caminhada. *Revista Brasileira de Medicina do Esporte,* Vol.11, N°3, (Maio/Junho 2005), pp.(181-186), ISSN 1517-8692.

Davison, K.K.; Markey, C.N. & Birch, L.L. (2000). Etiology of body dissatisfaction and weight concerns among 5-year-old girls. *Appetite,* Vol.35, N°2, (October 2000), pp.(143-151), ISSN 0195-6663.

Davison, K.K. & Birch, L.L. (2001). Weight status, parent reaction, and self-concept in five-year-old girls. *Pediatrics,* Vol.107, N°1, (January 2001), pp.(46-53), ISSN 0031-4005.

Duquin, M.E. (1989). Fashion and fitness: Images in women's magazine advertisement. *Arena Review,* Vol.13, N°2, (December 1989), pp. (97-109), ISSN 0735-1267.

Erling, A. & Hwang, C. (2004). Body-esteem in Swedish 10-year-old children. *Perceptual and motor skills,* Vol. 99, N°2, (Octuber 2004), pp.(437-444), ISSN 0031-5125.

Ferrando, D.B.; Blanco, M.G.; Masó, J.P.; Gurnés, C.S. & Avellí, M.F. (2002). Eating attitudes and body satisfactions in adolescents: a prevalence study. *Actas españolas de psiquiatria,* Vol.30, N°4, (July/August 2002), pp.(207-212), ISSN 1139-9287.

Ferriani, M.G.C.; Dias, T.S.; Silva, K.Z. & Martins, C.S. (2005). Autoimagem corporal de adolescentes atendidos em um programa multidisciplinar de assistência ao adolescente obeso. *Revista Brasileira de Saúde Materno-Infantil,* Vol.5, N°1, (Janeiro/Março 2005), pp. (27-33), ISSN 1519-3829.

Field, A.E.; Austin, S.B.; Taylor, C.B. Malspeis, S.; Rosner, B.; Rockett, H.R.; Gillman, M.W. & Colditz, G.A. (2003). Relation between dieting and weight change among preadolesce and adolescents. *Pediatrics,* Vol.112, N°4, (October 2003), pp.(900-906), ISSN 0031-4005.

Finger, C. (2003). Brazilian beauty. *Lancet,* Vol.362, N°9395, p.1560, ISSN 0140-6736.

Fonseca, H. & Matos, M.G. (2005). Perception of overweight and obesity among Portuguese adolescents: an overview of associated factors. *European Journal of Public Health,* Vol.15, N°3, (June 2005), pp.(323-328), ISSN 1101-1262.

Freitas, S.; Gorenstein, C. & Appolinario, J.C. (2002). Instrumentos para a avaliação dos transtornos alimentares. *Revista Brasileira Psiquiatria,* Vol.24, N°3, (December 2002), pp.(34-8), ISSN 1516-4446.

Friestad, C. & Rise, J. (2004). A longitudinal study of the relationship between body image, self-esteem and dieting among 15-21 year olds in Norway. *European eating disorders review,* Vol.12 N°4, (July/August 2004), pp.(247-255), ISSN 1072-4133.

Gardner. R.M.; Friedman, B.N. & Jackson, N.A. (1998). Methodological concerns when using silhouettes to measure body image. *Perceptual and motor skills,* Vol.86, N°2, (April 1998), pp.(387-395), ISSN 0031-5125.

Gardner, R.M.; Stark, K.; Jackson, N.A. & Friedman, B.N. (1999). Development and validation of two new scales for assessment of body image. *Perceptual and motor skills,* Vol.89, N°3 (December1999), pp.(981-993), ISSN 0031-5125.

Gardner, R.M.; Stark, K.; Friedman, B.N. & Jackson, N.A. (2002. Predictors of eating disorders scores in children ages 6 through 14: a longitudinal study. *Journal of psychosomatic research,* Vol. 49, N°3, (September 2002), pp.(199-205), ISSN 0022-3999.

Gleaves, D.H.; Williamson, D.A.; Eberenz, K.P.; Sebastian, S.B. & Barker, S.E. (1995). Clarifying body image disturbance: Analysis of a multidimensional model using structural modeling. *Journal of Personality Assessment,* Vol.64, N°3, (June 1995) pp.(478-493), ISSN 0022-3891.

Granner, M.L.; Black, D.R. & Abood, D.A. (2002). Levels of cigarette and alcohol use related to eating-disorder attitude. *American journal of health behavior*, Vol.26, N°1, (February 2002), pp.(43-55), ISSN 1087-3244.

Grigg, M.; Bowman, J. & Redman, S. (1996). Disordered eating and unhealthy weight reduction practices among adolescent females. *Preventive medicine,* Vol.25, N°6 (November/December 1996), pp. (748-756), ISSN 0091-7435.

Grillo, E. & Silva, R.J.M. (2004). Early manifestations of behavioral disorders in children and adolescents. *Jornal de Pediatria,* Vol.80, N°2, (Abril 2004), pp.(21-27), ISSN 0021-7557.

Gucciardi, E.; Celasun, N.; Ahmad, F., Stewart, D.E. (2004). Eating disorders. *BMC Women´s Health,* Vol.4, suppl.1, (August 2004) pp. (S21), ISSN 1472-6874.

Heinberg, L.J. & Thompson, J.K. (1992). Social comparison: gender, target importance rating, and relation to body-image disturbance. *Journal of social behavior and personality,* Vol.7, N°2, pp.(335-344), ISSN 0886-1641.

Hesse-Biber, S.; Clayton-Matthews, A. & Downey, J.A. (1987). The differential importance of weight and body-image among college men and women. *Genetic, social, and general psychology monographs.* Vol.113, N°4, (November 1987), pp.(509-528), ISSN 8756-7547.

Hill, A.J. & Franklin, J.A. (1998). Mothers, daughters, and dieting: investigating the transmission of weight control. *The British journal of clinical psychology,* Vol.37, N°1, (February 1998), pp.(3-13), ISSN 0144-6657.

Irving, L.M. (1990). Mirror images: Effects of the standard of beauty on the self and body-esteem of women exhibiting varying levels of bulimic symptoms. *Journal of social and clinical psychology,* Vol.9, N°2, pp.(230-242), ISSN 0736-7236.

Jauregui-Lobera, I., Polo, I.M., González, M.T. & Millán, M.T. (2008). Percepción de La obesidad em jóvenes universitários y pacientes com trastornos de la conducta alimentaria. Nutrición hospitalaria Vol. 23, N°3, (May/June 2008), pp. (226-233), ISSN 0212-1611.

Johnson, F. & Wardle, J. (2005). Dietary restraint, body dissatisfaction, and psychological distress: a prospective analysis. *Journal of abnormal psychology,* Vol.114, N°1, (February 2005), pp.(119-125), ISSN 0021-843X.

Kakeshita, I.S. & Almeida, S.S. (2006). Relação entre índice de massa corporal e a percepção da auto-imagem em universitários. *Revista de Saúde Pública,* Vol.40, N°3, (Junho 2006), pp.(497-504), ISSN 0034-8410.

Kakeshita, I.S. (2004). Estudo das relações entre o estado nutricional, a percepção da imagem corporal e o comportamento alimentar em adultos. [Master´s dissertation]. Ribeirão Preto: Faculdade de Filosofia, Ciências e Letras - USP.

Kaufman, A. (2000). Transtornos alimentares na adolescência. *Revista Brasileira de Medicina,* Vol.57, N°1, (Janeiro 2000), pp.(8), ISSN 0034-7264.

Keel, P.K.; Heatherton, T.F.; Harnden, J.L. & Hornig, C.D. (1997). Mothers, fathers, and daughters: dieting and disordered eating. *Eating disorders: The Journal of Treatment & Prevention,* Vol.5, N° 3, pp.(216-228), ISSN 1064-0266

Kelly, A. M., Wall, M., Eisenberg, M. E., Story, M. & Neumark-Sztainer, D. (2005). Adolescent girls with high body satisfaction: Who are they and what can they teach us? *Journal of adolescent health care*, Vol.37, N°5, (November 2005), pp.(391-396). ISSN 0197-0070.

Killen, J.D.; Taylor, C.B.; Halyward, C.; Wilson, D.M.; Haydel, K.F.; Hammer, L.D.; Simmonds, B.; Robinson, T. N.; Litt, I.; Varady, A.. & Kraemer, H. (1994). Persuit of thinness and onset of eating disorder symptom in a community sample of adolescent girls: a three-year prospective analysis. *The International journal of eating disorders,* Vol.16, N°3, (November 1994), pp.(227-238), ISSN 0276-3478.

Kjelsas, E., Bjornstrom, C. & Gotestam, K.G. (2004). Prevalence of eating disorders in female and male adolescents (14-15 years). *Eating behaviors,* Vol.5, N°1, (January 2004), pp.(13-25), ISSN 1471-0153.

Lattimore, P.J. & Butterworth, M. (1999). A test of the structural model of initiation of dieting among adolescent girls. *Journal of psychosomatic research,* Vol.46, N°3, (March 1999), pp.(295-299), ISSN 0022-3999.

Lemes, S.O.; Valverde, M.A.; Fisberg, P.I.P. & Franques, A.M. (2001). Percepção de imagem corporal em adultos (obesos e sobrepeso) do "Spa Médico São Pedro/Sorocaba-SP". *A Folha Medica,* Vol.120, N°4, (Outubro/Dezembro 2001), pp.(229-234), ISSN 0015-5454.

Leonhard, M.L. & Barry, N.J. (1998). Body image and obesity: effects of gender and weight on perceptual measures of body image. *Addictive behaviors.* Vol.23, N°1, (January/February 1998), pp.(31–34). ISSN 0306-4603.

Lowes, J. & Tiggemann, M. (2003). Body dissatisfaction, dieting awareness and the impact of parental influence in young children. *British journal of health psychology,* Vol.8, N°2, (May 2003), pp.(135-47), ISSN 1359-107X.

Luz, S.S. (2003). Avaliação de sintomas de transtornos alimentares em universitários de Belo Horizonte [Master´s dissertation]. São Paulo: Faculdade de Ciências Farmacêuticas, Universidade de São Paulo.

Madrigal, H.; Sanches-Villegas, A.; Martinez-Gonzalez, M.A.; Kearney, J.; Gibney, M.J.; Irala, J. & Martinez, J.Á. (2000). Underestimation of body index through perceived body image as compared to self-reported body mass index in the European Union. *Public Health* Vol.114, N°6, (November 2000), pp.(468-473), ISSN 0033-3506.

Martin, M.C. & Kennedy, P.F. (1993). Advertising and social comparison: Consequences for female preadolescents and adolescents. *Psychology and Marketing,* Vol.10, N°6, (November/December 1993), pp.(513-30), ISSN 1520-6793.

McCabe, M. P., & Ricciardelli, L. A. (2004a). Body image dissatisfaction among males across the lifespan: a review of past literature. *Journal of Psychosomatic Research,* Vol.56, N°6, (June 2004), pp.(675-685), ISSN 0022-3999.

McCabe, M. P., & Ricciardelli, L. A. (2004b). Longitudinal study of pubertal timing and extreme body change behaviors among adolescent boys and girls. *Adolescence,* Vol.39, N°153, pp.(145-166), ISSN 0001-8449.

Mendelson, B.K.; McLaren, L.; Gauvin, L. & Steiger, H. (2002). The relationship of selfesteem and body esteem in women with and without eating disorders. *The International Journal of Eating Disorders,* Vol.31, N°3, (April 2002), pp.(318-323), ISSN 0276-3478.

Miranda, M.R. (2000). Anorexia nervosa e bulimia à luz da psicanálise - a complexidade da relação mãe-filha. *Pediatria Moderna,* Vol.36, N° 6, (Novembro/Dezembro 2000), pp.(396-401), ISSN 0031-3920.

Mond, J.M., Hay, P.J., Rodgers, B., Owen, C. & Beumont, P.J. (2004). Beliefs of women concerning causes and risk factors for bulimia nervosa. *The Australian and New Zealand journal of psychiatry*, Vol.38, N°6, (June 2004) pp.(463-469), ISSN 0004-8674.

Morgan, C.M.; Vecchiatti, I.R. & Negrão, A.B. (2002). Etiologia dos transtornos alimentares: aspectos biológicos, psicológicos e socioculturais. *Revista Brasileira de Psiquiatria*, Vol.24, Supl3, (Dezembro 2002), pp.(18-23), ISSN 1516-4446.

Morrison, T.G.; Kalin, R. & Morrison, M.A. (2004). Body-image evaluation and body-image investment among adolescents: A test of sociocultural and social comparison theories. *Adolescence*, Vol.39, N°155, (Fall 2004), pp.(571-592), ISSN 0001-8449.

Mukai, T. (1996). Mothers, peers, and perceived pressure to diet among Japanese adolescent girls. *Journal of research on adolescent*, Vol.6, N°3, pp.(309-324), ISSN 1050-8392.

Murray, S.H.; Touyz, S.W. & Beumont, P.J.V. (1996). Awareness and perceived influence of body ideals in media: A comparison of eating disorder patients and the general community. *Eating disorders: A Journal of Treatment and Prevention*, Vol.4, N°1, pp.(33-46). ISSN 1064-0266.

Neumark-Sztainer, D.; Paxton, S.J.; Hannan, P.J.; STAT, M.; Haines, J. & Story, M. (2006). Does body satisfaction matter? Five-year longitudinal associations between body satisfaction and health behaviors in adolescent females and males. *The Journal of adolescent health*, Vol.39, N°2 (August 2006), pp.(244-251), ISSN 1054-139X.

Norton, R.; Olds, T.; Olive, S. & Dank, S. (1996). Ken and Barbie at life size. *Sex Roles*, Vol.34, N°3-4 (February 1996), pp.(287-294). ISSN 0360-0025.

Nunes, M.A.; Olinto, M.T.A.; Barrosa, F.C. & Camey, S. (2001). Influência da percepção do peso e do índice de massa corporal nos comportamentos alimentares anormais. *Revista Brasileira de Psiquiatria*, Vol.23, N°1, (Março 2001), pp.21-27, ISSN 1516-4446.

Nunes, M.A.; Barros, F.C.; Olinto, M.T.A.; Camey, S. & Mari, J.D. (2003). Prevalence of abnormal eating behaviors and inappropiate methods of weight control in young women from Brazil: a population-based study. *Eating and weight disorders*, Vol.8, N°2, (June 2003), pp.(100-106), ISSN 1124-4909.

O'Brien, K.; Venn, B.J.; Perry, T.; Green, T.J.; Aitken, W.; Bradshaw, A. & Thomson, R. (2007). Reasons for wanting to lose weight: different strokes for different folks. *Eating Behaviors*, Vol.8, N°1, (January 2007), pp.(132-135), ISSN 1471-0153.

O'Koon, J. (1997). Attachment to parents and peers in late adolescence and their relationship with self image. *Adolescence*, Vol.32, N°126, pp.(471-482), ISSN 0001-8449.

Ogden, J. & Thomas, D. (1999). The role of familial values in understanding the impact of social class on weight concern. *The International journal of eating disorders*, Vol.25, N°3, (April 1999), pp.(273-279), ISSN 0276-3478.

Ohring, R.; Graber, J.A. & Brooks-Gunn, J. (2002). Girls' recurrent and concurrent body dissatisfaction: correlates and consequences over 8 years. *The International journal of eating disorders*, Vol.31, N°4, (May 2002), pp.(404-415), ISSN 0276-3478.

Oliveira, F.P.; Bosi, M.L.M.; Vigário O.S.; Vieira, R.S. (2003). Comportamento alimentar e imagem corporal em atletas. *Revista Brasileira de Medicina e Esporte*, Vol.9, N°6 (Novembro/Dezembro 2003), pp.(348-356), ISSN 1517-8692.

Paxton, S. J.; Wertheim, E. H.; Gibbons, K.; Szmukler, G. I.; Hillier, L. & Petrovich, J. L. (1991). Body image satisfaction, dieting beliefs, and weight loss behaviors in adolescent girls and boys. *Journal of Youth and Adolescence*, Vol.20, N°3, (June 1991), pp.(161-379), ISSN 0047-2891.

Pedrinola, F. (2002) Nutrição e transtornos alimentares na adolescência. *Pediatria Moderna,* Vol.38, N°8, (Agosto 2002), pp.(377-380), ISSN 0031-3920.

Pesa, J.A.; Syre, T.R. & Jones, E. (2000). Psychosocial differences associated with body weight among female adolescents: the importance of body image. *The Journal of adolescent health.* Vol.26, N°5, (May 2000), pp.(330-337), ISSN 1054-139X.

Petrie, T.A.; Austin, L.J.; Crowley, B.J.; Helmcamp, A.; Johnson C.E.; Lester, R.; Rogers, R.; Turner, J. & Walbrick, K. (1996). Sociocultural expectations of attractiveness for males. *Sex Roles,* Vol.35, N°9-10, (November 1996), pp.(581-602), ISSN 0360-0025.

Pinheiro, A.P. (2003). Insatisfação com o corpo, auto-estima e preocupações com o peso em escolares de 8 a 11 anos de Porto Alegre [Master´s dissertation]. Porto Alegre: Universidade Federal do Rio Grande do Sul.

Pinheiro, A.P. & Giugliani, E.R.J. (2006a) Quem são as crianças que se sentem gordas apesar de terem peso adequado? *Jornal de Pediatria,* Vol.82, N°3, (Maio/Junho 2006), pp.(232-235), ISSN 0021-7557.

Pinheiro, A.P. & Giugliani, E.R. (2006b). Body dissatisfaction in Brazilian schoolchildren: prevalence and associated factors. *Revista de Saude Publica,* Vol.40, N°3, (June 2006), pp.(489-496), ISSN 0034-8910.

Pope, H.G.; Olivardia, R.; Gruber, A. & Borowiescki, J. (1999). Evolving ideals of male body image as seen through action toys. *The International journal of eating disorders.* Vol.26, N°1, (July 1999), pp.(65-72), ISSN 0276-3478.

Raudenbush, B. & Zellner, D.A. (1997). Nobody's satisfied: effect of abnormal eating behaviors and perceived and actual weight status on body image satisfaction in males and females. *Journal of social and clinical psychology,* Vol.16, N°1, (Spring 1997), pp.(95-110), ISSN 0736-7236.

Reato, L.F.N.; Azevedo, M.R.D.; Nogueira, F.C.; Ribeiro, C. & Souza, S. (2000). Distúrbio alimentar em adolescente. *Sinopse de Pediatria,* Vol.6, N°3, (Setembro 2000), pp.(69-72), ISSN 0100-9281.

Reato, L.F.N. (2002). Imagem corporal na adolescência e meios de comunicação. *Pediatria Moderna,* Vol.38, N°8, (Agosto 2002), pp.(362-366), ISSN 0031-3920.

Ricciardelli, L.A.; Mccabe, M.P. & Banfield, S. (2000). Body image and body change methods in adolescent boys: a role of parents, friends, and the media. *Journal of psychosomatic research,* Vol.49 N°3, (September 2000), pp.(189-197), ISSN 0022-3999.

Ricciardelli, L.A. & McCabe, M. (2001). Children's body image concerns and eating disturbance: a review of the literature. *Clinical psychology review,* Vol.21, N°3, (April 2001), pp.(325-344), ISSN 0272-7358.

Rierdan, J. & Koff, E. (1997). Weight, weight-related aspects of body image and depression in early adolescent girls. *Adolescence,* Vol.32, N°127, (Fall 1997), pp.(615-624), ISSN 0001-8449.

Robinson, T.N. (2001). Television viewing and childhood obesity. *Pediatric clinics of North America,* Vol.48, N°4, (August 2001), pp.(1017-1025), ISSN 0031-3955.

Robinson, T.N.; Chang, J.Y.; Haydel, K.F. & Killen, J.D. (2001). Overweight concerns and body dissatisfaction among third-grade children: the impacts of ethnicity and socioeconomic status. *The Journal of pediatrics.* Vol.138, N°2, (February 2001), pp.(181-187), ISSN 0022-3476.

Rodin, J.; Silberstein, L. & Striegel-Moore, R. (1985) Women and weight: a normative discontent. In: *Psychology and gender*, Sonderegger, T.B. (Ed), pp.267-307, University of Nebraska Press, ISBN 0803291507, Lincoln, NE.

Rosen, J.C.; Jones, A.; Ramirez, E. & Waxman, S. (1996). Body shape questionnaire: studies of validity and reliability. *The International journal of eating disorders*, Vol.20, N°3, (November 1996), pp.(315-319), ISSN 0276-3478.

Saikali, C.J.; Soubhia, C.S.; Scalfaro, B.M. & Cordás TA. (2004). Imagem corporal nos transtornos alimentares. *Revista de Psiquiatria Clínica*, Vol.31, N°4, (Julho/Agosto 2004), pp.(154-156), ISSN 0101-6083.

Sands, E.R. & Wardle, J. (2003). Internalization of ideal body shapes in 9-12-year-old girls. *The International journal of eating disorders.*, Vol.33, N°2, (March 2003), pp.(193-204), ISSN 0276-3478.

Savage, J. S.; Dinallo, J. M. & Downs, D. S. (2009). Adolescent body satisfaction: the role of perceived parental encouragement for physical activity. *The International Journal of Behavioral Nutrition and Physical Activity*, Vol.6, N°90, Published online 2009 December 9. doi: 10.1186/1479-5868-6-90, ISSN 1479-5868.

Scagliusi, F.B.; Polacow, V.O.; Cordas, T.A.; Coelho, D.; Alvarenga, M.; Philippi, S.T. & Lancha Junior, A.H. (2006). Tradução, adaptação e avaliação psicométrica da Escala de Conhecimento Nutricional do National Health Interview Survey Câncer Epidemiology. *Revista de Nutrição*, Vol.19, N°4, (Julho/Agosto 2006), pp.(425-436), ISSN 1415-5273.

Schwartz, M.B. & Brownell, K.D. (2004). Obesity and body image. *Body Image*, Vol.1, N°1, (January 2004), pp.(43-56), ISSN 1740-1445

Secord, P. F. & Jourard, S. M. (1953). The appraisal of body cathexis: body-cathexis and the self. *Journal of Consulting Phychology*. Vol.17, N°5, (Octuber 1953), pp.(343-347), ISSN 0095-8891.

Silva, C.G.; Teixeira, A.S. & Goldberg, T.B.L. (2003). O esporte e suas implicações na saúde óssea de atletas adolescentes. *Revista Brasileira de Medicina do Esporte*, Vol.9, N°6, (November/December 2003), pp.(426-432), ISSN 1517-8692.

Silverstein, B.; Perdue, L.; Peterson, B. & Kelly, E. (1986). The role of the mass media in promoting a thin standard of bodily attractiveness for women. *Sex Roles*, Vol.14, N°9-10, (May 1986), pp.(519-33), ISSN 0360-0025.

Smolak, L. (2004). Body image in children and adolescents: Where do we go from here? *Body Image*, Vol.1, N°1, (January 2004), pp.15-28, ISSN 1740-1445.

Smolak, L.; Levine, M.P. & Schermer, F. (1999). Parental input and weight concerns among elementary school children. *The International journal of eating disorders*, Vol.25, N° 3, (April 1999), pp.(263-271), ISSN 0276-3478.

Smolak, L. & Levine, M.P. (2001). Body image in children. In: *Body image, eating disorders and obesity in youth: assessment, prevention and treatment*. Thompson JK, Smolak L, (Eds.), pp.41-66, American Psychological Association, ISBN 978-1-55798-758-7, Washington (DC).

Sommers-Flanagan, R.; Sommers-Flanagan, J. & Davis, B. (1993). What's happening on music television? A gender role content analyses. *Sex Roles*, Vol.28, N°11-12, (June 1993), pp.745-53, ISSN 0360-0025.

Souza-Kaneshima, A.M.; França, A.A.; Kneube, D.P.F. & Kaneshima, E.N. (2006). Ocorrência de anorexia nervosa e distúrbio de imagem corporal em estudantes do ensino médio de uma escola da rede pública da cidade de Maringá, Estado do Paraná. *Acta Scientiarum Health Sciences,* Vol.28, N°2, (Julho/Dezembro 2006), pp.(119-127), ISSN 1679-9291.

Souza-Kaneshima, A.M.; França, A.A.; Kneube, D.P.F. & Kaneshima, E.N. (2008). Identificação de distúrbios da imagem corporal e comportamentos favoráveis ao desenvolvimento da bulimia nervosa em adolescentes de uma Escola Pública do Ensino Médio de Maringá, Estado do Paraná. *Acta Scientiarum Health Sciences,* Vol.30, N°2, (Julho/Dezembro 2008), pp.(167-173), ISSN 1679-9291.

Stein, S.; Chalhoub, N. & Hodes, M. (1998). Very early-onset bulimia nervosa: report of two cases. *The International journal of eating disorders.* Vol.24, N°3, (November 1998), pp.(323-327), ISSN 0276-3478.

Stettler, N. (2004). Comment the global epidemic of childhood obesity: is there a role for the paediatrician? *Obesity reviews,* Vol.5; N° 1, (May 2004), pp.(1-3), ISSN 1467-7881.

Stice, E.; Schupak-Neuberg, E.; Shaw, H.E. & Stein, R.I. (1994). Relation of media exposure to eating disorder symptomatology: An examination of mediating mechanisms. *Journal of Abnormal Psychology,* Vol.103, N°4, pp.(836-840), ISSN 0021-843X.

Stice, E.; Nemeroff, C. & Shaw, H.E. (1996). Test of the dual pathway model of bulimia nervosa: Evidence of dietary restraint and affect regulation mechanism. *Journal of Social and Clinical Psychology.* Vol.15, N°3, (Fall 1996), pp.(340-363), ISSN 0736-7236.

Stice, E.; Cameron, R.P.; Killen, J.D.; Hayward C. & Taylor, C.B. (1999). Naturalistic weight-reduction efforts prospectively predict growth in relative weight and onset of obesity among female adolescents. *Journal of consulting and clinical psychology,* Vol.67, N°6, (December 1999), pp.(967-674), ISSN 0022-006X.

Stice, E.; Hayward, C.; Cameron, R.; Killen, J. & Taylor, C. (2000). Body image and eating disturbances predict onset of depression among female adolescents: a longitudinal study. *Journal of Abnormal Psychology,* Vol.109, N°3, (August 2000), pp.(438-444), ISSN 0021-843X.

Stice, E.; Presnell, K. & Spangler, D. (2002). Risk factors for binge eating onset in adolescent girls: a 2-years prospective investigation. *Health psychology,* Vol.21, N°2, (March 2002), pp.(131-138), ISSN 0278-6133.

Stice, E. & Whitenton, K. (2002). Risk factors for body dissatisfaction in adolescent girls: a longitudinal investigation. *Developmental psychology,* Vol.38, N°5, (September 2002), pp.(669-678), ISSN 0012-1649.

Stice, E. & Shaw, H.E. (2002). Role of body dissatisfaction in the onset and maintenance of eating pathology: a synthesis of research findings. *Journal of psychosomatic research,* Vol.53, N°5, (November 2002), pp.(985-993), ISSN 0022-3999.

Stormer, S.M. & Thompson, J.K. (1996). Explanations of body image disturbance: A test of maturational status, negative verbal commentary, social comparison, and sociocultural hypotheses. *The International journal of eating disorders,* Vol.19, N°2, (March 1996), pp.(193-202), ISSN: 0276-3478.

Striegel-Moore, R. (2001). Body image concerns among children. *The Journal of pediatrics,* Vol.138, N°2, (February 2001), pp.(158-160), ISSN 0022-3476.

Striegel-Moore, R.H.; Schreiber, G.; LO, A.; Crawford, P.B.; Obarzanek, E. & Rodin, J. (2000). Eating disorder symptoms in a sample of 11 to 16 year-old black girls and white girls: The NHLBI growth and health study. *The International journal of eating disorders,* Vol.27, N°1, (January 2000), pp.(49-66), ISSN 0276-3478.

Stunkard, A.J.; Sorenson, T. & Schlusinger, F. (1983). Use of the Danish adoption register for the study of obesity and thinness, In: *Genetics of neurological and psychiatric disorders,* Kety, S.S.; Rowland, L.P.; Sidman, R.L. & Matthysse, S.W., pp 115-120, Raven Press, ISBN 0890046263, New York.

Tanaka, S.; Itoh, Y. & Hattori, K. (2002). Relationship of body composition to body-fatness estimation in Japanese university students. *Obesity research,* Vol.10, N°7, (July 2002), pp.(590-596), ISSN 1071-7323.

Tavares, M.C.G.C. (2003). *Imagem corporal: conceito e desenvolvimento.* Editora Manole, ISBN 8520416373, Barueri-SP.

Taylor, C.B.; Sharpe, T.; Shisstak, C.; Byrson, S.; Estes, L.S. & Gray, N. (1998). Factors associated with weight concerns in adolescent girls. *The International journal of eating disorders,* Vol.24, N°1, (July 1998), pp.(31-42), ISSN 0276-3478.

Thompson, M.A. & Gray, J.J. (1995). Development and validation of a new body-image assessment scale. *Journal of personality assessment,* Vol.64, N°2, (April 1995), pp.(258-269), ISSN 0022-3891.

Thompson, A.M. & Chad, K.E. (2000). The relationship of pubertal status to body image, social physique anxiety, preoccupation with weight and nutritional status in young females. *Canadian journal of public health,* Vol.91, N°3, (May/June 2000), pp.(207-211), ISSN 0008-4263.

Thompson, J.K. & Smolak, L. (2001). *Body image, eating disorders and obesity in youth: assessment, prevention, and treatment,* American Psychological Association, ISBN 978-1-55798-758-7 Washington (DC).

Thornton, B. & Moore, S. (1993). Physical attractiveness contrast effect: Implications for self-esteem and evaluations of the social self. *Personality & social psychology bulletin,* Vol.19, N°4, (August 1993), pp.(474-480), ISSN 0146-1672.

Tiggemann, M. (1994). Gender differences in the interrelationships between weight dissatisfaction, restraint, and self esteem. *Sex Roles,* Vol.30, N°5-6, (March 1994), pp.(319-330), ISSN 0360-0025.

Tribess, S.; Virtuoso Junior, J. S. & Petroski, E. L. (2010). Estado nutricional e percepção da imagem corporal de mulheres idosas residentes no nordeste do Brasil. *Ciência & Saúde Coletiva,* Vol.15, N°1, (Janeiro 2010), pp.(31-38), ISSN 1413-8123.

Triches, R.M. & Giugliani, E.R.J. (2007). Insatisfação corporal em escolares de dois municípios da região Sul do Brasil. *Revista de Nutrição,* Vol.20, N°2, (Março/Abril 2007), pp.(119-128), ISSN 1415-5273.

Vigarello, G. (Ed.). (2006). *História da beleza: o corpo e a arte de se embelezar, do Renascimento aos dias de hoje,* Ediouro, ISBN 8500018666, Rio de Janeiro, RJ.

Vilela, J.E.; Lamounier, J.A.; Dellaretti Filho, M.A.; Barros Neto, J.R. & Horta, G.M. (2004). Eating disorders in school children. *Jornal de Pediatria.* Vol.80, N°1, (January/February. 2004), pp.(49-54), ISSN 0021-7557.

Wang, Z.; Byrne, N.M.; Kenardy, J.A. & Hills, A.P. (2005). Influences of ethnicity and socioeconomic status on the body dissatisfaction and eating behaviour of Australian children and adolescents. *Eating Behaviors.* Vol.6, N°1, (January 2005), pp.(23-33), ISSN 1471-0153.

Wardle, J. & Cooke, L. (2005). The impact of obesity on psychological well-being. *Best practice & research: Clinical endocrinology & metabolism.* Vol.19, N°3, (September 2005), pp.(421-440), ISSN 1521-690X.

Wheeler, L. & Miyake, K. (1992). Social comparison in everyday life. *Journal of Personality and Social Psychology,* Vol.62, N°5, (May 1992), pp.(760-773), ISSN 0022-3514.

Wichstrom, L. (1995). Social, psychological and physical correlates of eating problems: a study of the general adolescent population in Norway. *Psychological medicine,* Vol.25, N°3, (May 1995), pp.(567-579), ISSN 0033-2917.

Williamson, S. & Delin, C. (2001). Young children's figural selections: accuracy of reporting and body size dissatisfaction. *The International journal of eating disorders,* Vol.29, N°1, (January 2001), pp.(80-84), ISSN 0276-3478.

Winstead, B.A., & Cash, T.F. (1984, March). *Reliability and validity of the Body-Self Relations Questionnaire.* Paper presented at the annual meeting of the Southeastern Psychological Association, New Orleans, LA.

Part 3

Predisposing and Maintaining Factors

8

The Quality of Depressive Experience as a Prognostic Factor in Eating Disorders

Mario Speranza, Anne Revah-Levy, Elisabetta Canetta, Maurice Corcos and Frederic Atger
Centre Hospitalier de Versailles. Service de Pédopsychiatrie. Le Chesnay
INSERM U669, Université Paris-Sud et Université Paris Descartes, France

1. Introduction

There is overwhelming evidence that depression is one of the most common experiences of eating disorder patients (Herzog et al., 1992; Touchette et al., 2010). Individuals with anorexia or bulimia nervosa commonly display high levels of dysphoric affects, feelings of emptiness and ineffectiveness and emotions such as loneliness and desperation (Bruch 1973). Self-depreciating emotions associated with pathological eating behaviors may probably trigger depressive episodes (Nolen-Hoesema et al., 2007). However, several authors have suggested that eating behaviors themselves (whether starving, bingeing or purging) may serve as adaptive strategies to regulate negative emotions, such as those associated with identity and interpersonal disturbances, frequently seen in these patients (Heatherton et Baumeister, 1991).

For these reasons, it seems worthwhile, in eating disorders, to look for depression not only in a categorical way but also in a dimensional way and to explore the subjective experience of depression of these patients. This is in line with recent conceptualizations on depression from different theoretical perspectives which converge towards the identification of two types of fundamental depressive experiences framed by personality development: the first one focused on concerns associated with disruption in relationships with others (with feelings of loss, abandonment and loneliness) and the second one centered on problems concerning identity (associated with low self-esteem, feelings of failure, culpability, lack of self-confidence) (Blatt and Zuroff 1992). According to Blatt (Blatt, 2004), maladaptive behaviors would emanate directly from an overemphasis and exaggeration of one of the two essential developmental lines of the personality: the Dependent/Anaclitic line, which concerns the establishment of satisfying interpersonal relationships, and the Self-critical/Introjective line, which focuses on the achievement of a positive and cohesive sense of self (Blatt and Zuroff 1992).

Blatt and colleagues have initially developed the Depressive Experience Questionnaire (DEQ) to assess these two dimensions which emerge as independent factors in analytic studies (Blatt et al., 1976). However, subsequent theoretical developments have suggested that different levels could be indentified, each following a developmental trajectory from immature to more mature forms of interpersonal relatedness and self-definition.

Investigations using the Depressive Experience Questionnaire (DEQ) have thus identified two levels within the Dependency factor (relabeled more appropriately, Interpersonal Concerns): a first sub-factor, labeled *Neediness,* assesses feelings of loneliness and insecurity as well as a marked vulnerability to nonspecific experiences of loss, rejection, and abandonment. The second sub-factor, labeled *Relatedness,* appears to assess a more mature level of interpersonal relatedness, including valuing intimate relationships and being concerned about disruptions of particularly meaningful, specific, interpersonal relationships (Blatt 2004). In a similar way, the development of a sense of self seems to follow an analogous progression. Research conducted with the DEQ has identified two levels within the development of self-definition: a first level, which corresponds to the Self-critical factor of the DEQ, assesses concerns about self-worth and failure to meet self and externally imposed standards. The second level contains more positive, proactive expressions of competence and confidence in one's self and in the future. Items corresponding to this more mature level of self-definition load mostly on the Efficacy factor already identified within the DEQ. Thus, the DEQ appears to measure adaptive and maladaptive dimensions of interpersonal relatedness (Neediness and Relatedness)(McBride et al., 2006), as well as adaptive and maladaptive dimension of self-definition (Self-Criticism and Efficacy)(Blatt 2004).

Blatt and colleagues in their initial conceptualization largely emphasized the link between the personality dimension of self-criticism and the clinical expression of depression. However, they hypothesized the existence of several forms of introjective and anaclitic psychopathology, not just limited to depression. Several authors since have reported high levels of both self-criticism and dependency in disorders such as depression (Bagby et al., 1994), panic disorder (Bagby et al., 1992) or social phobia (Cox et al., 2000). The exploration of the depressive experience of eating disorder patients has only recently brought attention (Speranza et al., 2003), notwithstanding the fact that the clinical features of these disorders may imply a specific psychopathology of the developmental processes involving interpersonal relatedness and self-definition. In fact, current theorization on eating behaviors considers these disorders as a reflection of a specific developmental arrest in the separation–individuation process due to the primary caregiver's failure to provide essential functions during development (Corcos and Jeammet 2001). The eating disorder symptoms could be an attempt to cope with needs stemming from this incomplete self-development or to an interruption of the separation–individuation process (Goodsit 1997). Moreover, it can be hypothesized that the level of maturation of interpersonal relationships and/or identity could differentially characterize and influence the outcome of eating disorders according to the different subtypes.

The aim of this paper was to reach a better understanding of the impact of personality development on the clinical outcome of patients with eating disorders. We specifically sought to explore if anorexic or bulimic patients presenting more immature forms of interpersonal relatedness and/or self-definition would present a worst outcome. As relational maturation and identity formation are special duties of adolescence, we focused our investigation on a sample of adolescents and young female with eating disorders.

2. Methods

2.1 Participants

The participants of this study were derived from a multicentre research project investigating the psychopathological features of eating disorders (Inserm Network No. 494013). The overall design of the Network was a cross-sectional investigation, with only a subset of research centres involved in a prospective follow-up study at 30 months. The recruitment centres were academic psychiatric hospitals specialized in adolescents and young adults (age range for reception: 15–30 years). For this study, only female participants who had requested care for an eating disorder were screened for inclusion. At the first assessment and at outcome, patients included in the sample completed a research protocol that consisted of a clinical interview (for sociodemographic and diagnostic data) and a self-report questionnaire eliciting psychopathological features. Eating disorder diagnoses, whether of Anorexia Nervosa or Bulimia Nervosa, were made by a psychiatrist or a clinical psychologist specialized in the field of eating disorders using DSM-IV diagnostic criteria (APA 2000). Diagnostic assessment was made using the Mini International Neuropsychiatric Interview (MINI) which is a structured, validated diagnostic instrument that explores each criterion necessary for the establishment of current and lifetime DSM-IV axis I main diagnoses (eating disorders, anxiety and depressive disorders, substance-related disorders)(Sheehan et al., 1998). Patients were invited to participate in the follow-up study 3 years later. At 18 months, a reminder letter was sent to all participants. A second letter was sent just before contacting them by phone to plan the second assessment. Only patients with complete files at follow-up were included in the study.

2.2 Measures at baseline

The quality of the depressive experience was assessed with the Depressive Experience Questionnaire (Blatt et al., 1976). The DEQ is a 66-item self-report scale rated on a 7-point Likert scale ranging from 1 (strongly disagree) to 7 (strongly agree). This questionnaire was designed to assess the personality dimensions hypothesized by Blatt and Zuroff (Blatt and Zuroff 1992) to underlie different forms of depression. The instrument was developed by assembling a pool of items describing experiences frequently reported by depressed individuals. Factor analyses of the 66 items in normal and clinical samples have yielded three orthogonal factors matching the constructs of Interpersonal Concerns, Self-Criticism, and Efficacy (Blatt et al., 1976; Kuperminc et al., 1997). Subsequent factor analyses have identified two sub-factors within the Interpersonal Concerns factor, namely Neediness and Relatedness corresponding to different levels of maturation of interpersonal relatedness (Blatt et al., 1995; Rude and Burnham 1995). The DEQ has been shown to have high internal consistency and test-retest reliability (Mongrain and Zuroff 1994), high convergent and discriminant validity (Blaney and Kutcher 1991), as well as a high level of construct validity (Blatt and Zuroff 1992; Mongrain and Zuroff 1994). For the present study, we calculated the factor scores for Self-Criticism and Efficacy using the factor-weighting procedure provided by Blatt and colleagues (Blatt et al., 1976) and adapted in French by Atger and colleagues (Atger et al., 2003). We also calculated the sub-factor scores for the Neediness and Relatedness subscales of the Interpersonal Concerns factor using the scoring program for SPSS developed by Besser & Babchoock (Besser and Babchoock 2001).
Depression severity was measured with the French translation of the abridged version of the Beck Depression Inventory (BDI-13). The BDI is a self-report inventory measuring characteristic attitudes and symptoms of depression (Beck 1961). An abridged version with 13 items selected within all the items showing a high correlation (≥.90) with the total score of the BDI-21 has been developed as a specific tool for epidemiological studies including clinical and non-clinical subjects (Beck and Beck 1972). The 21-item and the 13-item forms have shown correlations ranging from 0.89 to 0.97 and a similar factor structure indicating that the short form is an acceptable substitute for the long form (Beck et al., 1974). Both the

original version of the BDI-13 and the French translation have high internal consistency and substantial test-retest reliability (Beck et al., 1988; Bobon et al., 1981).

Binge eating behaviors were assessed with questions issued from the MINI diagnostic interview (Sheehan et al., 1998). Binge eating behaviors (defined as the consumption of large amounts of food in a short period of time associated with a sense of lack of control during the episode) were considered as present if they were currently used, independently of their frequency.

At the end of the assessment procedure, the clinician rated the severity of the illness with the Clinical Global Impression scale (CGI)(Guy 1976). The CGI requires the clinician to rate on a 7 point scale (1=normal to 7=extremely ill) the severity of the patient's illness at the time of assessment, relative to the clinician's past experience and training with patients with the same diagnosis.

2.3 Outcome criteria

A clinical interview was realized at follow-up. The clinical outcome at 3 years was approached categorically according to presence or absence of an eating disorder on the basis of the Psychiatric Status Rating Scale (PSRS) for anorexia nervosa or bulimia nervosa (Herzog et al., 1996; Herzog et al., 1993). The PSRS, which is part of the diagnostic assessment LIFE Eat II, is based on DSM-IV diagnostic criteria for eating disorders. It defines six levels of severity according to the presence and the degree of clinical symptoms. A score at least of 5 means that the patient fulfills all the diagnostic criteria for an eating disorder (whether R-AN, P-AN or BN)(Fichter and Quadflieg 1999). Treatments received during follow-up were recorded (types of treatment, duration). The types of treatment were recoded in dichotomous answers (yes/no) according to Honkalampi and colleagues (Honkalampi et al., 2000) as follows: (1) Pharmacotherapy: antidepressants: treatment was considered as correct if prescribed at least for 3 months at a usual dosage; (2) Psychotherapy: any psychotherapy was recorded as positive, independently from the type, if duration was at least 6 months weekly. (3) Hospitalisation: (full or partial admission). Social outcome was assessed with the Groningen Social Disability Scale (GSDSII) at the end of the clinical interview (Wiersma et al., 1990). Patients were considered as having an unfavorable social outcome for scores in the moderate or severe range on the GSDSII.

2.4 Procedure

Diagnostic interviews were conducted by a research team of master's level clinicians (psychologists or psychiatrists) familiar with DSM-IV Axis-I/II disorders and experienced in assessment and/or treatment of psychiatric adolescents. To reach high levels of reliability, the research evaluation team participated in several training sessions, including commented scoring of videotaped interviews. Final research diagnoses were established by the best-estimate method on the basis of the interviews and any additional relevant data from the clinical record according to the LEAD standard (Pilkonis et al., 1991). The protocol was approved by the local ethics committee (Paris-Cochin Hospital). After full information had been provided, all subjects gave written consent to participate in the study.

2.5 Statistical analysis

Comparisons between anorexic and bulimic participants at baseline were calculated with a chi^2 test for categorical variables and with an analysis of variance (ANOVA) test for continuous variables, as appropriate. Following these tests, a priori pairwise contrasts were performed with alpha level adjusted using the Bonferroni procedure. Relationships between variables were calculated using Pearson's correlations. To evaluate the predictive power of depression (in terms of severity of depression and in terms of the quality of the depressive experience) on the long-term outcome of eating disorder patients, we performed a logistic regression analysis. Presence or absence of an eating disorder at outcome was the dependent variable. Age, BMI, severity of the illness, presence of binge eating behaviors, severity of depression (BDI) and quality of the depressive experience (Self-criticism, Efficacy, Neediness and Relatedness subscales of the DEQ) at inclusion were the independent variables. We used a stepwise method to identify the best model predicting the clinical outcome of eating disorders. Differences in treatments delivered during the study period were secondarily added to the model. Finally, a logistic regression analysis was performed to identify the clinical variables at inclusion who best predicted social outcome measured with the Groningen scale. Results are presented as mean ± standard deviation. Statistical analyses were performed with the 10.1 version of the Statistical Package for Social Sciences.

Variables	R-AN (N=42)	P-AN (N=19)	BN (N=33)	Total (N=94)	Statistics *		
					F	*P<*	≠
SOCIO-DEMOGRAPHICS AT INCLUSION							
AGE (M±SD)	19.4±3.0	20.7±3.0	23.2±3.8	21.0±3.7	12.7	<0.001	BN>R-AN/P-AN
EDUCATION (BACHELOR DEGREE)(N, %)	25 (59)	14 (74)	25 (76)	65 (68)	2.90	ns	
LIFE SITUATION (STILL LEAVING IN FAMILY)(N, %)	33 (79)	12 (63)	9 (27)	54 (57)	24.8	<0.001	BN<R-AN/P-AN
CLINICAL CHARACTERISTICS AT INCLUSION							
INPATIENT STATUS (N, %)	37 (88)	13 (68)	5 (12)	55 (58)	41.5	<0.001	BN<R-AN/P-AN
BODY MASS INDEX (M±SD)	15.0±1.6	15.2±2.3	20.8±3.6	17.1±3.8	50.6	<0.001	BN>R-AN/P-AN
BINGE EATING BEHAVIORS (N, %)	2 (5)	15 (79)	33 (100)	50 (53)	73.7	<0.001	R-AN<P-AN/BN
CLINICAL GLOBAL IMPRESSION (M±SD)	5.1±1.0	4.9±1.0	4.4±0.9	4.8±1.0	4.18	<0.05	R-AN<BN
BECK DEPRESSION INVENTORY (M±SD)	12.1±8.0	18.5±6.9	12.7±8.9	13.6±8.5	4.28	<0.05	P-AN>R-AN/BN
DEQ SELF-CRITICISM (M±SD)	1.2±1.1	1.6±0.9	1.0±0.9	1.2±1.0	2.60	ns	-
DEQ EFFICACY (M±SD)	-0.84±1.0	-0.68±0.8	-0.47±1.0	-0.67±1.0	1.19	ns	-
DEQ RELATEDNESS (M±SD)	40.4±6.0	41.2±8.1	43.7±6.2	41.7±6.6	2.36	ns	-
DEQ NEEDINESS (M±SD)	47.3±9.2	48.5±10.5	47.8±10.4	47.7±9.8	0.09	ns	-

R-AN=Restricting Anorexia nervosa. P-AN=Purging Anorexia Nervosa.
BN=Bulimia Nervosa. DEQ = Depressive Experience Questionnaire

Table 1. Socio-demographic and clinical characteristics of the sample at inclusion

3. Results

From the initial sample of the Inserm Network on eating disorders, 118 patients fulfilling the inclusion criteria of this study were selected to be included in the follow-up and retraced 3 years later. Among these subjects, 19 refused to participate or were unavailable. 99 subjects were directly interviewed, of whom 4 had to be excluded because they did not completely answered the self-questionnaire. Statistical analyses were performed on a final sample of 94 subjects (79.7% of the initial sample). Subtypes were represented as follow: 42 restricting anorexics, 19 purging anorexics and 33 bulimics. The mean age of the sample was 21.0±3.7.

Bulimic participants were slightly older than anorexic participants and lived more often outside the family. The level of education was similar between groups. Anorexic participants were more often recruited as inpatients and showed a more severe clinical picture compared to bulimics. Comparisons between groups on depression measures at inclusion show a differential picture. Purging anorexics had significant higher scores than restricting anorexics and bulimics concerning the severity of depression assessed with the BDI. On the contrary, we did not observe any significant differences between groups in levels of self-definition (Self-critical and Efficacy) and interpersonal relatedness (Neediness and Relatedness). The negative scores on the Efficacy factor (calculated according to factor scores of the control group) highlights that this factor seems to measure a developmental more mature capacity. Socio-demographic and clinical characteristics of the sample at inclusion are presented in table 1.

	(1)	(2)	(3)	(4)	(5)	(6)	(7)	(8)
Body Mass Index (1)	-							
Clinical Global Impression (2)	-0.19	-						
Binge eating behaviors (3)	0.55**	-0.20	-					
Beck Depression Inventory (4)	-0.01	0.22	0.11	-				
DEQ Self-Criticism (5)	-0.03	0.19	0.09	0.46**	-			
DEQ Efficacy (6)	0.12	0.03	0.11	-0.21*	0.25*	-		
DEQ Relatedness (7)	0.24*	0.15	0.18	0.37**	0.31**	-0.02	-	
DEQ Neediness (8)	0.11	0.17	0.30	0.44**	0.41**	-0.08	0.69**	-

DEQ = Depressive Experience Questionnaire;

Table 2. Correlations between variables at inclusion (* $p < 0.05$. ** $p < 0.05$).

Correlations between variables at inclusion showed that the clinical severity of the eating disorder and the presence of binge eating behaviors were unrelated with BDI and with the subscales of the DEQ. The BDI showed a positive correlation with all DEQ subscales (correlations were in the medium range going from 0.37 to 0.46) with the exception of the Efficacy factor that was negatively correlated to depression (-0.21). These moderate correlations indicate that the DEQ scales are not equivalent to severity scales but identify specific personality traits (Table 2).

The mean duration of the follow-up was 30.6±6 months. According to the Psychiatric Status Rating Scale (PSRS), 44% (N=41) of the initial sample still presented an eating disorder fulfilling DSM-IV criteria. A higher proportion of patients (63%) still presented symptoms of an eating disorder (PSRS≥3). The persistence of a diagnosis was independent from the initial subtype of eating disorder. The group of purging anorexics was the most instable in terms of the subtype of eating disorder presented at follow-up. 17% of the patients showed an unfavorable social outcome at follow-up without differences between groups. All patients received at the same rates a pharmacotherapy or a psychotherapy or a combination of the two. Restricting and purging anorexics were more often rehospitalized during the follow-up compared to bulimics (Table 3).

Considering that eating disorder subtypes did not show any difference in DEQ measures at inclusion, the regression analysis was conducted on the entire simple of eating disorders (N= 94). The logistic regression analysis significantly discriminated between participants with (N=41) and without (N=53) a persisting diagnosis of eating disorder (2log$L$ = 111.0, Model F(df =3)= 12.1 , p=0.01, Nagelkerke R^2 0.17). The model included the severity of the eating disorder (CGI), the Neediness subscale and the Relatedness subscales of the DEQ at inclusion. The Neediness subscale (Wald Z=6.19, p=0.013; OR=1.09, IC 1.02-1.17) and the severity of the eating disorder (Wald Z=4.00, p=0.045; OR=1.62, IC 1.01-2.61) at inclusion were significantly associated with the persistence of an eating disorder. The Relatedness subscale, which was negatively associated with diagnostic persistency, just missed the level of significance (Wald Z=3.74, p=0.053, OR=0.91, IC 0.82-1.00)(Table 4). Treatments delivered during the follow-up had no impact on the results. Finally, social outcome was significantly predicted by a model including the severity of depression and the Relatedness subscale of the DEQ (2log*L* = 58.0, Model F(df =2)= 17.7, p=0.003, Nagelkerke R^2 0.32). BDI was positively associated with the social outcome (B=0.14, Wald Z=7.87, p=0.01; OR=1.15, IC 1.04-1.26); Relatedness was negatively associated with the social outcome (B=-0.017, Wald Z=4.63, p=0.03; OR=0.84, IC 0.72-0.98).

Outcome variables	R-AN (N=42)	P-AN (N=19)	BN (N=33)	Total (N=94)	Statistics χ^2 /ANOVA with Bonferroni		
					F	*P<*	≠
DURATION OF THE FOLLOW-UP (M±SD)	31.2±6	28.8±5	31.2±6	30±6	0.81	ns	-
ED SYMPTOMS (PSRS≥3)(N, %)	26 (62)	12 (63)	21 (64)	59 (63)	0.02	ns	-
ED DIAGNOSIS (PSRS≥5)(N, %)	19 (45)	9 (47)	13 (39)	41 (44)	0.39	ns	-
SUBTYPES OF ED (N, %)					26.2	<0.001	
- RESTRICTING ANOREXIA	16 (84)	2 (22)	0	18 (37)			
- PURGING ANOREXIA	0	3 (33)	5 (38)	8 (19)			
- BULIMIA NERVOSA	3 (16)	4 (44)	8 (61)	15 (37)			
SOCIAL FUNCTIONING (GSDSII)(N,%)	8 (20)	3 (18)	4 (12)	15 (17)	0.91	ns	-
TREATMENT RECEIVED (N, %)							
- ANTIDEPRESSANTS	17 (40)	10 (53)	10 (30)	37 (39)	2.60	ns	-
- PSYCHOTHERAPY	23 (55)	12 (63)	18 (54)	53 (56)	0.44	ns	-
- HOSPITALISATION	22 (52)	11 (58)	8 (24)	41 (44)	7.91	<0.05	BN<R-AN/P-AN
- PHARMACO AND PSYCHOTHERAPY	8 (19)	5 (26)	4 (12)	17 (18)	1.70	ns	-

R-AN=Restricting Anorexia nervosa. P-AN=Purging Anorexia Nervosa. BN=Bulimia Nervosa. ED=Eating Disorders. PRSR= Psychiatric Status Rating Scale. GSDSII= Groningen Social Disability Scale . DEQ = Depressive Experience Questionnaire

Table 3. Description of the clinical outcome of the sample

Predicting variables	B	S.E.	Wald	Sig.	Exp(B)	IC per Exp(B) 95%	
Clinical Global Impression	0.48	0.24	4.00	0.045	1.62	1.01	2.61
DEQ Relatedness	-0.97	0.05	3.74	0.053	0.91	0.82	1.00
DEQ Neediness	0.09	0.03	6.19	0.013	1.09	1.02	1.17

DEQ = Depressive Experience Questionnaire

Table 4. Prediction of the diagnostic outcome according to the severity and the quality of the depressive experience

4. Discussion

At our knowledge, this is the first research investigating the relationships between the development levels of interpersonal relatedness and self-definition and the clinical outcome of adolescents and young adults with an eating disorder. Two main findings should be highlighted: first, a less mature level of interpersonal relatedness at inclusion (as assessed by the Neediness sub-factor of the DEQ) was a significant predictor of the persistence of an eating disorder diagnosis at 3-year follow-up, independently from the severity of the eating disorder, which also appeared as a significant predictor. Second, a more mature level of interpersonal relatedness (as assessed by the Relatedness sub-factor of the DEQ) appeared as a protective factor of a poor social outcome three years later. On the contrary, the severity of depression was a negative predictor of the social outcome, result that agrees with other studies from the literature (Godart et al., 2004). The other variables, such as the BMI, the presence of binge eating behaviors or the other sub-factors of the DEQ at inclusion, had no direct influence over the clinical and social outcome of eating disorders.

Personality factors have already been identified as significant predictors of diagnostic status and social outcome in eating disorders. For example, obsessive-compulsive personality traits have been repeatedly associated with poor diagnostic outcome in anorexia nervosa (Crane et al., 2007; Steinhausen 2009). Furthermore, impulsivity (Fichter et al., 2006) and low self-directedness (Rowe et al., 2011) have been related to poor outcome in bulimia nervosa. Results from our study add some interesting data from a developmental perspective showing that personality features reflecting the maturational level of interpersonal relationships may play a significant role in the outcome of eating disorders.

There are several ways in which the developmental level of interpersonal relationships can negatively impact the clinical outcome of eating disorders: via the influence it exerts on the clinical expression of the disorders and via the reduced efficacy of the therapeutic interventions. As Blatt and coworkers have largely described (Blatt 2004; Zuroff et al., 1999b), the establishment of increasingly mature and satisfying interpersonal relationships is an essential component of personality development. Interpersonal relationships are dynamic systems that change continuously throughout development following a trajectory ranging from dependency to more mature expressions of mutuality and reciprocity, including intimacy. Flourishing relationships also allow a dynamic balance between focus on intimate relationships and focus on other social relationships (Fincham and Beach 2010). Subjects with an immature development of interpersonal relationships may feel less competent in social interactions and may experience them as unpleasent and distressing. Investigations in samples of normal adolescents have shown that the Neediness sub-factor of the DEQ correlates negatively with measures of interpersonal competence (Henrich et al., 2001) and is associated to dysphoria, anxiety over loss, introversion, and discomfort with depending on others (Zuroff et al., 2004). Intense separation distress is a common feature among eating disorders (Touchette et al., 2010) and many patients demonstrate marked separation anxiety when confronted to real or imagined abandonments. High scores on the Neediness sub-factor of the DEQ in eating disorders may reflect the disconfort of these patients in social relationships (Zuroff et al., 1999a; Zuroff et al., 2004).

A personality profile characterized by high dependency may have direct implications for therapeutic relationships in eating disorders. As pointed by Zuroff and colleagues (Zuroff et al., 2004), dependent people expect to be hurt in relationships and adopt submissive interpersonal style to forestall conflict and to elicit protection and support (Zuroff et al.,

2004). This interpersonal style may foster ambivalent feelings toward the therapeutic situation perceived as dangerous and may interfere with the subject's ability to engage in psychotherapy. On the contrary, as witnessed in our study by the protecting value of high levels of Relatedness, valuing intimate relationships and being able of positively use interpersonal and social resources are essential factors that can positively promote the development of therapeutic relationships. Relatedness seems to capture personality features that correspond to a greater level of psychological maturity, indicating a sensitivity to the feelings and need of others and a regard for a symmetrical relationships rather than need gratification only (Zuroff et al., 1999b). As pointed by Greenberg and Bornstein, relational trust, insight and psychological mindedness are tightly related to interpersonal development (Greenberg and Bornstein 1988) as it is the case for therapeutic change. As Blatt and colleagues have highlighted, depressed patients can differently react to treatments (whether psychotherapy or pharmacotherapy) according to the quality and development of interpersonal relatedness and self-definition dimensions (Blatt et al., 1995). Using data from the National Institute of Mental Health Treatment for Depression Collaborative Research Program, Zuroff and Blatt (Zuroff and Blatt 2006) have shown that, independent of type of treatment, a perceived positive therapeutic relationship early in treatment predicts a better adjustment as well a greater enhanced adaptive capacities throughout the 18-month follow-up. If therapeutic relationships contribute directly to positive therapeutic outcome, it should deserve special attention as a specific mechanism involved in change. As pointed by Fonagy and Target (Fonagy and Target 2002), treatment research should begin with the identification of key dysfunctions associated with a particular disorder and by establishing a conceptual link between the method of treatment and the dysfunctional mechanism identified in connection with the disorder.

According to our results, relational and interpersonal issues should be considered as key dysfunctions in eating disorders and should deserve specific attention. In fact, if symptom control is often a vital aim at the beginning of the therapy, elaborating relational experiences and family dynamics seem essential for the long term care of eating disorders. It is not surprising that interest in family interventions in eating disorders has increased over the past 5 years. A recent metanalysis of RCT studies has shown that systemic family therapy appears efficacious for the treatment of adult eating disorders (von Sydow et al., 2010). Family interventions are the current first-line treatment for adolescent anorexia nervosa and promising for adolescent bulimia nervosa (Le Grange and Eisler 2009; Lock 2011). Familiy treatment would be effective not only for weight restoration, but also in improving some psychological symptoms including dietary restraint, interoceptive deficits, and maturity fears (Couturier et al., 2010). Although encouraging, however these conclusions are based on few trials that included only small numbers of participants with several issues regarding potential bias. The field would benefit from large, well-conducted trials (Fisher et al., 2010).

There are several limitations to this study that must be acknowledged. First, the sample was composed of young women with medium to high levels of education recruited from university hospitals specialized in adolescents and young adults with severe disorders. It is possible that the sample contained patients with specific clinical and socio-demographic profiles that may reduce the generalisability of the results. Second, the study had a naturalistic design, with therapeutic interventions freely chosen on the basis of usual practices. Although we controlled treatments in all statistical analyses, differences in treatments received may have influenced the evolution of patients over time. A final limitation is the middling rate of follow-up. A certain number of refusals can be explained by the young age at inclusion and the duration of the study. However, we made the choice of directly collecting data and retaining only patients with complete files to ensure a good quality of the sample.

5. Conclusions

Aside from these limitations, the results of our study indicate that an immature development of interpersonal relatedness can act as a negative prognostic factor of the long-term outcome of patients with eating disorders. This result implies that relational issues should deserve specific attention in eating disorders and indirectly supports the interest of family approaches for these patients. More generally, this study highlights the interest of a person-centered approach focusing on the subjective experience of patients. As Fonagy and Target (Fonagy and Target 2002) have outlined, the majority of studies do not explore the subjective experience and the psychological distress of patients, although this may be critically different among subjects. The investigation of the subjective experience can deepen our understanding of psychiatric disturbances as categorized by the DSM-IV and refine our prediction about treatment outcomes for a variety of different types of psychological disturbances (Fonagy 2004). This approach is also in line with the recommendations issued by the working group on personality disorders for the future DSM-V. The working group, arguing that personality psychopathology fundamentally emanates from disturbances in thinking about self and others, and that these features influence treatment strategies, has proposed to include an assessment of the levels of self (including identity and self-direction) and interpersonal functioning (including empathy and intimacy) to describe the personality characteristics of all patients, independently from the presence of a personality disorder (APA 2011). Professionals should carefully monitor interpersonal concerns when assessing eating disorder patients and should develop specific therapeutic strategies to handle the negative relational expectancies frequently experienced by these patients (Goodsit 1997).

6. Acknowledgments

This work was conducted within the clinical research project "Dependence Network 1994-2000". The Network received the support of the Institut National de la Santé et de la Recherche Médicale (Réseau Inserm n° 494013) and of the Fondation de France. The promoter of the project is the Institut Mutualiste Montsouris. All the centres participating in the project should be acknowledged: Department of Adolescent and Young Adult Psychiatry, Institut Mutualiste Montsouris, Paris, France ; Department of Psychiatry, Hôpital Pinel, Amiens, France ; Department of Psychiatry, Hôpital Saint-Jacques, Nantes, France ; Department of Psychiatry Hôpital Universitaire, Besançon, France ; Department of Child and Adolescent Psychiatry, SUPEA, Lausanne, Switzerland.

7. References

APA. (2000). *Diagnostic and Statistical Manual of Mental Disorders, Fourth Edition, Text Revision.* (American Psychiatric Association, Washington, DC).

APA. (2011). http://www.dsm5.org/ProposedRevisions/Pages/proposedrevision.aspx?rid=397

Atger F, Frasson G, Loas G, Guibourge S, Corcos M, Perez Diaz F, Speranza M, Venisse JL, Lang F, Stephan P et al.,. (2003). [Validation study of the Depressive Experience Questionnaire]. Encephale 29,445-55.

Bagby RM, Cox BJ, Schuller DR, Levitt AJ, Swinson RP, Joffe RT. (1992). Diagnostic specificity of the dependent and self-critical personality dimensions in major depression. J Affect Disord 26,59-63.

Bagby RM, Schuller DR, Parker JD, Levitt A, Joffe RT, Shafir MS. (1994). Major depression and the self-criticism and dependency personality dimensions. Am J Psychiatry 151,597-9.

Beck AT. (1961). A systematic investigation of depression. Compr Psychiatry 2,163-70.

Beck AT, Beck RW. (1972). Screening depressed patients in family practice. A rapid technic. Postgrad Med 52,81-5.

Beck AT, Rial WY, Rickels K. (1974). Short form of depression inventory: cross-validation. Psychol Rep 34,1184-6.

Beck AT, Steer RA, Garbin MG. (1988). Psychometric properties of the Beck Depression Inventory: twenty-five years of evaluation. Clinical Psychology Review 8,77- 100.

Besser A, Babchoock A. (2001). DEQ scoring program for SPSS.

Blaney PH, Kutcher GS. (1991). Measures of depressive symptoms: Are they interchangeable? Journal of Personality Assessment 56,502–512.

Blatt SJ. (2004). *Experiences of depression. Theoretical, clinical, and research perspectives.* (American Psychological Association, Washington, DC).

Blatt SJ, D'Affliti SJ, Quinlan DM. (1976). *Depressive experiences questionnaire.* (Yale University Press, New Haven, CT).

Blatt SJ, Zohar AH, Quinlan DM, Zuroff DC, Mongrain M. (1995). Subscales within the dependency factor of the Depressive Experiences Questionnaire. J Pers Assess 64,319-39.

Blatt SJ, Zuroff DC. (1992). Interpersonal relatedness and self-definition: two prototypes for depression. Clin Psychol Rev,527-62.

Bobon DP, Sanchez-Blanque A, Von Franckell D. (1981). Comparison between the short form of the Beck Depression Inventory and the combined Beck Pichot Inventory. Journal de Psychiatrie Biologique et Therapeutique 1,211- 218.

Bruch H. (1973). *Eating disorders: obesity, anorexia nervosa and the person within.* (Basic Books, New York).

Corcos M, Jeammet P. (2001). Eating disorders: psychodynamic approach and practice. Biomed Pharmacother 55,479-88.

Couturier J, Isserlin L, Lock J. (2010). Family-based treatment for adolescents with anorexia nervosa: a dissemination study. Eat Disord 18,199-209.

Cox BJ, Rector NA, Bagby RM, Swinson RP, Levitt AJ, Joffe RT. (2000). Is self-criticism unique for depression? A comparison with social phobia. J Affect Disord 57,223-8.

Crane AM, Roberts ME, Treasure J. (2007). Are obsessive-compulsive personality traits associated with a poor outcome in anorexia nervosa? A systematic review of randomized controlled trials and naturalistic outcome studies. Int J Eat Disord 40,581-8.

Fichter MM, Quadflieg N. (1999). Six-year course and outcome of anorexia 541 nervosa. Int J Eat Disord 26,359–85.

Fichter MM, Quadflieg N, Hedlund S. (2006). Twelve-year course and outcome predictors of anorexia nervosa. Int J Eat Disord 39,87-100.

Fincham FD, Beach SRH. (2010). Of memes and marriage: Toward a positive relationship science. Journal of Family Theory & Review,4-24.

Fisher CA, Hetrick SE, Rushford N. (2010). Family therapy for anorexia nervosa. Cochrane Database Syst Rev,CD004780.

Fonagy P. (2004). Foreward. In *Experiences of depression. Theoretical, clinical, and research perspectives*. Blatt SJ, ed. (American Psychological Association, Washington, DC.

Fonagy P, Target M. (2002). The place of psychodynamic theory in developmental psychopathology. Dev Psychopathol 12,407–25.

Godart NT, Perdereau F, Curt F, Lang F, Venisse JL, Halfon O, Bizouard P, Loas G, Corcos M, Jeammet P et al.,. (2004). Predictive factors of social disability in anorexic and bulimic patients. Eat Weight Disord 9,249-57.

Goodsit A. (1997). Eating disorders a self psychological perspective. In *Handbook of treatment for eating disorders*. Garner DM, Garfinkel PE, eds. (Guilford, New York). pp 205-28.

Greenberg RP, Bornstein RF. (1988). The dependent personality: II. Risk for psychological disorders. J Pers Assess,136-43.

Guy W. (1976). *Clinical Global Impressions, ECDEU Assessment Manual for Psychopharmacology, revised*. (Rockville, MD).

Heatherton TF, Baumeister RF. (1991). Binge-eating as escape from self-awareness. Psychol Bull 110, 86-108.

Henrich CC, Blatt SJ, Kuperminc GP, Zohar A, Leadbeater BJ. (2001). Levels of interpersonal concerns and social functioning in early adolescent boys and girls. J Pers Assess 76,48-67.

Herzog DB, Field AE, Keller MB, West JC, Robbins WM, Staley J, Colditz GA. (1996). Subtyping eating disorders: is it justified? J Am Acad Child Adolesc Psychiatry 35,928-36.

Herzog DB, Keller MB, Sacks NR, Yeh CJ, Lavori PW. (1992). Psychiatric comorbidity in treatment-seeking anorexics and bulimics. J Am Acad Child Adolesc Psychiatry 31,810-8.

Herzog DB, Sacks NR, Keller MB, Lavori PW, von Ranson KB, Gray HM. (1993). Patterns and predictors of recovery in anorexia nervosa and bulimia nervosa. J Am Acad Child Adolesc Psychiatry 32,835-42.

Honkalampi K, Hintikka J, Saarinen P, Lehtonen J, Viinamaki H. (2000). Is alexithymia a permanent feature in depressed patients? Results from a 6-month follow-up study. Psychother Psychosom 69,303-8.

Kuperminc GP, Blatt SJ, Leadbeater BJ. (1997). Relatedness, self-definition, and early adolescent adjustment. Cognitive Therapy and Research 21,301–320.

Le Grange D, Eisler I. (2009). Family interventions in adolescent anorexia nervosa. Child Adolesc Psychiatr Clin N Am 18,159-73.

Lock J. (2011). Evaluation of family treatment models for eating disorders. Curr Opin Psychiatry.

McBride C, Zuroff D, Bacchiochi J, Bagby MR. (2006). Depressive Experiences Questionnaire: Does it measure maladaptive and adaptive forms of dependency? Soc Behav and Pers 34, 1, 1-16.

Mongrain M, Zuroff DC. (1994). Ambivalence over emotional expression and negative life events: Mediators of depressive symptoms in dependent and self-critical individuals. Journal of Personality and Individual Differences 16,447-458.

Nolen-Hoesema S, Stice E, Wade E, Bohon C. (2007). Reciprocal Relations Between Rumination and Bulimic, Substance Abuse, and Depressive Symptoms in Female Adolescents. J of Abnorm Psychology, 116, 1, 198–207.

Pilkonis PA, Heape CL, Ruddy J, Serrao P. (1991). Validity in the diagnosis of personality disorders: The use of the LEAD standard. Psychol Assessment 31,46-54.

Rowe S, Jordan J, McIntosh V, Carter F, Frampton C, Bulik C, Joyce P. (2011). Dimensional measures of personality as a predictor of outcome at 5-year follow-up in women with bulimia nervosa. Psychiatry Res 185,414-20.

Rude SS, Burnham BL. (1995). Connectedness and neediness: Factors of the DEQ and SAS Dependency scales. Cognitive Therapy and Research 19,323–340.

Sheehan DV, Lecrubier Y, Sheehan KH, Amorim P, Janavs J, Weiller E, Hergueta T, Baker R, Dunbar GC. (1998). The Mini-International Neuropsychiatric Interview (M.I.N.I.): the development and validation of a structured diagnostic psychiatric interview for DSM-IV and ICD-10. J Clin Psychiatry 59 Suppl 20,22-33; quiz 34-57.

Speranza M, Atger F, Corcos M, Loas G, Guilbaud O, Stephan P, Perez-Diaz F, Halfon O, Venisse JL, Bizouard P et al.,. (2003). Depressive psychopathology and adverse childhood experiences in eating disorders. Eur Psychiatry 18,377-83.

Steinhausen HC. (2009). Outcome of eating disorders. Child Adolesc Psychiatr Clin N Am 18,225-42.

Touchette E, Henegar A, Godart NT, Pryor L, Falissard B, Tremblay RE, Cote SM. (2010). Subclinical eating disorders and their comorbidity with mood and anxiety disorders in adolescent girls. Psychiatry Res 185,185-92.

von Sydow K, Beher S, Schweitzer J, Retzlaff R. (2010). The efficacy of systemic therapy with adult patients: a meta-content analysis of 38 randomized controlled trials. Fam Process 49,457-85.

Wiersma D, de Jong A, Kraaijkamp HJM, Ormel J. (1990). *GSDSII. The Groningen Social Disabilities Schedule*. (University of Groningen, Department of Social Psychiatry).

Zuroff DC, Blatt SJ. (2006). The therapeutic relationship in the brief treatment of depression: contributions to clinical improvement and enhanced adaptive capacities. J Consult Clin Psychol 74,130-40.

Zuroff DC, Blatt SJ, Sanislow CA, 3rd, Bondi CM, Pilkonis PA. (1999a). Vulnerability to depression: reexamining state dependence and relative stability. J Abnorm Psychol 108,76-89.

Zuroff DC, Mongrain M, Santor DA. (2004). Conceptualizing and measuring personality vulnerability to depression: comment on Coyne and Whiffen (1995). Psychol Bull 130,489-511; discussion 512-22.

Zuroff DC, Moskowitz DS, Cote S. (1999b). Dependency, self-criticism, interpersonal behaviour and affect: evolutionary perspectives. Br J Clin Psychol 38 (Pt 3),231-50.

9

Bulimia Nervosa and Personality: A Review

Ignacio Jáuregui Lobera
Pablo de Olavide University, Seville, Spain

1. Introduction

A relatively new approach, which tends to be applied in order to subtype eating disorders, is based on the study of personality and its disturbances. A well-known statement is that anorexia nervosa and bulimia nervosa are disorders with a high level of heterogeneity in terms of personality variables. Clinical observation has long found a link between personality and eating disorders. Despite the fact that a lot of personality profiles have been described among eating disorder patients, in case of anorexia nervosa and bulimia nervosa the personality traits tend to be described within a dimension of impulsivity-compulsivity. The study of personality in eating disorder patients seems to be useful as a subtyping strategy, this being more effective than the traditional symptoms-based categorization (diagnostic criteria), mainly in order to predict the psychosocial functioning and different clinical features (Abbott, Wonderlich, et al., 2001; Steiger & Stotland, 1996; Westen & Harnden-Fischer, 2001; Wonderlich & Mitchell, 2001).

The association between eating disorders and personality disorders has been studying mainly from the moment in which the personality disorders were included in the axis II of DSM. An improvement with regards to the study of personality disorders was the development of specific structured interviews and self-reported questionnaires in order to assess personality traits and its disturbances (Echeburúa & Marañón, 2001; Loranger, 1995; Matsunaga, Kiriike, et al., 1998; Millon & Ávila, 1998; Spitzer, Williams, et al., 1992).

Personality disorders constitute rigid and maladaptive thoughts, feelings and behaviours, all related with poor learning of effective coping strategies. As a result, patients suffering from personality disorders usually have interpersonal conflicts and severe psychosocial limitations. Moreover, these disorders imply a psychological distress and they are stable throughout life (Echeburúa & Corral, 1999; Sarason & Sarason, 1996; Vázquez, Ring, et al., 1990).

There is a shortage of reliable studies on epidemiology of personality disorders due to several facts, as the heterogeneity of the studied populations and the scarce of valid and reliable instruments. Nevertheless, all the studies usually show a common conclusion, this being the high prevalence of personality disorders (ranging from 6% in general population to 20%-40% among psychiatric outpatients) and a slightly higher prevalence among women (Echeburúa & Corral, 1999).

The frequent comorbidity between personality disorders and other pathologies of the DSM axis I may be explained by different facts: a) personality disorders may be a risk factor for suffering from mental disorders; b) personality disorders may be a consequence of any mental disorders, and c) both, personality disorders and other mental disorders may follow an independent course (Medina & Moreno, 1998). In case of eating disorders the association with a personality disorder usually makes an early diagnostic difficult, makes the treatment more difficult, and usually is related with a poor prognostic (Díaz, Carrasco, et al., 1999).

Research has consistently linked anorexia (particularly restrictive type) to personality traits such as introversion, conformity, perfectionism, rigidity, and obsessive-compulsive features (Casper, 1990). The picture for bulimia is less clear and somehow mixed. Traits such as perfectionism, shyness, and compliance have consistently emerged in studies of individuals with bulimia or with anorexia, although research has often found bulimic patients to be extroverted, histrionic, and affectively unstable (Vitousek & Manke, 1994).

Different studies have been developed based on two points of view. As a result the focus may be on how many patients suffering from eating disorders have any personality disorders, or the focus could be how many patients with personality disorders suffer from any eating disorders. In the first case there is a wide range of comorbidity, from 21% to 97% (Dolan, Evans, et al., 1994; Skodol, Oldham, et al., 1993). Following Westen & Harnden-Fischer (2001), the comorbidity between eating disorders and personality disorders could reflect the possibility a) that many patients have the random misfortune of having two or more disorders, at least one of which is on axis I and another on axis II; b) that anorexic and bulimic behaviours are symptomatic expressions of personality pathology and hence distinctions regarding syndromes, states and traits embodied in the distinction between DSM axis I and axis II may be problematic with respect to eating disorders; or c) that some common genetic or environmental diathesis underlies both eating disorders and personality disorders.

With regards to the above-mentioned dimension of impulsivity-compulsivity, personality pathology in eating disorders is related with specific forms of neurotransmitter dysregulation, anorexia and bulimia lying at opposite ends of a personality continuum defined by compulsivity at the anorexic end and impulsivity at the bulimic (Skodol, Oldham, et al., 1993). Following this theory, patients with anorexia are most frequently diagnosed with cluster C (anxious/avoidant) personality disorders, whereas bulimic patients are more likely to receive cluster B (dramatic/erratic) diagnoses. Another usual finding refers to the association between bulimia and borderline personality disorder (Herzog, Keller, et al., 1992; Kennedy, McVey, et al., 1990; Skodol, Oldham, et al., 1993). Despite these findings, above and beyond there are a lot of studies, which fail to find a clear relationship between personality variables and eating disorders. So that, the research based on the relationships between eating disorders and personality is highly inconsistent (Gartner, Marcus, et al., 1989; Steiger, Liquornik, et al., 1991).

It is well known, that there is an extensive comorbidity of anorexic and bulimic symptoms with each other. If certain core personality traits are associated with, or contribute to, specific eating disordered behaviour, and these personality traits are in many respects polar opposites, how could one individual display both classes of symptoms, as it is represented in Figure 1? (Westen & Harnden-Fischer, 2001). In fact, patients who have a lifetime history of both disorders or who simultaneously have symptoms of both disorders more often receive a personality disorder diagnosis than patients with either bulimia or anorexia (restricting type). In addition, their personality disorder diagnoses are equally distributed in cluster B or cluster C. What could explain the inconsistency of the studies? It is possible that both, anorexia nervosa and bulimia nervosa may be linked to personality factors heterogeneously. So that, more than one type of personality could cause or contribute to the symptoms of the eating disorders (Sohlberg & Strober, 1994).

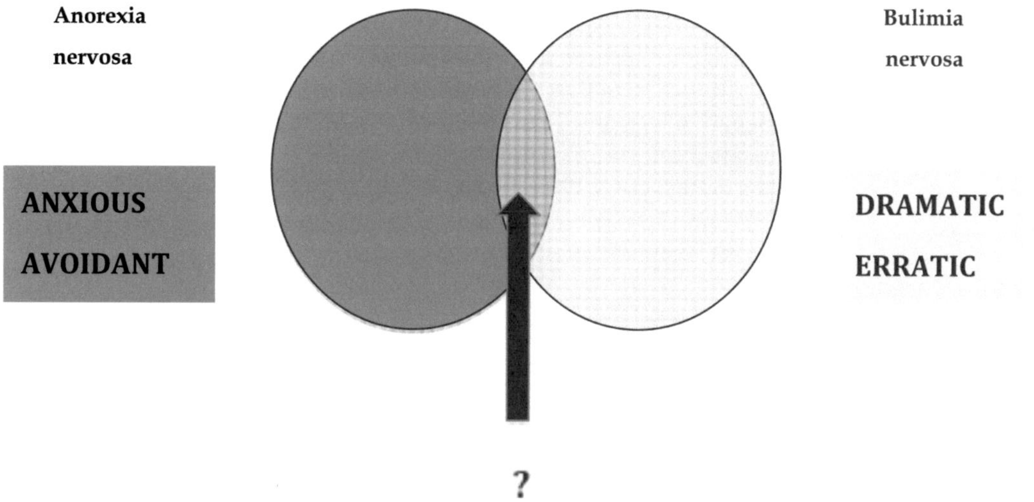

Fig. 1. Comorbidity of anorexic and bulimic symptoms with each other, and core personality traits in anorexia and bulimia.

Despite the inconsistencies across different studies, the understanding of the relation between eating disorders and personality disorders is relevant, because patients with comorbid personality pathology have a worse course, greater psychological distress, greater mood disturbances, and a slower recovery than those without comorbid personality disorders (Herzog, Keller, et al., 1992; Herzog, Keller, et al., 1992; Steiger, Leung, et al., 1993; Wonderlich & Swift, 1990).

The presence of obsessiveness, rigidity, perfectionism, dependency, social inhibition or low self-sufficiency is usual among patients with anorexia nervosa, while patients with purging-type anorexia nervosa and bulimia nervosa usually are more impulsive, and show high levels of sensitivity, emotional instability, and lower self-esteem. The association of bulimia nervosa and other disturbances (i.e., poor impulse control, self-injuries, aggressive behaviour, kleptomania, substance abuse, gambling, stealing or sexual promiscuity) is highly frequent (Braun, Sunday, et al., 1994; Gartner, Marcus, et al., 1989; Matsunaga, Kiriike, et al., 1998; Steiger & Stotland, 1996; Wonderlich & Swift, 1990).

With regards to bulimia nervosa, some researches have focused on the distinction between multi-impulsive versus uni-impulsive patients (Lacey & Evans, 1986). In case of uni-impulsive patients, binge eating is the only symptom or behaviour that could be described as impulsive. In case of multi-impulsive patients, there are a lot of symptoms or behaviours related to impulsivity (stealing, substance abuse, etc.). Multi-impulsive bulimic patients usually have significantly greater rates of borderline personality disorder and mood disorders than uni-impulsive bulimic patients (Lacey & Evans, 1986). These two groups of bulimic patients may represent very different kinds of patients, despite the fact that they have the same eating disorder symptoms. These two types of bulimic patients constitute an example of two possible subtypes within the general classification of bulimia nervosa that may not be easily differentiated by the eating symptoms. Nevertheless, they may differ in personality, aetiology, or function of symptoms (Westen & Harnden-Fischer, 2001).

The differences in personality style are related to clinical variables. Bulimic patients with borderline personality disorder (or any cluster B personality disorder of the DSM), display a poorer outcome across a wide range of treatments, including individual and group therapy, cognitive behaviour therapy, and pharmacotherapy. Compared to bulimic patients free of personality disorders, those with cluster B disorders show more general psychopathology, drug and alcohol use, self-destructive behaviour, suicide attempts, histories of sexual/physical abuse, negative appraisals of family functioning, greater hospitalization rates, and higher use of psychotropic medication (Herzog, Keller, et al., 1992; Johnson, Tobin, et al., 1989; Rossiter, Agras, et al, 1993; Steiger & Stotland, 1996; Wonderlich & Swift, 1990).

1.2 Summarising

- Clinical observation has long found a link between personality and eating disorders.
- In case of eating disorders the association with a personality disorder usually makes an early diagnostic difficult, makes the treatment more difficult, and usually is related with a poor prognostic.
- Research has often found bulimic patients to be extroverted, histrionic, and affectively unstable.
- It is possible that both, anorexia nervosa and bulimia nervosa may be linked to personality factors heterogeneously. So that, more than one type of personality could cause or contribute to the symptoms of the eating disorders.
- Patients with purging-type anorexia nervosa and bulimia nervosa usually are more impulsive, and show high levels of sensitivity, emotional instability, and lower self-esteem.
- With regards to bulimia nervosa, some researches have focused on the distinction between multi-impulsive versus uni-impulsive patients. In case of uni-impulsive patients, binge eating is the only symptom or behaviour that could be described as impulsive. In case of multi-impulsive patients, there are a lot of symptoms or behaviours related to impulsivity (stealing, substance abuse, etc.).

2. Bulimia nervosa and personality

A lot of studies have found a high prevalence of disorders included in the axis II of DSM among patients with bulimia nervosa, the term co-diagnostic being more appropriate than the concept of comorbidity. This is due to the fact that the latter means the concurrence of two different disorders, which does not respond to the current knowledge about personality and its disturbances. The concept of co-diagnostic also refers to the idea of a cross-sectional and simultaneous evaluation, which could change over time, this highlighting a temporal but no stable association between the two disorders (Ponce de León, 2006).

Studies based on the association between bulimia nervosa and personality styles have been reported a great variability of results due to conceptual and methodological problems (Ponce de León, 2006). The evaluation of personality implies to assess the stability of the traits over time and in different contexts, and to control several variables closely related to the environment. Variables as age, gender, patterns of social relationships, etc., could influence the evaluation of the personality acting as confounders. The usual chronicity of bulimia nervosa may be another factor of confusion, due to the frequent changes that patients display overtime with regards to their symptoms, which could be understood as personality traits. The eating dysregulation showed by bulimic patients has neurobiological consequences and may induce changes in the environment. As a result, the evaluation should be difficult. Many times symptoms of the eating disorders and specific symptoms of personality disorders are overlapped, making difficult a proper evaluation of the association between both bulimia nervosa and personality disorder. Another point to take into account is the fact that the majority of the samples of bulimic patients usually comprise only women (or they have a low representation of men), so that is difficult to generalize the results of the evaluations. Finally diagnostic criteria for both bulimia nervosa and personality disorders have been modified in the past years and they are usually under discussion (Ponce de León, 2006; Westen, 1997; Westen & Shedler, 1999_a, 1999_b; Westen & Westen, 1998).

2.2 How may the results about studies based on the relationship between bulimia nervosa and personality disorders be interpreted?

As it has been mentioned the prevalence of personality disorders among eating disorder patients shows a wide range of results, and in case of bulimia nervosa ranges from 4% to 84%, despite the majority of studies report prevalence between 20% and 75%. By means of instruments as MMPI, EPQ and other similar scales, it has been reported that bulimic patients have higher scores in extraversion, poor impulse control, novelty seeking or low frustration tolerance, than anorectic patients (Gargallo, Fernández, et al., 2003; Ponce de León, 2006).

Despite the fact that bulimia nervosa seems to be closely related to personality disorders of cluster B of DSM (Jáuregui Lobera, Santiago Fernández, et al., 2009), there are studies finding close links between bulimia nervosa and obsessive syndromes and disorders of cluster C (von Ranson, Kaye, et al., 1999). This seems a surprising result taking into account the dimension impulsivity-compulsivity. This surprising finding is highlighted by the fact that a relatively frequent association between bulimia nervosa and obsessive-compulsive disorder has been found (8%-33%) (von Ranson, Kaye, et al., 1999). In addition, it has been reported that this link between bulimia nervosa and obsessiveness persists after the patients are recovered from their eating disorder or when they are recovered from other associated syndromes as anxiety or depression (von Ranson, Kaye, et al., 1999).

The relationship between bulimia nervosa and borderline personality disorder remains confusing. As opposite of the obsessiveness, borderline traits are present mainly at the beginning of the bulimic symptoms decreasing over time. More over the decrease of the bulimic symptoms usually is associated with a decrease of the borderline thoughts, feelings and behaviours (Ponce de León, 2006).

Despite the fact that the dimension impulsivity-compulsivity seems to be a useful tool to represent the two main eating disorders, it is difficult to explain the concurrence of bulimia nervosa and obsessiveness, or how an eating disorder as anorexia nervosa becomes another one as bulimia nervosa. So that, studies on the association between personality and eating disorders remain controversial. But there is a consensus about the fact that in case of a history of anorexia nervosa and bulimia nervosa, and in case of a purging type-anorexia it is possible to find the highest prevalence of associated personality disorders (mainly of clusters B and C), and the poorest outcome (Bulik, Sullivan et al., 1995; Bussolotti, Fernández-Aranda, et al., 2002; Rossiter, Agras, et al., 1993).

The co-occurrence between bulimia nervosa and personality disorders ranges from 4%-80%, mainly between 20%-75% of cases, and cluster B personality disorders (DSM), especially the borderline personality disorder, is the most frequently reported (Wonderlich & Swift, 1990). It is noted in the literature on eating disorders, that comorbid personality disorders are generally associated with various factors such as diagnosis, greater impulsivity and self-harm, more substance abuse/dependence, more suicide attempts, more frequent purging behaviours, mood disorders, sexual abuse, greater comorbidity and severity of the disorder. Also, personality disorders have been identified as predictors and worse prognosis associated with a higher frequency of treatment dropout (Herzog, Kelller et al., 1992; Steiger, Leung et al., 1993; Wonderlich & Swift, 1990).

It is possible to interpret the association between bulimia nervosa and personality in different ways as follows:

a. The association could be the result of an overlap between symptoms-traits, the result of methodological errors, or the concurrence of different syndromes (i.e., anxiety, depression) in bulimia nervosa.
b. Bulimia nervosa and some personality disorders could have links with regards to biology and/or environment. In this case it would be appropriate to take into account the dimension impulsivity-compulsivity.
c. It could be admitted that there are two different patients, from a clinical point of view: Those who hardly fit criteria of personality disorders (these being more closely related to compulsivity), and those more closely related to impulsivity and usually suffering from personality disorders (mainly of cluster B).

2.3 Summarising

- Studies based on the association between bulimia nervosa and personality styles have reported a great variability of results due to conceptual and methodological problems.
- Many times symptoms of the eating disorder and specific symptoms of personality disorders are overlapped, making difficult a proper evaluation of the association between both bulimia nervosa and personality disorder.
- The prevalence of personality disorders among eating disorder patients shows a wide range of results, and in case of bulimia nervosa the majority of studies report prevalence between 20% and 75%.
- Despite the fact that the dimension impulsivity-compulsivity seems to be a useful tool to represent the two main eating disorders, it is difficult to explain the concurrence of bulimia nervosa and obsessiveness, or how an eating disorder as anorexia nervosa becomes another one as bulimia nervosa.
- Comorbid personality disorders are generally associated with various factors such as diagnosis, greater impulsivity and self-harm, more substance abuse/dependence, more suicide attempts, more frequent purging behaviours, mood disorders, sexual abuse, greater comorbidity and severity of the eating disorder.

3. Impulsivity and bulimia nervosa

In bulimic patients, the association between the specific eating disorder symptoms and many psychopathological disorders whose core seems to be the poor impulse control, such as suicide attempts, hetero-aggressive behaviour, kleptomania, alcohol abuse/dependence, substance abuse/dependence, gambling or sexual promiscuity, has long been described. The study of Clinton & Glant (1992) may be illustrative due to the fact that it reports the presence of alcohol abuse in 22.2%, drug abuse in 14.4%, and suicide attempts in 21.4% (7.1 % having performed more than one attempt) of bulimic patients. Some authors state that studies of neurotransmitters in eating disorders suggest that in both the purging type anorexic patients and bulimic patients, as well as in the binge eating disorder, exist a deficit of the serotonergic function, which, in turn, is observed often in the above-mentioned psychopathological disorders (Diaz Marsá, 1999; Steiger, Young et al., 2001). So that, it seems that impairment (primary or secondary) in the brain function would be common to these disorders, which would explain the frequency with which they appear jointly. Studies of some authors could even pose to understand bulimia as a variant of impulse control disorder that would have its outer manifestation in eating behaviour, as there are several similarities in the structure of both psychopathological disorders: the inclination to carry out a detrimental act to themselves or others, inability to resist the impulsive act, feelings of restlessness or anxiety that increases progressively before the impulsive act, which are relieved when this is done to give way to feelings of shame or guilt (Fahy & Eisler, 1993; Newton, Freeman, et al., 1993; Westen & Harnden-Fischer, 2001).

There are different points of view with respect to the relationship between bulimia nervosa and impulsivity. One of them is based on the observed prevalence of the association between bulimia nervosa and impulsivity assessed by clinical interviews. These studies propose that impulsivity among bulimic patients would be a specific eating disorder subtype. Another proposal of these studies is that impulsivity could be reflecting the association between bulimia nervosa and other psychopathological disorders. The second type of studies (mainly based on psychometric assessments) states that impulsivity and bulimia nervosa would have a common base, which would be a specific type of personality. The third group of studies relates symptoms more than diagnostics, in order to explore the possible association between bulimic symptoms and impulsivity based on biological and psychosocial common roots, in both clinical and non-clinical samples (Peñas Lledó, 2006).

The relationship between bulimia nervosa and impulsivity leads to two different diagnostics, which are usually involved in bulimic patients. Up to date, the multi-impulsive bulimia (Lacey & Evans, 1986) is not accepted as different type of bulimia nervosa, despite many authors state its undoubted clinical presence (Fichter, Quadflieg, et al., 1994; Welch & Fairburn, 1996). The use of very different criteria to assess this multi-impulsive bulimia leads to great differences of prevalence (Cook Myers, Wonderlich, et al., 2006), ranging from 18% to 80%. Despite the discussion on the real existence of this form of bulimia nervosa, there is a consensus on the fact that the more impulsive the behaviours are the worst is the prognostic of bulimic patients (Fichter, Quadflieg, et al., 1994). Another diagnostic usually involved in this field of study is the borderline personality disorder. In this personality disorder the disordered eating behaviour is only one of the criteria for the diagnostic, the rest being described as different impulse control deficits. The prevalence of this personality disorder among bulimic patients ranges from 2%-50% approximately (Marino & Zanarini, 2001; Peñas Lledó, 2006; Wonderlich & Swift, 1990). Finally a question emerges: How many patients with a borderline personality disorder and bulimia nervosa could really suffer from a multi-impulsive bulimia? (And vice versa). Some facts orientate the possible response: comparing bulimic patients with and without a borderline personality disorder, there are more impulsive behaviours (other than eating-related behaviours) among the patients with the associated personality disorder. On the other hand, comparing multi-impulsive bulimic patients and non-multi-impulsive bulimic patients the first group shows a higher prevalence of borderline personality disorder (63% vs. 13%) (Peñas Lledó, 2006).

Different psychometric studies on impulsivity as a dimension of personality usually (but non always) show that bulimic patients have higher scores on impulsivity than control participants do.

Regarding the impulsivity symptoms and bulimic symptoms, may be that both have a common base. On the other hand these symptoms would have a function, which could be the seeking of well-being and/or the avoidance of negative thoughts/emotions. Many times this function reaches a high psychopathological severity due to its self-destructive power. Impulsive behaviours as well as bingeing are usually related to intolerable negative emotions, and many times both people who binge and those with other impulsive behaviours present higher scores on coping strategies focused on emotions (Peñas Lledó, 2006; Peñas Lledó & Waller, 2001)

As it was mentioned above, a neurobiological base of the impulsivity has been proposed, this being based on the serotoninergic regulation. In all disorders with this type of dysregulation, pharmacological treatments which act on serotoninergic receptors has shown proved efficacy.

3.1 Summarising

- Some authors state that studies of neurotransmitters in eating disorders suggest that in both the purging type anorexic patients and bulimic patients, as well as in the binge eating disorder, exist a deficit of the serotonergic function.
- The same is referred to some psychopathological disorders whose core seems to be a poor impulse control, such as suicide attempts, hetero-aggressive behaviour, kleptomania, alcohol and other substance abuse/dependence, gambling or sexual promiscuity among others.
- Some authors propose to understand bulimia as a variant of an impulse control disorder, which would have its outer manifestation in eating behaviour.
- Some studies propose that impulsivity among bulimic patients would be a specific eating disorder subtype. Another proposal is that impulsivity could be reflecting the association between bulimia nervosa and other psychopathological disorders.
- Another type of studies (mainly based on psychometric assessments) states that impulsivity and bulimia nervosa would have a common base, which would be a specific type of personality.
- Up to date, the multi-impulsive bulimia is not accepted as a different type of bulimia nervosa despite many authors state its undoubted clinical presence.

4. Multi-impulsive bulimia nervosa

The high impulsivity associated with bulimia nervosa leads to a worse prognostic, and patients with different impulsive behaviours linked to bulimic symptoms were said to comprise a subgroup, which was named as multi-impulsive bulimia nervosa. In this concept (Lacey & Evans, 1986) were included some impulsive behaviours as aggressiveness (self/hetero) expressed by suicide attempts, purging behaviours, self mutilations, burns, other forms of self-harm, sexual promiscuity, stealing, substance abuse/dependence, reckless driving or physical aggressions. In addition to the absence of consensus with regards to the reality of this type of bulimia nervosa as a clinical subgroup, there are a lot of methodological problems for its conceptualization, the main being the weak consensus on the definition of the different involved behaviours and the heterogeneity of the samples in which the studies have been based on.

Fichter et al. (1994) defined the characteristics of multi-impulsivity, by the fact that bulimic patients should have three or more of the following impulsive behaviours:

a. One or more suicide attempts
b. One or more self-harm episodes
c. One or more stealing episodes (other than those related to food)
d. Alcohol abuse/dependence
e. Substance abuse/dependence
f. Sexual promiscuity (having sexual relations with five or more different partners in the two last years, or ten or more since the puberty)

Besides these behaviours, patients with multi-impulsive bulimia nervosa show interpersonal relations, which are unstable (fluctuating between idealization and devaluation), self-identity problems, labile emotions, low frustration tolerance, empty feelings, etc. (Fernández Aranda, 2006).

As it was said, the biological base of the impulsivity highlights the role of the serotoninergic system, and despite the research on candidate genes, there are no relevant conclusions up to date. The prevalence of this multi-impulsive bulimia nervosa ranges from 16%-80%. Such a wide range is due to severe methodological problems, which make it difficult to obtain a clearer conclusion. It seems that after applying the Fichter's criteria we would obtain 18%-30% of multi-impulsive bulimia nervosa among the bulimic patients (Fernández Aranda, 2006; Fichter, Quadflieg, et al., 1994; Lacey & Evans, 1986). With regards to the personality characteristics of these patients, they show a poorer self-esteem, low level of assertiveness, and high levels of hostility among others less relevant ones. A relevant point with respect to multi-impulsive bulimia nervosa is the fact that these patients show less treatment adherence and, in general, a worse prognostic.

4.1 Summarising

- With regards to the reality of this type of bulimia nervosa as a clinical subgroup, there is no consensus up to the date.
- Besides impulsive behaviours, patients with multi-impulsive bulimia nervosa show interpersonal relationships, which are unstable (fluctuating between idealization and devaluation), self-identity problems, labile emotions, low frustration tolerance, and empty feelings.
- It is accepted that applying the Fichter's criteria we would obtain 18%-30% of multi-impulsive bulimia nervosa among the bulimic patients.
- Patients with multi-impulsive bulimia nervosa usually show less treatment adherence and, in general, a worse prognostic.

5. Bulimia nervosa and substance abuse/dependence

Patients with bulimia nervosa and substance abuse/dependence usually show high levels of psychopathology, impulsivity (expressed by the previously commented different behaviours), more physical problems, more hospitalizations, and poorer treatment adherence and prognostic. The risk for substance abuse/dependence among bulimic patients is much higher when bulimia nervosa is associated with other psychopathological disorders. Depending on the associated disorder that risk may be increased from 2 (depression) to 7 times (bipolar disorder) (Bulik, Sullivan, et al., 1997; Holderness, Brooks-Gunn, et al., 1994).

In general, the rates of substance abuse/dependence are higher among patients with eating disorders and this association is greater among women with bulimia nervosa and anorexia nervosa purging-type, for both alcohol and illicit drug disorders. With respect to the onset of each disorder, it seems that there is a bidirectional association. Some patients report the onset of a substance abuse/dependence to precede the eating disorder and vice versa (Baker, Mitchell, et al., 2010).

Up to date the reason of such a frequent association remains unclear, and different biological and psychological explanations have been proposed. As a result of families and twin studies, it seems that there are shared genetic influences between bulimia nervosa and substance abuse/dependence. With respect to bulimia nervosa and alcohol abuse/dependence distinct genetic factors have been reported. In addition to the diagnostics, some common genetic factors have been described for the covariance between bulimic symptoms and substance abuse/dependence symptoms, and this relationship could be more relevant than the relation between diagnostics is. In fact, the more severe the eating disorder symptoms, the greater the number of substance types used (Baker, Mitchell, et al., 2010).

Recent literature has shown that patients with bulimia nervosa are two to three times more likely to have an alcohol or illicit drug abuse/dependence. In many cases bulimia nervosa manifests before a substance abuse/dependence, binge eating preceding symptoms of substance abuse/dependence. With respect to specific symptoms, the concern about weight and shape in women with a history of binge eating is usually associated with different substance abuse/dependence (increasing risk by 2). It seems that binge eating, purging behaviours, and body image would be associated with alcohol use disorder and that purging behaviours would be associated with illicit drug use disorders. Some results on the association between symptoms of bulimia nervosa and substance abuse/dependence have lead to the hypothesis of bulimia nervosa as an addictive disorder, and it could be that there is a general vulnerability to bulimia nervosa and substances misuse and that additional factors (e.g., personality) determine which behaviours arise. (Bulik, 1987; Holderness, Brooks-Gunn et al., 1994; Kaye, Lilenfeld, et al., 1996).

5.1 Summarising

- Patients with bulimia nervosa and substance abuse/dependence usually show high levels of psychopathology, impulsivity, more physical problems, more hospitalizations, and poorer treatment adherence and prognostic.
- The rates of substance abuse/dependence are higher among patients with eating disorders and this association is greater among women with bulimia nervosa and anorexia nervosa purging-type.
- Up to date the reason of such a frequent association remains unclear, and different biological and psychological explanations have been proposed.
- Some results on the association between symptoms of bulimia nervosa and substance abuse/dependence have lead to the hypothesis of bulimia nervosa as an addictive disorder.

6. Bulimia nervosa and self-harm

Among causes for death, suicide and medical problems related to the nutritional status are the most relevant in bulimia nervosa. It is said that mortality in bulimia nervosa (mean 0.3%) is lower than in anorexia nervosa. Having bulimia nervosa a shorter course than anorexia nervosa, it is difficult to state clear conclusions about mortality because the rates of mortality increase when the periods of follow-up are longer. The suicide, as cause of death in bulimia nervosa, represents the 20% of mortality. Among the patients with bulimia nervosa, almost 30% commit life-long suicide attempts. These patients seem to be different from the rest of patients with bulimia nervosa with respect to their personality and psychopathological symptoms other than the specific eating disorder symptoms (Bulik, Sullivan, et al., 1999; Corcos, Taieb, et al., 2002; Favaro & Santoanastaso, 1996).

The relationship between self-harm behaviours and bulimia nervosa shows that the more frequent the presence of self-harms is the higher is the prevalence of bulimic symptoms. Some studies have found increased rates of self-harm associated with bulimia nervosa, but the same rate of self-harm in bulimia nervosa and in binge eating disorder. That could mean that self-harm may be associated with some common symptoms (e.g. bingeing) more than with a specific diagnostic. Among patients who binge, the presence of self-harm seems to be higher in those who have a history of physical or sexual abuse. In fact, different studies have found higher levels of impulsive behaviour (substance abuse, self-harm) in individuals who have been abused, and a high likelihood of physical or sexual abuse in individuals with eating disorders (Mitchell, Hatsukami, et al., 1988; Schmidt, Hodes et al., 1992; Suzuki, Takeda et al., 1995; Welch & Fairburn, 1996).

The relationships between eating disorders and suicidal behaviour and non-suicidal self-harm have been examined primarily in eating disorder samples. Some studies suggest that suicide attempts and non-suicidal self-harm are found in more than half of bulimic patients (Franko & Keel, 2006; Svirko & Hawton, 2007). These rates appear higher in bulimia nervosa compared to anorexia nervosa, although it seems that there are similar rates of this behaviour in the anorexia nervosa purging-type as in bulimia nervosa (Favaro & Santonastaso, 2000; Nagata, Kawarada et al., 2000). In binge eating disorder, suicidal behaviour appears higher than that in obese non-binge eating disorder controls (Grucza, Przybeck, et al., 2007). Anorectic and bulimic patients with suicidal behaviour or non-suicidal self-harm usually report greater numbers of other disorders such as drug or alcohol abuse/dependence, anxiety disorders and depression (Fedorowicz, Falissard, et al., 2007; Franko, Keel, et al., 2004). Other studies with eating disorder patients have found that anorexia and bulimia are associated with major depression (Berkman, Lohr, et al., 2007), and anorexia nervosa purging-type and bulimia nervosa are frequently associated with alcohol use disorders (Bulik, Klump, et al., 2004).

Empirical studies confirm that there is a strong correlation between self-harm and eating disorders despite there are wide variations in prevalence. In fact, the reported incidence of self-harm in eating disorder patients varies in a range of 13%-68%. A higher incidence of self-harm in bulimia nervosa and anorexia nervosa purging-type than in the anorexia nervosa restrictive type has been reported. Possible common factors are impulsivity, obsessive-compulsive traits, dissociation, trauma, conflict in the family environment and sensitivity to cultural factors, among others. Both self-harm and eating disorders may represent failures in emotion regulation, and both forms of body practices could act as an attempt to a more affective coping (Dohm, Striegel-Moore, et al., 2002; Franko & Keel, 2006; Levitt, Sansone, et al., 2004; Svirko & Hawton, 2007).

6.1 Summarising

- The suicide, as cause of death in bulimia nervosa, represents 20% of mortality. Among the patients with bulimia nervosa, almost 30% commit life-long suicide attempts.
- The more frequent the presence of self-harms is the higher is the prevalence of bulimic symptoms.
- Self-harm may be associated with some common symptoms (e.g. bingeing) more than with a specific diagnostic.
- Different studies have found higher levels of impulsive behaviour (substance abuse, self-harm) in individuals who have been abused, and a high likelihood of physical or sexual abuse in individuals with eating disorders.
- A higher incidence of self-harm in bulimia nervosa and anorexia nervosa purging-type than in the anorexia nervosa restrictive type has been reported.

7. Bulimia nervosa and borderline personality disorder

It seems to have a consensus on the fact that borderline personality disorder (BPD) is the most characteristic in patients with eating disorders, mainly in those with bulimia nervosa with a range of prevalence between 2%-50%. Such a wide range has lead to state that there might be a conceptual confusion between BPD and bulimia nervosa, due to the frequent overlap of their symptoms. With regards to anorexia nervosa, this BPD is more frequent in the purging-type. Different behaviours, which are frequent among bulimic patients (e.g., impulsivity, lack of control, self-harm), also are common in the BPD, this suggesting the possible conceptual confusion between the two disorders.

The presence of BPD in bulimic patients causes a poor prognostic, and this BPD has been mainly related to the presence of purging behaviours (bulimia nervosa and anorexia nervosa purging-type) (Gargallo, Fernández Aranda, et al., 2003).

7.1 Main facts with regards to the association between bulimia nervosa and BPD

a. BPD is the most frequently associated with bulimia nervosa.
b. Patients with bulimia nervosa and BPD show a high level of psychopathology.
c. Patients with bulimia nervosa and BPD have a poor prognostic.
d. Patients with both disorders show a poor treatment adherence.
e. The wide range of co-occurrence between bulimia nervosa and BPD could indicate severe methodological problems, as well as conceptual confusion.
f. In those patients with bulimia nervosa and BPD, the association with other disorders (e.g., depression, substance abuse/dependence) is frequent.
g. Patients with bulimia nervosa and BPD usually refer a history of sexual abuse, self-harm during their adolescence and hostile family environment.

8. Bulimia nervosa and personality disorders. Brief conclusions

- There is a high comorbidity between bulimia nervosa and personality disorders.
- The high variability observed with respect to this comorbidity is usually associated with methodological biases and the used diagnostic criteria, as well as with the biases introduced by the heterogeneity of the analysed samples.
- The presence of a personality disorder in these patients is associated with a higher severity of the disorder, being indicative of a worse prognosis.

- The type of personality disorder most frequently observed in patients diagnosed with bulimia nervosa is the borderline personality disorder.
- Impulsivity is the most consistent distinguishing finding described in bulimia nervosa.
- Patients with bulimia nervosa and personality disorders often have an additional Axis I disorder, the most common being major depression and/or substance abuse/dependence.

9. A model of a new approach: Eating disorders and coping strategies

In initial studies it was considered that the role played by coping strategies in eating behaviours was not clear (Wolff, Crosby, et al., 2000). Later on, it has been indicated that difficulties on emotion control explain better the occurrence of binge eating than eating restriction or weight and corporal image overestimation do (Whiteside, Chen, et al., 2007), so that in a binge disorder explanatory model emotional vulnerability and deficient strategies for the regulation of emotions would be included. Patients with eating disorders are more inclined to avoid affection than to the acceptance and control of emotions (Corstorphine, Mountford, et al., 2007).

Coping strategies have been related to the prognostic of eating disorders and it has been observed that impulsiveness, present in some of its forms, is connected to maladaptive strategies of emotional regulation (Nagata, Matsuyama, et al., 2000).

The specificity of deficient coping strategies found in patients with eating disorders has also been discussed. With respect to bulimia nervosa, it has been observed that the tendency to avoidance, understood as a coping strategy, could be more related to a depressive than to a bulimic symptomatology. However, other strategies such as problem solving or cognitive restructuring do not seem to differ depending on depressive symptoms (Tobin & Griffing, 1995).

The problem to be confronted when it´s time to assess how different coping strategies with a determined symptomatology or personality styles relate to each other lies in the fact that interrelations among different strategies are very frequent. (Folkman & Moskovitz, 2004). The studies which have related coping strategies and personality usually conclude that emotionally stable, extrovert and responsible people tend to solve situations or change the meaning of these situations perceiving their coping as efficient, while unstable and introvert people are used to withdraw from society and usually wish the situation had not occurred, perceiving little efficiency in their coping (Bouchard, 2003; Cano, Rodríguez, et al., 2007; David & Suls, 1999).

Knowledge about coping strategies in patients with eating disorders is relevant and this relevance does not only lie in a theoretical interest or in its relationship with comorbidity or personality characteristics but also in a therapeutic interest. Hence, learning of new and more adaptive forms of coping with problems and emotions is essential in some treatment forms for these pathologies (Foa & Wilson, 1991; Peterson, Wonderlich, et al., 2004).

In a recent study (Jáuregui Lobera, Estébanez, et al., 2009), it was observed that patients with eating disorders showed more self-criticism, social withdrawal, inadequate control centred upon emotions and inadequate control in general. On the contrary, a group of students showed bigger scores at problem solving, social support, cognitive restructuring, adequate control centred upon problems, and adequate control in general. Perceived self-efficacy was greater in the student group too. Regarding personality features in the group of patients, punctuation in introversion was significantly greater, while in the group of students punctuations are greater in the trustful, convincing and impulsive scales. The comparison between two groups of patients (eating disorders and other mental disorders) did not reveal the existence of differences in coping styles except at self-criticism, style in which patients' scores with eating disorders were relevantly greater than those obtained in other mental disorders. Regarding personality styles, punctuations at inhibited and impulsive personalities were greater in the patients with other mental disorders than in the group of eating disorders.

Comparing patients with anorexia and bulimia, patients with anorexia nervosa obtained higher scores at self-criticism, and also at convincing, respectful and sensitive personality. Patients with bulimia nervosa scored more at impulsive personality.

In the same study, a cluster analysis revealed the existence of two groups of patients. One group showed greater self-criticism, wishful thinking, social withdrawal, inadequate control centred upon emotions and inadequate control in general. In this group introversion, inhibition, sensitivity and impulsivity prevailed. In this group, 53.1% of the patients suffered from bulimia and 69% suffered from anorexia. In the other group, scores were higher in problem solving, social support, perceived self-efficacy, adequate control centred upon problems and adequate control in general. In this group scores at sociable, trustful, convincing and respectful personality were higher. In this group, 46.5% of the patients suffered from bulimia and 31% suffered from anorexia.

With respect to personality features, this study confirmed what has been highlighted by other authors (Cano, Rodríguez, et al., 2007) in the sense that stability-extroversion is associated to more adequate coping strategies, while unstable-introvert people present greater inadequacy. However, studies on personality and eating disorders have proven controversial because they have serious methodological deficiencies (Echeburúa & Marañón, 2001). For the future, coping strategies studies could be proposed as something more operative than the idea of associating eating disorders to this or that personality style and making prognostic inferences on the basis of it. In fact, the result of the cluster analysis executed, using the dispositional (personality) as well as the contextual (coping strategies) ratify such findings as those of other authors (Strober, Salkin, et al., 1982; Westen & Harnden-Fischer, 2001) in the sense that there is presence of subgroups of patients with eating disorders with worse coping strategies and prevailing of introversion-instability.

10. Main conclusions of the chapter

- Research has often found bulimic patients to be extroverted, histrionic, and affectively unstable. It is possible that both, anorexia nervosa and bulimia nervosa may be linked to personality factors heterogeneously. So that, more than one type of personality could cause or contribute to the symptoms of the eating disorders.
- Despite the fact that the dimension impulsivity-compulsivity seems to be a useful tool to represent the two main eating disorders, it is difficult to explain the concurrence of bulimia nervosa and obsessiveness, or how an eating disorder as anorexia nervosa becomes another one as bulimia nervosa.
- Up to now, the multi-impulsive bulimia is not accepted as a different type of bulimia nervosa despite many authors state its undoubted clinical presence.
- Some results on the association between symptoms of bulimia nervosa and substance abuse/dependence have lead to the hypothesis of bulimia nervosa as an addictive disorder.

- A higher incidence of self-harm in bulimia nervosa and anorexia nervosa purging-type than in the anorexia nervosa restrictive type has been reported.
- The presence of borderline personality disorder in bulimic patients causes a poor prognostic, and this BPD has been mainly related to the presence of purging behaviours (bulimia nervosa and anorexia nervosa purging-type).
- For the future, coping strategies studies could be proposed as something more operative than the idea of associating eating disorders to this or that personality style and making prognostic inferences on the basis of it.

11. References

Abbot, DW.; Wonderlich, SA. & Mitchell JE (2001). Treatment implications of comorbid personality disorders. In: *The outpatient treatment of eating disorders: A guide for therapists, dietitians and physicians*, JE Mitchell (Ed), pp. 173-186. University of Minnesota Press, ISBN 978-0816637188, Minneapolis.

Baker, JH.; Mitchell, KS.; Neale, MC. & Kendler, KS. (2010). Eating disorder symptomatology and substance use disorders: prevalence and shared risk in a population based twin sample. *International Journal of Eating Disorders*, Vol 43., pp. 648–658, ISSN 0276-3478.

Berkman, ND.; Lohr, KN. & Bulik, CM. (2007). Outcomes of eating disorders: a systematic review of the literature. *International Journal of Eating Disorders*, Vol 40., pp. 293-309, ISSN 0276-3478.

Bouchard, G. (2003). Cognitive appraisals, neuroticism, and openness as correlates of coping strategies: An integrative model of adaptation to marital difficulties. *Canadian Journal of Behavioral Sciences*, Vol 35., pp. 1–12. ISSN 0008-400X.

Braun, DL.; Sunday, SR. & Halmi, KA. (1994). Psychiatric comorbidity in patients with eating disorders. *Psychological Medicine*, Vol 24., pp. 859-867. ISSN 0033-2917.

Bulik, C.; Sullivan, P.; Joyce, P. & Carter, F. (1995). Temperament character, and, personality disorder in bulimia nervosa. *The Journal of Nervous and Mental Disease*, Vol 183., pp. 593-598, ISSN 0022-3018.

Bulik, CM. (1987). Drug and alcohol abuse by bulimic females and their families. *American Journal of Psychiatry*, Vol 144., pp. 1604–1606, ISSN 0002-953X.

Bulik, CM.; Klump, KL.; Thornton, L.; Kaplan, AS.; Devlin, B.; Fichter, MM.; Halmi, KA.; Strober, M.; Woodside, DB.; Crow, S.; Mitchell, JE.; Rotondo, A.; Mauri, M.; Cassano, GB.; Keel, PK.; Berrettini, WH. & Kaye, WH. (2004). Alcohol use disorder comorbidity in eating disorders: a multicenter study. *Journal of Clinical Psychiatry*, Vol 65., pp. 1000–1007. ISSN 0160-6689.

Bulik, CM.; Sullivan, PF. & Joyce, PR. (1999). Temperament, character and suicide attempts in anorexia nervosa, bulimia nervosa and major depression. *Acta Psychiatrica Scandinavica*, Vol 100., pp. 27-32. ISSN 0001-690X.

Bulik, CM.; Sullivan, PF.; Fear, J. & Pickering, A. (1997). Predictors of the development of bulimia nervosa in women with anorexia nervosa. *The Journal of Nervous and Mental Disease*, Vol 185., pp. 704-707, ISSN 0022-3018.

Bussolotti, D.; Fernández-Aranda, F.; Solano, R.; Jiménez-Murcia, S.; Turón, V. & Vallejo, J. (2002). Marital status and eating disorders: an analysis of its relevance. *Journal of Psychosomatic Research*, Vol 53., pp. 1139-1145. ISSN 0022-3999.

Cano García, FJ.; Rodríguez Franco, L. & García Martínez, J. (2007). Spanish version of the Coping Strategies Inventory. *Actas Españolas de Psiquiatría*, Vol 35., pp. 29–39. ISSN 1139-9287.

Casper, R. (1990) Personality features of women with good outcome from restricting anorexia nervosa. *Psychosomatic Medicine*, Vol 52., pp. 156–170. ISSN 0033-3174.

Clinton, DN. & Glant, R. (1992). The eating disorders spectrum of DSM-III-R. Clinical features and psychosocial concomitants of 86 consecutive cases from a Swedish urban catchment area *The Journal of Nervous and Mental Disease*, Vol 180., pp. 244-50, ISSN 0022-3018.

Cook Myers, T.; Wonderlich, SA.; Crosby, R.; Mitchell, JE.; Steffen, KJ.; Smyth, J. & Miltenberger, R. (2006). Is multi-impulsive bulimia a distinct type of bulimia nervosa: Psychopathology and EMA findings. *International Journal of Eating Disorders*, Vol 39., pp. 655-661, ISSN 0276-3478.

Corcos, M.; Taïeb, O.; Benoit-Lamy, S.; Paterniti, S.; Jeammet, P. & Flament, MF. (2002). Suicide attempts in women with bulimia nervosa: frequency and characteristics. *Acta Psychiatrica Scandinavica*, Vol 106., pp. 381-386. ISSN 0001-690X.

Corstorphine, E.; Mountford, V.; Tomlinson, S.; Waller, G. & Meyer, C. (2007). Distress tolerance in the eating disorders. *Eating Behaviors*, Vol 8., pp. 91-97. ISSN 471-0153.

David, JP. & Suls, J. (1999). Coping efforts in daily life: role of big five traits and problem appraisals. *Journal of Personality*, Vol 67., pp. 265-94. ISSN 1467-6494.

Diaz Marsá, M. (1999). Psicobiología de los trastornos alimentarios. *Aula Médica Psiquiatría*, Vol 1., pp. 219-238.

Díaz, M.; Carrasco, JL.; Prieto, R. & Saiz, J. (1999). El papel de la personalidad en los trastornos de la conducta alimentaria. *Actas Españolas de Psiquiatría*, Vol 27., pp. 43-50. ISSN 1139-9287.

Dohm, FA.; Striegel-Moore, RH.; Wilfley, DE.; Pike, KM.; Hook, J. & Fairburn, CG. (2002). Self-harm and substance use in a community sample of Black and White women with binge eating disorder or bulimia nervosa. *International Journal of Eating Disorders*, Vol 32., pp. 389-400, ISSN 0276-3478.

Dolan, B.; Evans, C. & Norton, K. (1994). Disordered eating behaviour and attitudes in Female and Male Patients with Personality Disorders. *Journal of Personality Disorders*, Vol 8., pp. 17-27. ISSN 0021-843X.

Echeburúa, E. & Corral, P. (1999). Avances en el tratamiento, cognitivo-conductual de los trastornos de personalidad. *Análisis y Modificación de Conducta*, Vol 25., pp. 585-614, ISSN 211-7339.

Echeburúa, E. & Marañón, I. (2001). Comorbilidad de las alteraciones de la conducta alimentaria con los trastornos de personalidad. *Psicología Conductual*, Vol 9., pp. 513-525. ISSN 1132-9483.

Fahy, T. & Eisler, I. (1993). Impulsivity and eating disorders. *British Journal of Psychiatry*, Vol 162., pp. 193-197.

Favaro, A. & Santonastaso, P. (1996). Purging behaviors, suicide attempts, and psychiatric symptoms in 398 eating disordered subjects. *International Journal of Eating Disorders*, Vol 20., pp. 99-103, ISSN 0276-3478.

Favaro, A. & Santonastaso, P. (2000). Self-injurious behavior in anorexia nervosa. *The Journal of Nervous and Mental Disease*, Vol 188., pp. 537-542, ISSN 0022-3018.

Fedorowicz, VJ.; Falissard, B.; Foulon, C.; Dardennes, R.; Divac, SM.; Guelfi, JD. & Rouillon, F. (2007). Factors associated with suicidal behaviors in a large French sample of inpatients with eating disorders. *International Journal of Eating Disorders*, Vol 40., pp. 589–595, ISSN 0276-3478.

Fernández Aranda F. (2006). Poblaciones especiales: bulimia multi-impulsiva. In: *Bulimia nerviosa. Perspectivas clínicas actuales*, FJ. Vaz (Coord), pp. 241-247. Ergon, ISBN 978-84-8473-416-1, Madrid.

Fichter, MM.; Quadflieg, N. & Rief, W. (1994). Course of multi-impulsive bulimia. *Psychological Medicine*, Vol 24., pp. 591–604. ISSN 0033-2917.

Foa, E. & Wilson, R. (1991). *Stop obsessing: How to overcome your obsessions and compulsions*. Bantam Books, ISBN 978-0553381177, New York.

Folkman, S. & Moskowitz, JT. (2004). Coping: Pitfalls and promise. *Annual Review of Psychology*, Vol 55., pp. 745-774. ISSN 0066-4308.

Franko, DL. & Keel, PK. (2006). Suicidality in eating disorders: Occurrence, correlates, and clinical implications. *Clinical Psychology Review*, Vol 26., pp. 769–782. ISSN 0272-7358.

Franko, DL.; Keel, PK.; Dorer, DJ.; Blais, MA.; Delinsky, SS.; Eddy, KT.; Charat, V.; Renn, R. & Herzog, DB. (2004). What predicts suicide attempts in women with eating disorders? *Psychological Medicine*, Vol 34., pp. 843-853. ISSN 0033-2917.

Gargallo, M.; Fernández Aranda, F. & Raich, RM. (2003) Bulimia nerviosa y trastornos de la personalidad. Una revisión teórica de la literatura. *International Journal of Clinical and Health Psychology*, Vol 3., pp. 335-349. ISSN 1697-2600.

Gartner, AF.; Marcus, RN.; Halmi, K. & Loranger, AW. (1989). DSM-III-R Personality Disorders in Patients with Eating Disorders. *American Journal of Psychiatry*, Vol 146., pp. 1585-1591, ISSN 0002-953X.

Grucza, RA.; Przybeck, TR. & Cloninger, CR. (2007). Prevalence and correlates of binge eating disorder in a community sample. *Comprehensive Psychiatry*, Vol 48., pp. 124–131. ISSN 0010-440X.

Herzog DB.; Keller, MB.; Sacks, NR.; Yeh, CJ. & Lavori, PW. (1992). Psychiatric morbidity in treatment seeking anorexics and bulimics. *Journal of the American Academy of Child and Adolescent Psychiatry*, Vol 31., pp. 810-818. ISSN 021-9630.

Herzog, DB.; Keller, MB.; Lavori, PW.; Kenny, GM. & Sacks, NR. (1992). The Prevalence of Personality Disorders in 210 women with Eating Disorders. *Journal of Clinical Psychiatry*, Vol 53., pp. 147-152. ISSN 0160-6689.

Holderness, CC.; Brooks-Gunn, J. & Warren, MP. (1994). Co-morbidity of eating disorders and substance abuse review of the literature. *Interantional Journal of Eating Disorders*, Vol 16., pp. 1–34, ISSN 0276-3478.

Jáuregui Lobera, I.; Estébanez, S.; Santiago Fernández, MJ.; Alvarez Bautista, E. & Garrido, O. (2009). Coping strategies in eating disorders. *European Eating Disorders Review*, Vol 17., pp. 220-226. ISSN 1072-4133.

Jáuregui Lobera, I.; Santiago Fernández, MJ. & Estébanez Humanes, S. (2009). Eating behaviour disorders and personality. A study using MCMI-II. *Atención Primaria*, Vol 41., pp. 201-206. ISSN 0212-6567.

Johnson, C.; Tobin, D. & Enright, A. (1989). Prevalence and clinical characteristics of borderline patients in an eating-disordered population. *Journal of Clinical Psychiatry*, Vol 50., pp. 9-15. ISSN 0160-6689.

Kaye, WH.; Lilenfeld, LR.; Plotnicov, K.; Merikangas, KR.; Nagy, L.; Strober M, Bulik CM.; Moss, H. & Greeno, CG. (1996). Bulimia nervosa and substance dependence: Association and family transmission. *Alcoholism: Clinical and Experimental Research,* Vol 20., pp. 878–881. ISSN 0145-6008.

Kennedy, SH.; McVey, G. & Kata, R. (1990). Personality Disorders in Anorexia Nervosa and Bulimia Nervosa. *Journal of Psychiatry Research,* Vol 24., pp. 259-269. ISSN 0022-3956.

Lacey, JH. & Evans, CDH. (1986). The impulsivist: a multi-impulsive personality disorder. *British Journal of Addiction,* Vol 81., pp. 641–649. ISSN 0952-0481.

Levitt, JL.; Sansone, RA. & Cohn, L. (2004). *Self-harm behavior and eating disorders.* Brunner-Routledge, ISBN 9780415946988, New York.

Loranger, AW. (1995). *International Personality Disorder Examination (IPDE).* Organización Mundial de la Salud, ISBN 978-0880489171, Ginebra:

Marino, MF. & Zanarini, MC. (2001). Relationship between EDNOS and its subtypes and Borderline Personality Disorder. *International Journal of Eating Disorders,* Vol 29., pp. 349-353, ISSN 0276-3478.

Matsunaga, H.; Kiriike, N.; Nagata, T. & Yamagami, S. (1998). Personality disorders in patients with eating disorders in Japan. *International Journal of Eating Disorders,* Vol 23., pp. 399-408., ISSN 0276-3478.

Medina, A. & Moreno, MJ. (1998). *Los trastornos de la personalidad. Un estudio médico-filosófico.* Nanuk, ISBN 978-84-923902-0-5, Córdoba.

Millon, T. & Ávila, A. (1998). *Inventario clínico multiaxial de Millon-II: manual.* TEA Ediciones, ISBN 84-7174-491-0, Madrid.

Mitchell, JE.; Hatsukami, D.; Pyle, R. % Eckert, E. (1988). Bulimia with and without a family history of drug abuse. *Addictive Behaviors,* Vol 13., pp. 245-51. ISSN 0306-4603.

Nagata, T.; Kawarada, Y.; Kiriike, N. & Iketani, T. (2000). Multi-impulsivity of Japanese patients with eating disorders: primary and secondary impulsivity. *Psychiatry Research,* Vol 94., pp. 239–250. ISSN 0165-1781.

Nagata, T.; Matsuyama, M.; Kiriike, N.; Iketani, T. & Oshima, J. (2000). Stress coping strategy in Japanese patients with eating disorders: relationship with bulimic and impulsive behaviors. *The Journal of Nervous and Mental Disease,* Vol 188., pp. 280-286, ISSN 0022-3018.

Newton, JR.; Freeman, CP. & Munro, J. (1993). Impulsivity and dyscontrol in bulimia nervosa: is impulsivity an independent phenomenon or a marker of severity? *Acta Psychiatrica Scandinavica,* Vol 87., pp. 389-394. ISSN 0001-690X.

Peñas Lledó, EM. (2006). Impulsividad y bulimia nerviosa. In: Bulimia nerviosa. Perspectivas clínicas actuals, FJ. Vaz (Coord), pp. 63-69. Ergon, ISBN 978-84-8473-416-1, Madrid.

Peñas-Lledó, E. & Waller, G. (2001). Bulimic psychopathology and impulsive behaviors among nonclinical women. *International Journal of Eating Disorders,* Vol 29., pp. 71-75, ISSN 0276-3478.

Peterson, CB.; Wonderlich, SA.; Mitchell, JE. & Crow, SJ. (2004). Integrative cognitive therapy for bulimia nervosa. In: Handbook of eating disorders and obesity, JK. Thompson (Ed.), pp. 245–262. John Wiley & Sons, ISBN 78-0-471-23073-1, Hoboken, New Jersey.

Ponce de León, C. (2006). Bulimia nerviosa y personalidad. In: *Bulimia nerviosa. Perspectivas clínicas actuales,* FJ. Vaz (Coord), pp. 49-56. Ergon, ISBN 978-84-8473-416-1, Madrid.

Rossiter, EM.; Agras, WS.; Telch, CF. & Schneider JA. (1993). Cluster B personality disorder characteristics predict outcome in the treatment of bulimia nervosa. *International Journal of Eating Disorders,* Vol 13., pp. 349-357, ISSN 0276-3478.

Sarason, IG. & Sarason, BR. (1996). *Psicología anormal.* Prentice-Hall, ISBN 968-880-538-6, México.

Schmidt, U.; Hodes, M. & Treasure, J. (1992). Early onset bulimia nervosa: who is at risk? A retrospective case-control study. *Psychological Medicine,* Vol 22., pp 623-628. ISSN 0033-2917.

Skodol, AE.; Oldham, JM.; Hyler, SE.; Kellman, HD.; Doidge, N. & Dacies, M. (1993). Comorbidity of DSM-III-R Eating Disorders and Personality Disorders. *International Journal of Eating Disorders,* Vol 14., pp. 403-416, ISSN 0276-3478.

Sohlberg, S. & Strober, M. (1994). Personality in anorexia nervosa: an update and a theoretical integration. *Acta Psychiatrica Scandinavica,* Vol 89., pp. 1–15. ISSN 0001-690X.

Spitzer, RL.; Williams, JB.; Gibbon, M. & First, MB. (1992). *The Structured Clinical Interview for DSM-III-R (SCID).* Archives of General Psychiatry, Vol 49., pp. 624-629, ISSN 0003-990X.

Steiger, H. & Stotland, S. (1996). Prospective study of outcome in bulimics as a function of Axis-II comorbidity: Long-term responses on eating and Psychiatric symptoms. *International Journal of Eating Disorders,* Vol 20., pp. 149-161, ISSN 0276-3478.

Steiger, H. & Stotland, S. (1996). Prospective study of outcome in bulimics as a function of Axis-II comorbidity: Long-term responses on eating and Psychiatric symptoms. *International Journal of Eating Disorders,* Vol 20., pp. 149-161, ISSN 0276-3478.

Steiger, H.; Leung, F.; Thibaudeau, J. & Houle, L. (1993). Prognostic utility subcomponents of the borderline personality construct in bulimia nervosa. *British Journal of Clinical Psychology,* Vol 32., pp. 187-197. ISSN 0144-6657.

Steiger, H.; Liquornik, K.; Chapman, J. & Hussain N. (1991). Personality and family disturbances in eating-disorder patients: comparison of "restricters" and "bingers" to normal controls. *International Journal of Eating Disorders,* Vol 10., pp. 501–512, ISSN 0276-3478.

Steiger, H.; Young, SN.; Ng Ying Kin, NMK.; Koerner, N.; Israel, M.; Lageix, P. & Paris, J. (2001). Implications of impulsive and affective symptoms for serotonin function in bulimia nervosa. *Psychological Medicine,* Vol 31., pp. 85-95. ISSN 0033-2917.

Strober, M.; Salkin, B.; Burroughs, J. & Morrell, W. (1982). Validity of the bulimia-restricter distinction in anorexia nervosa. Parental personality characteristics and family psychiatric morbidity. *The Journal of Nervous and Mental Disease,* Vol 170., pp. 345-51, ISSN 0022-3018.

Suzuki, K.; Takeda, A. & Matsushita, S. (1995). Coprevalence of bulimia with alcohol abuse and smoking among Japanese male and female high school students. *Addiction,* Vol 90., pp. 971-975. ISSN 1360-0443.

Svirko, E. & Hawton, K. (2007). Self-injurious behavior and eating disorders: The extent and nature of the association. *Suicide and Life-Threatening Behavior,* Vol 37., pp. 409–421. ISSN 0363-0234.

Tobin, DL. & Griffing, AS. (1995). Coping and depression in bulimia nervosa. *International Journal of Eating Disorders*, Vol 18., pp. 359-363, ISSN 0276-3478.

Vázquez, C.; Ring, J. & Avia, MD. (1990). Trastornos de la personalidad. In: *Psicología Médica, Psicopatología y Psiquiatría*, F. Fuentenebro & C. Vázquez (Dirs.), Interamericana-McGraw Hill, ISBN 978-84-7615-586-8, Madrid.

Vitousek, K. & Manke, F. (1994). Personality variables and disorders in anorexia nervosa and bulimia nervosa. *Journal of Abnormal Psychology*, Vol 103., pp. 137–147

von Ranson, KM.; Kaye, WH.; Weltzin, TE.; Rao, R. & Matsunaga, H. (1999). Obsessive-compulsive disorder symptoms before and after recovery from bulimia nervosa. *American Journal of Psychiatry*, Vol 156., pp. 1703-1708, ISSN 0002-953X.

Welch, SL. & Fairburn, CG. (1996). Impulsivity or comorbidity in bulimia nervosa: A controlled study of deliberate self-harm and alcohol and drug misuse in a community sample. *British Journal of Psychiatry*, Vol 169., pp. 451–458. ISSN 0007-1250.

Westen, D. (1997). Divergences between clinical and research methods for assessing personality disorders: implications for research and the evolution of axis II. *American Journal of Psychiatry*, Vol 154., pp. 895–903. ISSN 0002-953X.

Westen, D. & Harnden-Fischer, J. (2001). Personality profiles in eating disorders: Rethinking the distinction between axis I and axis II. *American Journal of Psychiatry*, Vol 158., pp. 547–562. ISSN 0002-953X.

Westen, D. & Shedler, J. (1999_a). Revising and assessing axis II, part I: developing a clinically and empirically valid assessment method. *American Journal of Psychiatry*, Vol 156., pp. 258–272. ISSN 0002-953X.

Westen, D. & Shedler, J. (1999_b). Revising and assessing axis II, part II: toward an empirically based and clinically useful classification of personality disorders. *American Journal of Psychiatry*, Vol 156., pp. 273–285. ISSN 0002-953X.

Westen, D. & Westen, LA. (1998). Limitations of axis II in diagnosing personality pathology in clinical practice. *American Journal of Psychiatry*, Vol 155., pp. 1767–1771. ISSN 0002-953X.

Whiteside, U.; Chen, E.; Neighbors, C.; Hunter, D.; Lo, T. & Larimer, M. (2007). Difficulties regulating emotions: Do binge eaters have fewer strategies to modulate and tolerate negative affect? *Eating Behaviors*, Vol 8., pp. 162-169. ISSN 471-0153.

Wolff, GE.; Crosby, RD.; Roberts, JA. & Wittrock, DA. (2000). Differences in daily stress, mood, coping, and eating behavior in binge eating and nonbinge eating college women. *Addictive Behaviors*, Vol 25., pp. 205-16. ISSN 0306-4603.

Wonderlich, SA & Mitchell, JE. (2001). The role of personality in the onset of eating disorders and treatment implications. *Psychiatric Clinics of North America*, Vol 24., pp. 249-258. ISSN 0193953X.

Wonderlich, SA. & Swift, WJ. (1990). Borderline versus other Personality Disorders in the Eating Disorders: Clinical Description. *International Journal of Eating Disorders*, Vol 9., pp. 629- 638, ISSN 0276-3478.

10

A Psychological Profile of the Body Self Characteristics in Women Suffering from Bulimia Nervosa

Bernadetta Izydorczyk
Department of Clinical and Forensic Psychology, University of Silesia in Katowice, Poland

1. Introduction

Bulimia nervosa appears to be a significant medical condition and a serious social problem since it requires long term and multi-dimensional treatment, and its incidence rates among young generation (predominantly women), has incresed significantly in recent years. The results of scientific research described in psychological and psychiatric literature point to a variety of factors that contribute to development of this eating disorder [Fairburn, Harrison, Lacey, Evans, Thompson, Cash, Pruzinsky, Garner, Józefik, Głębocka, Rabe Jabłońska, Dunajska, Mikołajczyk, Samochowiec, Schier]. The most significant underlying factors include: biological disturbance of hunger and satiety sensing, familial factors (early childhood emotional deficits and traumatic experiences), socio-cultural factors (body image disturbances which develop as a consequence of the "terror" of a slim body, which is being promoted as the only way to success in life), as well as some individual factors such as impulse regulation disturbances, impulsivity, low frustration tolerance, neuroticism, perfectionism, obsessive-compulsive, borderline or histrionic personality disorders [Lacey, Mikołajczyk, Samochowiec]. Lacey and Evan, who defined the concept of Multi Impulsive Personality Disorder, included bulimia nervosa among its major symptoms [Lacey].

In the light of the recent psychological literature, cognitive and emotional body image disturbances are regarded as significant factors behind development of anorexia and bulimia nervosa [Thompson, Cash, Głębocka, Kulbat, Rabe Jabłońska, Schier]. However, far less scientific research is devoted to body image and the body self distortions in individuals suffering from bulimia nervosa [Rabe-Jabłońska, Dunajska]. The recently observed higher incidence of bulimia nervosa (especially among women), compared to anorexia nervosa, seems to point to a multitude of factors that determine development of this disorder. It also indicates the spread of the cultural cult of "ideal and perfect" body image, and the tendency to conform to social norms regarding physical appearance ("what I should look like") and to disapprove of one's current body shape, which is being promoted as a key to success in life. Thus it can be stated that adequate medical care as well as the quality of family, professional and social roles performed in life significantly support a psychological diagnosis of the body self structure, and determine effective therapy for bulimia nervosa.

It is a psychological diagnosis of body experiences and body image in anorexia and bulimia nervosa that I have focused on in my many years of scientific research and therapeutic work with bulimic and anorectic patients [Izydorczyk, Bieńkowska, Klimczyk].

In an attempt to provide a psychological profile of the body self characteristics, I have referred to cognitive [Fairburn, Thompson, Cash, Pruzinsky, Głebocka, Kulbat, Rabe-Jabłońska, Dunajska, Izydorczyk] as well as psychoanalytic concepts [Schier, Krueger, Lowen, Pervin, Tyson]. I have operationalized the body self variable and conducted statistical and clinical analysis of the research data using psychometric methods and a projective technique. I adopt terminology which is used in the field of cognitive psychology (e.g. body schema, body image, body self-evaluation, the actual self, the ideal self) and psychoanalysis (e.g. the body self, interoceptive awareness, acceptance of psychosexual development, maturity fear).

2. The body self – a definition and specification of the body self dysfunctions in bulimia nervosa, based on selected elements of the psychoanalytic theory

In psychology, a variety of terms are used to refer to the phenomenon of experiencing one's own self. They include such notions as the ego, the self, a sense of self, a sense of personal identity, self-awareness, self-knowledge, self-representation, and others. According to the definitions provided in psychological literature, it is possible to distinguish the following domains of the structure of the self: the self-as-agent vs. the self-as-subject, the real self vs. the ideal self, and the body self vs. the mental self. All of them constitute the major components of the so called psychological Self [Pervin].

The correlation between the body self and the individual's mental development has been clearly demonstrated and described in the psychoanalytic and cognitive theories regarding human functioning [Fairburn, Lacey, Thompson, Cash, Pruzinsky, Garner, Józefik, Głebocka, Kulbat, Rabe-Jabłońska, Mikołajczyk, Samochowiec, Schier, Brytek, Pervin, Tyson, Sugarman].

A review of psychoanalytic literature reveals that body image has a considerable impact on the development of an individual's personality. The ego, as conceived by Freud, denotes mainly the "body ego" [Krueger, Tyson, Schier]. Taking into consideration the psychoanalytic approach, an eating disorder is regarded as a pathology that occurs as a result of unsatisfied drives and desires, or as pathological development of the self and a sense of personal identity.

According to the fundamental assumptions of the object relations theory, the early childhood experiences significantly affect the separation-individuation process as well as the development of the self-as-subject and interpersonal relationships [Pervin].

As mentioned in Polish literature, the research results obtained in a group of bulimic females, using the Eating Disorder Inventory (EDI), prove that the women do not accept their psychosexual development, and exhibit incresed maturity fear as well as a tendency towards regression into childhood, which is a form of retreat, going back to a time when they felt safer than in adult life [Józefik]. Moreover, the findings reveal a low level of interoceptive awareness regarding body stimuli among the examined women. The level of difficulties related to psychosocial functioning turned out to be higher in this group, compared with the data received in the population of anorectic females [Józefik].

The findings of Sugarman's research on body image distortions in bulimia nervosa prove that the disturbances have their roots in the failure to carry out the process of separation of the object from the mother during the early practicing sub-phase of the separation-individuation process [Sugarman]. The author points out that women who suffer from bulimia nervosa find it difficult to differentiate and integrate the body self. Hence, they experience a number of neurotic conflicts and developmental deficits [Sugarman]. The

clinical analysis conducted by Sugarman demonstrates that bulimic females tend to encounter problems in relationships with their mothers. The daughter's ambivalent identification with the mother and her body and femininity, determines the development of pathological behaviours that affect the body such as uncontrolled binge eating and purging.
Sands, who represents the object relations perspective on the concept of the self, refers to Kohut's view and argues that bulimia nervosa "compensates" the deficits in the self-object functions that are initially provided by the mother [Sands]. She claims that a bulimic individual identifies him/herself by his or her symptoms with the false, perfectionist self, created under the influence of the person's narcissistic care-givers. Thus food becomes a substitute for the self-object. It is the bridge between the self and the self-object, and the significant transitional object whose role is to regulate the bulimic individual's affective states. The bulimic self (that is the body self) is expressed through body language and represents the primitive need for dependence and separation. Binge eating symbolically compensates for the need for care and dependence, and self-induced vomiting symbolizes the need for self-identity and for separation from the object [Sands].
Excessive preoccupation with body appearance, which is a natural consequence of developmental changes that occur during adolescence and emerging adulthood, may lead to body-size dissatisfaction among women with low self-esteem, who have experienced some developmental deficits. This in turn triggers the development of eating disorders such as bulimia nervosa.
According to the psychoanalytic approach, body experiences correlate with the development of an individual's sense of identity. Lowen clings to the opinion that "in fact, a person has a double identity - one of them stems from identification with the ego, the other is related to identification with the body and the feeling regarding it" [Lowen]. Meissner established the basic terminology regarding the body and its image. He defined the body as an actual physical organism. He used the term "the body self' to refer to a psychic structure that forms an integral component of the person's self system. Body image is, according to Meissner's definition, a system of images organized into representations of the body [Krueger]. When dealing with the issue of body experience, Bielefeld distinguished between the body schema and body image [Schier]. The body schema comprises the following components: body orientation which refers to the orientation towards the internal structure of the body as well as its surface; body size estimation (i.e. estimation of the volume, mass, length, and surface area of the *body);* body knowledge (i.e. the knowledge of the body structure and body parts) [Schier]. Body image, as described by Bielefeld, comprises such components as body consciousness which refers to a psychic representation of the body or its specified part perceived at a conscious level; body boundaries (i.e. a sense of separation between the body and the external world); body attitude, that is a person's attitude towards his or her body, measured in terms of positive or negative body perception (body image satisfaction and dissatisfaction) [Schier].
Krueger defines the notion of body image, at its early stage of development, as a system of primary bodily sensations. He shares Mahler's view that a sense of touch is the factor behind the emergence of a primitive sense of self. Tactile sensations facilitate the development of the primitive "skin ego" which forms the foundation of a sense of body self [Krueger]. A sense of body boundaries allows to differentiate self from non-self. Empathic resonance between the mother and the child stimulates the process of internalization of reciprocity and affirmation, and consequently determines the development of self-efficacy [Krueger, Schier]. The body boundaries form the foundation for psychological boundaries.

The body appears to be a "container" for the psychological self which integrates internal and external experiences, thereby stimulating the emergence of a coherent identity [Krueger].

Bulimic episodes of uncontrolled binge eating and destructive compensatory behaviours (e.g. self-induced vomiting, fasting, abuse of laxatives, diuretics or slimming pills, etc.) allow a bulimia sufferer to maintain his or her positive self-portrait and self-assessment which in turn are affected by the person's body experiences as well as the cognitive evaluation of his/her own physical appearance. Engaging in compulsive, self-destructive behaviours, a bulimic individual applies a variety of specific symbols related to the person's sensomotoric experiences, which is aimed at bridging the body and mind [Krueger]. Bulimic symptoms appear to represent the individual's attempt to satisfy his or her needs and compensate for developmental emotional deficits by resorting to substances (e.g. food, alcohol or drugs) or to certain activities (e.g. self-induced vomiting, purging, compulsive spending, impulsive sex, etc.). This can also be regarded as a form of escape from "painful" emotions [Krueger].

3. A cognitive perspective on body image disturbances in bulimia nervosa

The most common terms that cognitive theories refer to in their attempts to define body perception include such notions as: self-image, body image, self-knowledge and self-assessment. Body image is frequently defined as a cognitive self-schema construct, that is, a system of conscious generalizations regarding the body [Pervin]. According to cognitive psychologists, body image is one of the fundamental components of the body self. It is commonly referred to as sensual image of sizes, shapes and forms of the body as well as feelings regarding the mentioned features of the whole body or one of its specified parts [Thompson, Cash, Pruzinsky]. Thompson and his co-researchers made an attempt at systematizing the notions related to body image [Thompson, Cash, Pruzinsky]. Defining the feelings regarding the body, they identified the following aspects: weight satisfaction which can be measured in terms of a discrepancy between the actual (current) and the ideal (most desired) weight; body satisfaction which most frequently refers to the specified body parts (e.g. breast, thighs or hips); appearance satisfaction, that is, satisfaction with general appearance or its specified elements such as certain parts of the face, or the body parts that carry connotations of weight (e.g. the lower part of the body). Thompson and his co-researchers identified the phenomenon of inadequate body mass perception, and linked it to the concept of appearance orientation measured in terms of a degree of cognitive and behavioral involvement in physical appearance. Appearance anxiety seems to reflect the feelings of dissatisfaction and discomfort which occur as a result of excessive focus on body image [Thompson].

Garner and Garfinkel distinguished the following two forms of body image disturbances: inadequate body percept and body dissatisfaction [Rabe-Jabłońska,Dunajska]. In their studies the psychologists put forward the view that the former refers to inadequate perception of the body size; whereas the latter is related to an emotional attitude towards the body [Rabe-Jabłońska, Dunajska].

Developed by E.T. Higgins, Self-Discrepancy Theory provides a platform for understanding the development of body image. Higgins's theory posits that the structure of the body self determines an individual's self-perception and self-evaluation of his or her own body features (the actual self), as well as the person's thoughts and aspirations regarding the ideal body image (the ideal self), and the mental evaluation of the body features and characteristics which the person believes she or he should display (the ought self) [Higgins]. According to Higgins's theory, an individual aims at minimizing the actual-ideal or actual-ought self discrepancies.

Thompson refers to Higgins's theory of self-discrepancy in order to provide an explanation for body image disturbances. He claims that the constant comparison of an individual's actual body shape and the ideal body image has a negative effect on the development of a cognitive aspect of body image. The ideal-actual body image discrepancy underlies the state of body dissatisfaction, and determines development of an eating disorder [Cash, Pruzinsky, Thompson, Garner].

A cognitive model of eating disorders, developed by Fairburn, Cooper and Safran, points to a variety of interlinked factors which determine development of bulimia nervosa. The theory demonstrates that such factors as social pressure, dietary restriction, the feelings of hunger and inability to control it, trigger the onset of bulimia nervosa. Body image is considered to perform a significant regulatory role [Cash, Pruzinsky, Thompson].

A bulimic individual conducts subjective evaluation of his or her body attributes, which affects the person's cognitive functioning. A bulimia sufferer tends to be excessively concerned about body weight, shape and general physical appearance. This in turn leads to low self-esteem. The compensatory behaviours that a bulimic individual engages in (i.e. the bulimic symptoms) are aimed at improving hi or her self-assessment and reducing the consequent emotional tension and frustrations [Cash, Pruzinsky, Thompson].

4. A psychological profile of the body self characteristics in Polish women suffering from bulimia nervosa – an empirical analysis based on the author's own research results

An appropriate diagnosis of psychological mechanisms underlying eating disorders, including a diagnosis of the body self characteristics in adolescent girls and young females suffering from bulimia nervosa, proves to be a significant predictor of successful treatment. Hence, during many years of my scientific research, I focused on the above mentioned issues.

4.1 Research objectives and variables

The main aim of this research was to determine the strength level for the characteristics of the body self structure in a group of selected 30 young Polish females suffering from bulimia nervosa, and in the control population of females who were similar in age and social status, and were not revealing any eating disorders or mental disturbances. The main question addressed in this study was: "Do the examined women who suffer from bulimia nervosa significantly differ from the healthy females in terms of the strength level for the characteristics of their body self structure?"

The main independent variable in the research was clinically diagnosed bulimia nervosa in the examined females. Its indicators included bulimic symptomatology as well as a medical diagnosis code (F.50.02, according to the ICD-10 classification).The main variable was the structure of the body self, defined, referring to the subject literature, as a complex construct constituting the following configuration: emotional experience related to body and its functions, as well as mental concept (perception and thoughts) regarding physical appearance [Cash, Pruzinsky, Thompson,Garner]. The major components of the variable which were empirically examined in the study included:

1. A body schema (a degree of an individual's knowledge of one's own body, and the person's awareness of specific body parts),
2. A sense of body boundaries (the feeling of separating one's own body from the external world, which facilitates the process of perceiving oneself as a bodily creature, definite and different from others)
3. Interoceptive awareness, i.e. the feeling of perplexity accompanying the process of recognizing and responding to emotional states and body sensations; and also the fear of high affection and the prospect of losing control over it)
4. Experiences related to body functions (maturity fear experienced by an individual, that is, the person's approval of psychosexual development, which is related to the process of entering the stage of maturity, and to body image change as well as loss of the sense of childhood security),
5. Body image, i.e. a sensual image of sizes, shapes and forms of the body as well as the feelings regarding the body. The major aspects of body image include: adequate evaluation of body shape and size, as well as feelings regarding the body (satisfaction, acceptance or disapproval).
6. Self-evaluation and body satisfaction– the level of general satisfaction with one's own body, weight, body shape and physical appearance. Body self-evaluation includes assessment of an individual's current body shape (i.e. the "actual me"image) and evaluation of the ideal, most desired attributes which the person would like to have (i.e. the ideal body image - "what I would like to look like").

An additional control variable was body mass index BMI. It has been announced that individuals who fall into the BMI range of 19.5 to 24.5 have a healthy weight. A BMI of under 19.5 is usually referred to as underweight. A Body Mass Index reading over 24.5 is considered overweight.

4.2 Subjects

102 Polish females participated in the research. The subjects were selected intentionally. Clinical population No. I consisted of 52 females clinically diagnosed with bulimia nervosa (the F.50.02 code, according to the ICD criteria of psychiatric classification). Whereas clinical population No. II was comprised of 50 women with no history of past or present eating disorders or other mental disturbances (e.g. bulimia or anorexia nervosa, psychogenic binge eating). The additional criteria which excluded participation in the research included: improper intellectual development, chronic somatic conditions (visible disability and body distortions), and organic changes in the CNS. The data mentioned above was gathered by means of clinical interviews conducted among the examined individuals. The aforementioned factors may affect the development of body image. Hence, the females exhibiting any of the dysfunctions mentioned above were excluded from the group of research subjects. During the research, all bulimic participants remained under medical care. The mean duration of treatment in the group of the examined bulimic females ranged from 2 to 12 months. A mean age in the research sample ranged from 21 to 25 years. The research was conducted anonymously with the personal consent obtained from each participant, and with the approval of a Human Research Ethics Committee.

4.3 Research methods

The methods applied in the research included an inventory (i.e. the Eating Disorder Inventory (EDI) devised by Garner, and Thompson's Body Dissatisfaction Inventory) as well as projective techniques such as Thompson's Silhouette Test and a thematic drawing: "body image". The inventories and projective techniques applied in the research procedures, aimed at making a psychological diagnosis of the investigated variables, are fully described in the subject literature [Thompson, Hornowska, Paluchowski, Oster].

The Eating Disorder Inventory devised by Garner is one of the instruments most frequently used to measure the patterns of behaviour and attitudes dominating the clinical picture of anorexia and bulimia nervosa, including those related to the process of perceiving and experiencing body [Thompson]. The following 3 scales, considered the purposes they had been devised for, were applied in the research: the Body Dissatisfaction Scale, the Interoceptive Deficits Scale, and the Maturity Fear Scale.

The Body Dissatisfaction Scale was used to measure the indicators of the body self component called "body image". The scale allowed to evaluate the level of the overall body satisfaction, and ever increasing discreditation of one's own appearance, body shape and weight as well as the particular body parts. It consisted of ten items. Each research participant was rated on a 0 to 40 point scale. The score ranging from 40 to 36 was interpreted as a very high level of discreditation of one's own body shape and size as well as body dissatisfaction. The score ranging from 35 to 22 points to considerable dissatisfaction with body shape, size and weight, and to negative feelings regarding body parts. The score ranging between 21 and 0 denotes the norm [Higgins].

The "Interoceptive Deficits" Scale was applied to measure the level of interoceptive awareness in the group of examined females. It allowed to evaluate the level of perplexity, which occurs in the process of recognizing and responding to emotional states and body sensations, and helped to assess the level of fear of high affection and of losing control. The scale consisted of eight items. Each research participant was rated on a 0 to 32 scale. A high score (13-32 points) points to a high degree of perplexity and discreditation of the experienced emotions. It proves that instead of being experienced, emotions undergo intellectual evaluation aimed at checking whether they are well-grounded, desired and justified. It can be assumed that a high score on this scale is interpreted as a significant risk factor which contributes to development of an eating disorder. A low score (0-10 points) indicates a properly retained ability to deal with and accept positive and negative emotions regarding one's own body. It is also an indicator of mental health [Higgins].

The "Maturity Fear" scale served as an instrument for measuring the level of approval of psychosexual development. Maturity fear is related to the exhibited tendency, a desire to regain the pre-pubescent appearance [Higgins]. The examined subjects were rated on a 0 to 32 point scale. A high score (between 13 and 32) denotes a strong desire for being younger and regaining childhood security. It also proves the conviction that the requirements set during the period of maturity are too high. A low score (between 0 and 5) indicates a high level of psychosexual development acceptance, and mental transition to the stage of maturity [Higgins].

The second measurement instrument applied in the research was the Body Dissatisfaction Inventory devised by K. Thompson [Cash, Pruzinsky, Thompson]. It was used to measure the level of satisfaction and dissatisfaction with weight, body shape and appearance in the examined women. The research subjects rated themselves on a 10-point satisfaction-dissatisfaction continuum, which resulted in the scores ranging from 0 (a high level of satisfaction) to 10 (a high level of dissatisfaction). It was assumed that the score of 5 should be interpreted as an average level of body satisfaction.

Another instrument used in the research to measure body image was a projective technique - the Silhouette Test by Thompson [Cash, Pruzinsky, Thompson]. It allowed to make a comparison between the actual body image (the actual self image), perceived by the subject, and its ideal image (the ideal self image). The instrument consists of a set of nine male and nine female silhouettes ranging from very thin to very fat. The subjects' task was to select the figure which most closely matched their current body shape, and one image which they considered ideal. Additionally, the subjects were supposed to provide details concerning their age, current weight and height. The figure ratings obtained in the test were used to calculate the current-ideal discrepancy (the individual's perceived current body shape versus the ideal body image), and thus to examine the respondents' body image acceptance The scores received in the research ranged from 0 (lack of discrepancy, which indicates a high level of body image acceptance) to 8 (very high discrepancy, which proves a low level of body image acceptance).

Thematic drawing ("body image") was used to examine the level of body schema complexity as well as a sense of body boundaries (the feeling of separating one's own body from the external world, which allows to perceive oneself as a bodily creature, definite and different from others). It is a projective technique, in which the study subject's task is to draw a picture of body. The test is based on an assumption that the drawing is projection of the examined person's self image, especially such components of the body self as the body schema and body boundaries [Hornowska, Paluchowski, Oster]. In order to investigate the aforementioned elements, the test analysis focused on such aspects of the drawing as evaluating the number of body details as well as investigating formal and structural elements of the drawing (the size of the figures, the pencil stroke and pressure). Referring to theoretical assumptions concerning the role of the human figure drawing in a psychological diagnosis, it was assumed that the greater number of details corresponds with a higher level of the body schema complexity [Hornowska, Paluchowski, Oster].

Formal and structural analysis of the drawings focused on the size adequacy of the depicted figures. Both too small and extremely large figures seem to point to inadequate perception of body size. Such aspects of drawings as the presence of the main body parts (e.g. head, hair, nose, lips, eyes, neck, trunk, arms, hands, legs, and feet) and the characteristics of the body portrayal (e.g. the pencil stroke, the kinds of lines, body proportions, scaling the figure up or down) were taken into consideration in psychological interpretation of the indicators of a body schema and body boundaries. The pencil stroke analysis, based on the Goodenough-Harris Draw-A-Person Test, involved examining the kinds of lines drawn by the research subjects (e.g. unbroken, dotted, thick, thin, or not sharp). An unconnected, thin and blurred stroke can be interpreted as difficulties in establishing precise body boundaries in the examined person.

It was also assumed that the number of body parts the subject considered significant and included in her drawing corresponded with the level of the person's body schema and image complexity. The subject scored 1 point for each detail depicted in the drawing. Lack of the particular body part meant 0 points. The accuracy of classifying the particular indicators into the given categories was examined by five competent judges (clinical psychologists), on the basis of the following scale:

- 0 – a low (inadequate) score (lack of the particular body part in the drawing);
- 1 – a high (adequate) score (an element depicted in the drawing);
- 0.5 – an average score.

The research comprised two stages. The first phase involved psychological measurement of the examined indictors of the body self in the population of 102 Polish females, using clinical and test methods, as well as projective techniques (e.g. observation, a clinical interview, or thematic drawing: "body image").

The second stage of the research was aimed at conducting a statistical and clinical analysis of the research data, which involved the following steps:

- calculating the mean values for the strength level of the investigated body self indictors in the clinical population of women suffering from bulimia nervosa as well as in the control population of females;
- assessing the intra-group similarities and differences regarding the strength and configuration of the investigated indicators of the body self structure in the whole population of the research subjects (i.e. females suffering from bulimia nervosa and the individuals in the control population) using the k-means method [Stanisz]
- assessing significant differences between the clinical population and the control group of females in terms of the strength level for the investigated indicators of the body self structure, using Student's t-test for two independent samples.

5. A psychological profile of the body self characteristics in females suffering from bulimia nervosa

Statistical cluster analysis conducted using the k-means allowed to distinguish three clusters in the whole research population of 102 females. Cluster No. I and Cluster No. II consisted of women diagnosed with bulimia nervosa. Whereas cluster No. III was comprised of females revealing no mental disturbances or eating disorders.

The research data analysis demonstrated certain significant differences between the examined females in the aforementioned three clusters in terms of the strength level and configuration of the body self characteristics. Hence, the three clusters were referred to as: "Bulimic Type I (a socio-cultural type)", "Bulimic Type II (a separation type)", and Type III (an adequate type). Each of them referred to certain distinctive characteristics of the body self structure in the examined women.

Figure 1 displays a graphic illustration of significant differences regarding the emotional and cognitive characteristics of the body self in the examined 102 Polish females.

Statistical analysis of the research data reveals certain significant differences between the examined 102 females in terms of such indicators of the body self structure as: the level of satisfaction with one's own body (the quality of emotions regarding the body); the overall body self-assessment (acceptance or disapproval of the current body image; perception of body image (both current and ideal body shape); recognizing body sensations (interoceptive awareness, i.e. a degree of perplexity arousing in the process of recognizing and responding to the emotional states and body sensations); experiencing bodily functions (i.e. the level of maturity fear – accepting the level of psychosexual development related to the process of transition into adult life, body image transformation and loss of childhood security).

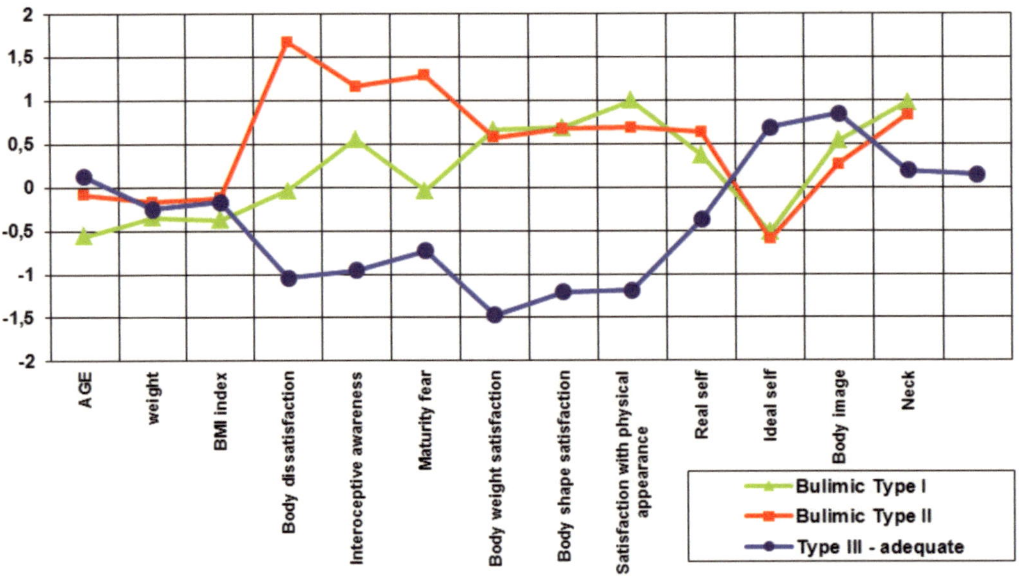

Legend
Bulimic Type I –a socio-cultural type
Bulimic Type II – a separation type
Type III- an adequate (normal) type
A Figure Test devised by Thompson and Gray (Contour drawing Rating Scale): Ideal self B, Real self A,
Thompson's Test: body weight satisfaction, body shape satisfaction, satisfaction with physical appearance, Thematic Drawing (scaling the figure up or down)
Garner's Eating Disorder Inventory – Body Dissatisfaction, Interoceptive Deficits and Maturity Fear.

Fig. 1. A graphic illustration of cluster analysis conducted using the k-means method. Specification of significant differences regarding the strength level for the body self characteristics between the bulimic subjects (Type I and Type II) and the examined females revealing no mental disturbances or eating disorders (Type III).

5.1 Psychological assessment of the body schema and body boundaries dysfunctions in women suffering from bulimia nervosa and in females exhibiting no eating disorders or mental disturbances

The indicators of the body schema and body boundaries among the examined females were examined using a projective technique, i.e. thematic drawing: "body image". Formal and structural analysis of the drawings focused on the characteristics of the body portrayal which included such aspects as: the size adequacy of the depicted figures (the tendency towards scaling the figures up or down; maintaining or losing body proportions), the number of details included in the drawing, the pencil stroke, and the kinds of lines drawn by the research subjects. The aforementioned elements were examined by five competent judges (psychologists) on the basis of the following criteria:

- 1-0.7 – a high score (a highly detailed drawing which depicts an elaborate figure, and includes more than 11 major body parts all of which are proportional and clearly outlined),
- 0.6-0.4 – an average score (a norm) – (a drawing which includes 11 major body parts all of which are proportional and appropriately outlined),

- 0.3-0 – a low score (a drawing which is not very detailed, and includes fewer than 11 major body parts which are not proportional; the figure is vaguely sketched, the line is unconnected and blurred).

The data gathered in the whole sample of 102 females (i.e. the women suffering from bulimia nervosa as well as the individuals exhibiting no eating disorders or mental disturbances) did not reveal any significant dysfunctions in terms of the body schema or body boundaries in any of the examined subjects. The mean values concerning the presence or absence of the major body parts in the participants' drawings turned out to be high or average in the majority of the examined females, which demonstrates the individuals' adequate (conforming to the norm) body schema complexity.

Cluster analysis of the data collected in the whole population of 102 females discovered that the subjects not suffering from bulimia nervosa (who comprised Cluster No. III) maintained a proper body schema and body boundaries. The individuals in this cluster did not present any distorted figures in their body drawings (the mean value for scaling the figures up and down reached 0.7). The bodies sketched by the females did not miss any parts, all of which were properly attached to the depicted figures (head featuring eyes, mouth, nose, hair; sharply drawn arms and legs with thighs and feet, connected to the body trunk). The mean values for the body proportions shown in the participants' drawings prove that the women in cluster No. III, maintained body proportions in their drawings: the proportion of arms to trunk, legs to trunk, and head to trunk. A sharp pencil stroke dominating in the drawings (the mean value = 0.84) as well as the so called average unbroken line (the mean value = 0.53) demonstrate maintained body boundaries. Cluster No. III was predominated by the females whose mean age was 23, and their average body weight reached 55.7 kg, at which level their BMI was 20.16 (within the normal range). Analysis of the mean values for the level of the women's satisfaction with their own body, its weight, shape and general physical appearance, points to the subjects' average (adequate) level of body acceptance and appearance satisfaction. The mean values in the "Body dissatisfaction" scale as well as those obtained as a result of Thompson's Figure Test also denote a high level of satisfaction with body shape and appearance among the females in cluster No. III. The mean values for evaluation of the current self image ("what I look like") and the ideal one ("what I would like to look like"), reaching the value of 3.95 and 3.63 respectively, also indicate adequacy in perceiving and experiencing body in this group of examined females. This in turn points to adequate (positive) self-assessment, as well as to one's own body satisfaction. A low mean value of 2.74 in the "Interoceptive awareness" scale (the EDI inventory) points to the fact that the non-bulimic subjects maintain a highly adequate ability to recognize and respond to the occurring emotional states and body sensations. It can also indicate that the women are able to accept and experience the feelings regarding the body, and they do not make any discrediting intellectual evaluation. The mean value of 4.58 in the"Maturity fear" scale (the EDI inventory) indicates a low level of emotional discreditation of body among the examined females. It also proves that they fully accept their body sexuality and transition into adult life, which is accompanied by mental acceptance of "farewell to childhood and childlike body image".

Summing up, the data obtained as a result of this research denote adequate self-perception and self-assessment as well as a high level of satisfaction with body shape and appearance in the group of non-bulimic females. Additionally, a certain tendency was detected: the females desired (ideal) body is thinner than their current body shape, which is proved by the mean BMI index value of 20.16 and the mean value of 3.63 for the ideal self in

Thompson's Figure Test. It appears that although the women would like to have a slimmer body, and seem to be rather dissatisfied with their real body image, their body self is not pathologically distorted. It might suggest the influence of the socio-cultural cult of thinness. However, the level of the examined women's mental maturity, their biological age (they constitute the oldest sample, compared with the other two clusters), and lack of emotional deficits or traumatic experience (especially in relationships with care-givers) can prove that they do not exhibit any symptoms of increased separation anxiety which usually impedes the separation-individuation process. The observed finding can be underpinned by the object relations theory which suggests that the quality of the infant's early relationship with a primary caregiver (an object) affects the individual's further development. According to the approach represented by Bruch, Mahler, Clein or Kruger, the mother's empathic resonance with the infant's internal experience allows the formation of the infant's primary body self, that is, a system of early bodily sensations, which in turn is a prerequisite for the further emergence of a sense of self and body boundaries that allow to differentiate self from non-self [Krueger]. The interview data prove that the examined females in cluster No.III did not experience any emotional deficits or psychic traumas in relationships with their mothers. Moreover, the subjects did not report any facts in their lives which could determine development of traumas in their interpersonal relationships (e.g. physical, sexual or mental abuse). Their biological age points to the fact that the women have already completed the process of separation, they have managed to shape their personal, social identity and the ability to establish a partner relationship based on a strong (emotional, sexual) bond. The females tend to yield to social pressure related to the "cult of thinness" and comply with the standards of attractiveness, which seems to affect the evolution of their body image. However, the socio-cultural factors are not strong enough to impede development of their female identity and thereby lead to pathological distortions of body image in the examined women.

Statistical analysis of the data obtained as a result of a Student's t-test demonstrates significant differences between the healthy females (Type III) and the bulimic subjects (Type I and Type II) in terms of body proportions in their figure drawings. Certain pathological tendencies were observed among the females suffering from bulimia nervosa. Significant disproportion of body parts (e.g. trunk-legs or trunk-head disproportion) was noticed in the figures drawn by the bulimic individuals. Additionally, certain body parts which they included in their drawings (e.g. stomach, hips, and breast) turned out to be excessively scaled up. The figure test was also applied by such researchers as Marike Tiggemann, Kevin Thompson, David Garner and Thomas Cash.

The research results described in the subject literature prove that body image dissatisfaction refers to certain attributes of physical appearance, predominantly to body shape and weight, as well as face, hair, stomach or breast. The data provided in Polish professional literature [8, 9, 11] indicate that women suffering from eating disorders show excessive (pathological) concern with the aforementioned body parts, and they tend to overestimate the influence of the specified body parts on their global self-assessment, and consequently discredit their bodies, and lower their self-esteem Excessive focus on body, and its negative evaluation constitute the major factors determining development of eating disorders, as it was pointed out by Cash [Cash, Pruzinsky, Thompson, Garner]. Lack of significant differences between the examined females comprising the three clusters, in terms of major body schema indicators seems to be justifiable since the body schema and the ability to recognize body boundaries are considered to be the primary (developed in the first two years of the person's life) function of the body which is not disturbed in women. With age, the knowledge concerning the body, related to developmental mechanisms and social influence, becomes more profound, which is accompanied by adequate body size perception. During adolescence, a distinct emotional attitude towards the body is shaped, and appearance proves to have increasingly significant influence on the person's self-assessment and self-esteem. The research subjects were young females in late adolescence, the final stage of development. This may provide an explanation for the trunk-legs or trunk-head disproportion noticed in the figures drawn by the subjects suffering from bulimia nervosa. The characteristic feature of their figure portrayals was the tendency towards scaling up the trunk which did not stay in proportion with the legs and head that were reduced in size. It can be presumed that the disproportions of body parts result from distorted body perception, which an individual develops in the course of his or her psychological development, as well as from the person's emotional experience regarding the body and his or her emotional attitude towards physical appearance, which is shaped during adolescence. As a result of psychosexual development occurring during the period of adolescence, the level of concern regarding body image increases. This, when coupled with social pressure concerning the body, may either stimulate development of proper characteristics of body image, or trigger its pathological distortions in bulimia sufferers.

5.2 Cognitive and emotional characteristics of the body self (i.e. emotions regarding the body, interoceptive awareness, body perception and self-assessment) – comparative analysis aimed at investigating the main differences between the bulimic subjects and the females exhibiting no mental disturbances or eating disorders

Statistical comparative analysis conducted using a student's t-test revealed significant differences between the examined women suffering from bulimia nervosa (N=52) and the non-bulimic subjects (N=50) in terms of such characteristics of the body self structure as the quality of emotions regarding the body, overall body self-assessment, perception of body image (both current and ideal appearance), recognizing bodily sensations (i.e. the deficits in interoceptive awareness), experiences related to bodily functions (i.e. the level of maturity fear and approval of psychosexual development which is related to the process of entering the stage of maturity, and to body image transformation as well as loss of the sense of childhood security).
The mean values for the level of body self-satisfaction, its weight, shape and appearance, obtained in the group of females exhibiting no eating disorders, indicate that the individuals in this cluster express rather positive feelings towards their own body and are satisfied with it. The mean value of 5.33 for the level of body dissatisfaction, received in the EDI inventory, as well as the mean values for body shape satisfaction (1.59), weight satisfaction (0.95) and appearance satisfaction (1.04), obtained in Thompson's silhouette test proved to be low, which suggests that the examined females in this sample do not exhibit any disturbances regarding their emotional body experience or cognitive body image.
The research results obtained in the group of females suffering from bulimia nervosa turned out to be significantly different. Analysis of the data collected in this sample revealed pathological (excessive) increase in the level of dissatisfaction with body, its shape and physical appearance. It is proved by the mean value of 23.06, obtained in the "Body dissatisfaction" scale (the EDI test), as well as by the mean values for body shape dissatisfaction (9.09), weight dissatisfaction (8.83) and appearance dissatisfaction (9.34), received in Thompson's silhouette test. The statistical significance of the differences between the bulimic and non-bulimic research subjects turned out to be considerably high (p=0.001).

The bulimia sufferers have been identified as having a decidedly higher, compared with the sample of healthy females, incidence of negative emotions regarding the body, and they reveal a higher level of body image dissatisfaction. The received finding seems to correlate positively with increased fear of gaining weight (the so called fat phobia) among the bulimic females. Low self-esteem and lack of body acceptance among bulimia sufferers, as well as their compensatory behaviours aimed at gaining the "perfect body" appear to have their roots in the fear of being fat, described in the subject literature [43], and regarded as a factor determining the onset of the eating disorder.

Analysis of the mean values for the level of interoceptive deficits regarding one's own body demonstrated statistically significant differences between the two groups of examined women. The mean value obtained by the bulimic subjects in the EDI test proved to be high (=16.55), which points to the females' high degree of discreditation of emotions regarding their own body. It indicates that instead of being experienced, their emotions undergo intellectual evaluation aimed at checking whether they are well-grounded, desired and justified. The low mean value of 2.74, received in the control population, indicates a properly maintained ability to deal with and accept positive and negative emotions regarding one's own body.

The mean values in the "Maturity fear" scale (the EDI inventory), obtained in the control population and in the clinical sample, as well as the data obtained as a result of statistical significance analysis conducted using a student's t-test reveal a considerable discrepancy between the two groups of examined females. The mean value of 12.45 for the level of maturity fear, obtained in the group of bulimic subjects, denotes the women's strong desire for being younger and regaining childhood security. It also proves the subjects' conviction that the requirements set during the period of maturity are too high. Whereas the low mean value of 4.58 in this scale, obtained in the sample of females exhibiting no eating disorders, can be interpreted as a low level of maturity fear among the individuals, and it indicates a high level of acceptance of psychosexual development and mental transition to the stage of maturity, that is, acceptance of feelings regarding the body and sexual functions of the body.

Analysis of the data obtained as a result of Thompson's Figure Test, aimed at examining the current self image ("what I look like") and the ideal one ("what I would like to look like"), revealed statistically significant differences between the bulimic and non-bulimic subjects. It was found that when evaluating their actual body image, the examined females in the control group tended to select the figure which most resembled their own body shape and weight (the average body weight in this group reached 55.7 kg, at which level the females' BMI was 20.16). The image they frequently opted for in Thompson's Figure Test was the so called slim silhouette to which a mean value of 3.95 was assigned. This indicates adequacy in perceiving body image. Whereas analysis of the data gathered in the group of females suffering from bulimia nervosa, who were close in age to the non-bulimic subjects, discovered that they perceive their bodies as fatter than they really are. A considerable discrepancy was revealed between the bulimic females' mean value for the current self rating (5.75) and the women's average body weight (55.43 kg) and BMI index value (19.81). It is surprising that although the mean values concerning body weight and BMI index were similar in the two groups of the examined females, the bulimia sufferers tended to exhibit distortions in perception of their current body image. It can be concluded that although the bulimic individuals weighed less than the healthy subjects, they tended to perceive their bodies as much fatter than they really were. The image they most frequently chose in Thompson's Figure Test to evaluate their current body image was a silhouette much fatter than their actual body. This seems to point to

distortions in cognitive body image, which is a distinguishing characteristic of body perception among individuals suffering from eating disorders, as was proved by the results of research conducted by Thompson and Cash [Cash, Pruzinsky, Thompson, Altabe].
Other significant differences between bulimic and non-bulimic females were discovered in terms of evaluation of the ideal body image ("what I would like to look like"). The data analysis revealed a tendency among the bulimic females which was dominated by a desire to have a much slimmer figure than their current body shape, which was proved by the mean value of 2.24 for the ideal self image, received in this group of women. This points to the individuals' "desire for slimness". An emaciated body shape turned out to be the image most frequently selected by the bulimic females in Thompson's Figure Test to represent their desired (ideal) body figure. A similar tendency is generally observed among anorectic individuals. The significant discrepancy between the current and ideal body image in the group of women suffering from anorexia nervosa may correlate with the fear of gaining weight, that is, fat phobia, which has been described in subject literature [Wilson].

5.3 Intra-group differences in terms of cognitive and emotional characteristics of the body self in the sample of females suffering from bulimia nervosa

Statistical analysis of the research data, conducted using a student's t-test (for two independent samples) revealed certain statistically significant differences between the examined females classified into the bulimic Type I and Type II. The following statistically different mean values were received in the EDI inventory, in Thompson's Body Dissatisfaction Inventory as well as in Thompson and Gray's Figure test:

- The EDI inventory- the Body Dissatisfaction Scale: Type I = 15.71,Type II = 32.00; the "Interoceptive Deficits" scale: Type I = 14.43, Type II = 19.13; the "Maturity Fear" scale: Type I = 8.89, Type II = 16.78;
- Thompson's Body Dissatisfaction Test - overall body shape satisfaction: Type I = 8.80, Type II = 8.86; weight satisfaction: Type I = 9.22, Type II = 8.94; physical appearance satisfaction: Type I = 9.89, Type II = 8.62;
- Thompson and Gray's Figure Test –Type I: current self-image =5.54, ideal self- image = 2.29; Type II: current self- image = 6.00, ideal self- image = 2.17.

The received data point to a considerably higher level of developmental dysfunctions and distortions in terms of body perception and emotions regarding the body in the subsample of bulimic females constituting Type II (the so called separation type). The subsample defined as Type I (socio-cultural) comprised 26 individuals who appeared to be slightly younger. A mean age in this group was 21 and 2 months. The females' average body weight was 54.5 kg, and a mean BMI in the investigated subsample reached the value of 19.38 (the lower limit of the norm). The real self-image score of 5.54, obtained in Thompson's silhouette test, proves that the bulimic females (Type I) have a realistic and adequate perception of their body. However, the man value of 2.29 for the ideal self rating, received in Thompson's figure test, points to the women's strong desire for an ideal body shape. This might mean that the need to yield to socio-cultural pressure related to the "cult of thinness" appears to be stronger among younger individuals who haven't completed the separation-individuation process yet.
The subsample of bulimic females classified into Type II (the separation type) was constituted by 23 individuals whose mean age was 22.6, average body weight was 56 kg, and a mean BMI in the investigated group reached the value of 20.32. During the clinical interview, it was discovered that the women had experienced emotional deficits and psychic traumas in their lives. The majority of the subjects in the sample reported childhood psychic traumas and

emotional deficits (e.g. physical or sexual abuse, some individuals were abandoned by significant objects - parents). As opposed to the females constituting the bulimic Type I, the individuals classified into Type II reported that their bulimic symptoms occurred in the early stages of the disease, and were preceded by several years of food restriction.
According to the information gathered during the clinical interview, the earliest onset of bulimia nervosa among the examined females classified into the separation Type II occurred shortly before they undertook treatment, having been self-motivated and encouraged by their family members. Remaining under medical supervision, the bulimics were able to control the cycles of binge eating and purging, and to reduce the frequency of the compensatory behaviours. The present findings seem to be consistent with other research investigating the role of trauma symptoms (especially sexual trauma experienced during childhood) in the development of eating disorders , which has been described in the subject literature [Rorty, Yager, Rossotto, Kent, Waller, Dagnan, Hartt]. Although the conducted studies do not provide evidence for a high correlation between childhood sexual trauma and the development of bulimia nervosa, they demonstrate that such traumatic experience is likely to increase the incidence of eating disorders, especially bulimia nervosa. According to the assumptions of the object relations theory, the real mother-child relationships are internalized during childhood, and provide a foundation for the emergence of personality and the ego identity [Tyson]. The mean values received in the EDI inventory, in Thompson's Body Dissatisfaction Inventory as well as in Thompson and Gray's Figure Test, obtained in the subsample of females constituting the bulimic Type II, indicate that the individuals exhibit a strong tendency towards emotional and cognitive devaluation of the body. The socio-cultural pressure related to the "cult of thinness" , coupled with growing fear of maturity and adulthood (the mean value of 16.78 in the EDI inventory), as well as incresed separation anxiety, reinforces the examined women's tendency towards discrediting their own bodies, which is stronger than among the bulimic females classified into Type I. A high (pathological) mean value in the "Interoceptive Deficits" scale (the EDI inventory), obtained in this subsample, points to the individuals' inadequate level of interoceptive awareness. It denotes a high degree of perplexity and discreditation of bodily sensations and emotions regarding the body. The data prove that instead of experiencing the emotions regarding their body perception, the examined bulimic females classified into the separation type conduct intellectual evaluation aimed at checking whether the emotions are well-grounded, desired and justified. The psychic mechanism of rationalization which prevails in this group of subjects impedes the individuals' ability to go through direct emotional experience. This finding supports the research conducted by Józefik, which has been described in Polish literature [Józefik]. The so called "bulimic self", as referred to in the subject literature, is reflected in the body self, i.e. it is expressed through body language. The bulimic self represents the primitive need for dependence as well as the need for autonomy and separation, which is manifested through binge eating and self-induced vomiting. These compensatory bahaviours allow an individual to establish his or her own identity, and to separate from a significant object [Sands].

6. A psychological profile and different configurations of the body self components distinguished in the population of females suffering from bulimia nervosa (conclusions drawn from the author's own research)

The data obtained as a result of this research revealed diversity in terms of the body self characteristics in the examined individuals suffering from bulimia nervosa. The subjects' life experience appeared to be the factor determining this diversity. It was found that some of the examined females had experienced emotional traumas which affected their psychological development. As a consequence of inadequate separation and individuation process, the examined individuals appear to exhibit considerable dysfunctions of the body self, and they will probably need long-term and multi-dimensional (psychological and medical) treatment. This group of bulimic females was referred to as bulimic Type II, the so called separation type. It was comprised of 23 subjects diagnosed with bulimia nervosa, whose mean age was 22 and 6 months. A diagnosis of the body self characteristics in this sample revealed significant dysfunctions in terms of all components of the body self structure. The main features that characterize this group of women include: strong emotional and cognitive disapproval of the current body image (i.e. body dissatisfaction and critical body self-assessment); a low level of interoceptive awareness of the body; and a discrepancy between the real and ideal self-image, accompanied by a tendency towards gaining an ideal emaciated figure which does not conform to the developmental norms. The subsample is predominated by females who have been experiencing increased separation anxiety, and at the same time they tend to completely discredit their bodies. The mean values for the level of body acceptance and experiencing emotions regarding the body, obtained in this group of the examined females, denote the individuals' strong tendency towards cognitive and emotional devaluation of the body. The mean values for the current and the ideal self rating, received in Thompson's Figure Test, point to a significant discrepancy between the two aspects. It can be concluded that the females' distorted perception of the actual body image, as well as their increased (pathological) perplexity and difficulties in recognizing and responding to emotional states and body sensations prove that the women exhibit certain dysfunctions of one of the body self components, i.e. interoceptive awareness. It is worth mentioning that the mean age and BMI values obtained in the group of bulimics classified into Type II conform to the age-appropriate norms. The question arises as to whether it is possible to provide an explanation for the fact that the females who exhibit a high degree of the body self dysfunctions have a normal body weight. The received data indicate that at the time of the research, the examined individuals in question had been participating in long term treatment for at least 12 months, and remained under regular medical supervision (e.g. they had been undergoing medical tests and were provided with medical and psychotherapeutic consultations), which was an obligation imposed by their therapeutic contracts. Hence, it can be concluded that the females' normal (adequate) body weight acts as "camouflage" or a "cover" for the considerable body self dysfunctions which they exhibit. This points to the existence of certain destructive psychological mechanisms aimed at camouflaging negative emotions regarding the body as well as cognitive body distortions. It appears that the individuals who enter nto a therapeutic contract try to observe its stipulations by maintaining an adequate body weight, but they still exhibit disturbances in their emotional and cognitive attitude towards the body. It is likely that the women's subordination is feigned, and they only pretend that they participate in the process of treatment. This might suggest that a long term and intensive psychotherapy aimed at eliminating body image distortions is an indispensable element of effective (not superficial) treatment of eating disorders. The childhood and adolescent relational (sexual) traumas reported by the examined females point to the necessity of introducing the treatment methods which would focus on dealing with psychological separation and individuation, and the problems related to the process of experiencing the body.

Another type of psychological profile distinguished among the examined females was defined as Type II - socio-cultural. It prevailed in the group of slightly older research subjects. It was discovered that evaluation of body image in this sample is determined by social-cultural factors and the cult of thinness. As a result of examination of the individuals' body self characteristics it was found that although the women do not exhibit any significant developmental dysfunctions (they display an average level of emotional and cognitive body acceptance, appropriate interoceptive awareness and adequate current body perception), they reveal a strong desire for a much slimmer (ideal) body. It is likely that the research data were affected by the fact that the examined females had been undergoing regular medical treatment and psychotherapy. The socio-cultural type is also characterized by an average sense of security related to the process of entering the stage of maturity and accepting "farewell to childhood". The research data demonstrate that the females are aware of their adequate feelings regarding the body, and they are generally satisfied with their actual appearance. However, a certain discrepancy was detected between the individuals' cognitive evaluation of their current body shape ("what I look like") and the so called ideal body image ("what I would like to look like"). This finding might point to slight distortions in the real body image observed in this group of research subjects.

7. Conclusions

Analysis of the data obtained as a result of this research revealed diversity in terms of the body self characteristics among bulimia sufferers experiencing a variety of destructive symptoms (e.g. episodes of binge eating and purging). Different configurations of the body self characteristics in bulimic individuals can be determined by a variety of major factors. They include socio-cultural determinants (e.g. the social pressure related to the commonly approved cult of thinness regarded as the key to success and positive self-assessment), which significantly contribute to development of bulimic tendencies. The major distortions in body perception and evaluation of physical appearance which develop in bulimia sufferers as a result of socio-cultural pressure, lead to developmental dysfunctions and disturbances of body experience. However, other components of the body self remain undisturbed (i.e. an appropriate body schema, an adequate level of interoceptive awareness and appropriate bodily functions, as well as lack of anxiety related to the process of transition into adult life and performing roles based on a female model of psychosexual maturity). The aforementioned dysfunctions are triggered by extrinsic (environmental) factors.

A different configuration of the body self characteristics emerges as a result of an inadequate process of psychological separation and individuation, disturbed by emotional deficits and psychological traumas during childhood. It is characterized by a higher, compared to the socio-cultural type, degree of cognitive and emotional dysfunctions of all the investigated components of the body self. The disturbances are determined by intrinsic (personality-based) factors, and correlate with inadequate separation and individuation in bulimic individuals.

A psychological differential diagnosis, aimed at distinguishing various types of the body self structure in the population of females suffering from bulimia nervosa, supports psychological diagnostic techniques, and thus improves the effectiveness of therapy in patients exhibiting this kind of disorder.

8. References

[1] FairburnCG.HarrisonP.J., Eating disorders.Lancet.1.Feb.2003, Vol.361, 9355, pp.407-16;

[2] FairburnCG. et al. The natural course of bulimia and binge eating disorder in young women. Arch. Gen. Psychiatry.Jul.2000, Vol. 27, pp.659-665

[3] Lacey, J.H., Evans, C.D.H...The impulsivist: A Multi - Impulsive Personality Disorder. British Journal of Addition, 2000, 81, pp.641-649
[4] Thompson J.K. Introduction: body image, eating disorders, and obesity - an emerging synthesis. In: Thompson J.K. ed. Body image, eating disorders, and obesity. An integrative guide for assessment and treatment. Washington: American Psychological Association DC; 1996, pp. 1-20.
[5] Cash, T. F., Pruzinsky T. Body image. A Handbook of Theory, Research and Clinical Practise. New York. London: The Guilford Press; 2004,
[6] Thompson J.K. (2004) Handboock of Disorders and Obesity. John Wiley/Sons, Inc.5, 6,], New York: Wiley; 2004, pp. 495-514.
[7] Garner D.M.EDI -3.Eating Disorders Inventory-3. Psychological Assessment Resources, Inc .USA; 2004
[8] Józefik B. Relacje rodzinne w anoreksji i bulimii psychicznej. Kraków: Wydawnictwo Uniwersytetu Jagiellońskiego, 2006, pp.33-34
[9] Józefik B. Anoreksja i bulimia psychiczna. Rozumienie i leczenie zaburzeń odżywiania się. Kraków: Wydawnictwo UniwersytetuJagiellońskiego,1999
[10] Głębocka A, Kulbat J., Czym jest wizerunek ciała? W: Głębocka A, Kulbat, J, ed. Wizerunek ciała: Portret Polek. Opole: Wydawnictwo UO; 2005, pp. 9-28.
[11] Rabe-Jabłońska J, Dunajska A. Poglądy na temat zniekształconego obrazu ciała dla powstawania i przebiegu zaburzeń odżywiania. Psychiatria Polska. 1997; 6: pp.723-738
[12] Mikołajczyk E. Samochowiec J. Cechy osobowości u pacjentek z zaburzeniami odżywiania. Psychiatria Via Medica 2004; Vol.1, No. 2, pp.91-95
[13] Schier K. Piękne brzydactwo. Psychologiczna problematyka obrazu ciała i jego zaburzeń. Warszawa: Wydawnictwo Naukowe Scholar,2009
[14] Izydorczyk B. Rybicka-Klimczyk A. Poznawcze aspekty obrazu ciała u kobiet a zaburzenia odżywiania. Endokrynologia Polska. Polish Journal of Endocrinology, 2008, Vol. 60, No. 4/2009,pp.1-8
[15] Izydorczyk B, Bieńkowska N. Obraz ja cielesnego - wybrane teoretyczne wątki rozumienia psychologicznych mechanizmów zjawiska. Part I Problemy Medycyny Rodzinnej, 2008, 4(25), pp.52-63
[16] Izydorczyk B., Bieńkowska N. Obraz ja cielesnego - wybrane teoretyczne wątki rozumienia psychologicznych mechanizmów zjawiska. Part II. Problemy Medycyny Rodzinnej; 2009, 1(26), pp.59 - 62
[17] Izydorczyk B., Rybicka-Klimczyk A. Środki masowego przekazu i ich rola w kształtowaniu wizerunku ciała u zróżnicowanych wiekiem życia kobiet polskich (analiza badań własnych). Problemy Medycyny Rodzinnej (2009), 3(28), pp.20-30
[18] Krueger D.W. Integrating Body Self and Psychological Self.Creating a New Story in Psychoanalysis and Psychotherapy. New York, London, Bruner-Routledge, 2002
[19] Lowen A. Narcyzm. Zaprzeczenie prawdziwemu ja. Warszawa Jacek Santorski, 1995.
[20] Pervin L.A.(2002) Pojęcie Ja W: Psychologia osobowości.Gdańsk GWP,2002
[21] Tyson P, Tyson R. Psychoanalytic Theories of Development and integration. Yale University Press. New Haven. London, 1990
[22] Schier K. Bez Tchu i Bez Słowa. Więź psychiczna, 2005
[23] Sugarman A. Bulimia: A. Displacement from Psychological Self to Body Self. In: J. Craig. Psychodynamic Treatment of Anorexia Nervosa and Bulimia. London. The Guilford Press.1991
[24] Sands S. Bulimia. Dissociation and Empathy: A Self-Psychological View. In: J. Craig Psychodynamic Treatment of Anorexia Nervosa and Bulimia. London. The Guilford Press.1991

[25] Higgins, T. Self-discrepancy: A theory relating self and affect. Psychological Review, 1987,(3), 319-340.
[26] Żechowski, C. Polska wersja Kwestionariusza Zaburzeń Odżywiania (EDI) - adaptacja i normalizacja. Psychiatria Polska, 2008, 2, pp.179 - 193.
[27] Hornowska, E., Paluchowski, W. J. Rysunek postaci ludzkiej według Goodenough - Harrisa. Poznań: Wydawnictwo Naukowe Uniwersytetu im. Adama Mickiewicza w Poznaniu,1987
[28] Oster G.D., GouldP. Rysunek w psychoterapii. Gdańsk: Gdańskie Wydawnictwo Psychologiczne,2005
[29] Thompson, J. K. Assessing body image disturbance: measures, methodology and implementation. In: J.K. Thompson (ed.), Body image, eating disorders, and obesity. An integrative guide for assessment and treatment (pp. 49-83). Washington: American Psychological Association DC.1996
[30] Thompson, J. K., Altabe, M. N. Psychometric qualities of the figure rating scale. International Journal of Eating Disorders, 1991, 5, pp.615-619.
[31] Thompson, J. K., Berg, P. (2002). Measuring body image attitudes among adolescents and adults. In: T.F.Cash, T. Pruzinsky (eds.), Body image. A handbook of theory, research, and clinical practice (pp.142- 153). New York, London: The Guilford Press 2002
[32] Tiggemann, M. Media Influences on Body Image Development. In: T.F.Cash, T. Pruzinsky (eds.), Body image. A handbook of theory, research, and clinical practice (pp. 91-98). New York, London: The Guilford Press.2002
[33] Tiggemann, M. Media exposure, body dissatisfaction and disordered eating: television and magazines are not the same. European Eating Disorders Review, 200311, 418-430.
[34] Garner, D.M., Olmsted, M.P., Bohr, Y., Garfinkel, P.E. *The Eating Attitudes Test: Psychometric features and clinical correlates.* Psychological Medicine, 1982, 12, pp.871-878. http://www.river-centre.org/abouteat26.html
[35] Cash, T. R., Pruzinsky, T. Future challenges for body image theory, research and clinical practice. In: T.F.Cash, T. Pruzinsky (eds.), Body image. A handbook of theory, research, and clinical practice (pp. 509-516). New York, London: The Guilford Press, 2002.
[36] Cash, T. F. (2002). Cognitive-Behavioral Perspectives on Body Image. In: T.F. Cash, T. Pruzinsky (eds.), Body image. A handbook of theory, research, and clinical practice. 2002
[37] Wilson C.P. Fear of Being Fat. The Treatment of Anorexia And Bulimia. New York: Jason Aronson Inc; 1985
[38] Rorty M., Yager J., Rossotto E. Childhood sexual, physical and psychological abuse in bulimia nervosa. Am J.Psychiatry.1994, Vol. 151, 8 pp.401-12.
[39] Kent A., Waller G., Childhood emotional abuse and eating psychopathology. Clinical Psychology Rev.2000.Vol. 20, 7, pp.887-903
[40] Waller G. Sexual abuse as a factor in eating disorders .Br J Psychiatry.Nov.1991, 159, pp. 664-71
[41] Kent A., Waller G.M, Dagnan D., A greater role of emotional than physical or sexual abuse in predicting disordered eating attitudes: the role of mediating variables. Int. J Eating Disorders 1999, Vol. 25, 2, pp.159- 67
[42] HarttJ., Waller G., Child abuse, dissociation and core beliefs in bulimic disorders. Child Abuse $ Neglect.Sep.2002, Vol. 26, 9, pp.923-38
[43] Wonderlich SA, et al. Eating disturbance and sexual trauma in childhood and adulthood. Int.J.Eat.Disorders2001,Vol. 30,4,pp. 4010-12]
[44] Stanisz A. (2007) Przystępny kurs statystyki z zastosowaniem STATISTICA PL

11

Physical Activity and Exercise in Bulimia Nervosa: The Two-Edged Sword

Solfrid Bratland-Sanda[1,2]
[1]*Department of Sport and Outdoor life sciences, Telemark University College, Bø in Telemark,*
[2]*Research Institute, Modum Bad Psychiatric Centre, Vikersund,*
Norway

1. Introduction

Physical activity and exercise has a widely known positive effect on various physiological and psychological variables, and lack of physical activity has been shown as an independent factor for obesity, type 2 diabetes, hypertension, certain types of cancer and other diseases (Pedersen & Saltin, 2006). However, in the Diagnostic and Statistical Manual for Mental Disorders version four (DSM-IV) (APA, 1994) excessive amounts of exercise is listed as one possible weight compensatory behavior among patients with bulimia nervosa (BN). In this chapter I will describe the effects of physical activity, and the motives for physical activity among patients with BN. Furthermore, the two-edged sword aspect of physical activity among patients with BN will be explored. This duality comes to show on one hand because of the excessiveness and the abuse of physical activity, and on the other hand the beneficial and therapeutic effects of correctly dosed physical activity in treatment of BN.

1.1 Definition of physical activity and exercise

Physical activity is defined as any type of bodily movement produced by skeletal muscles which results in an increased metabolism above resting level (Caspersen, Powell, & Christenson, 1985). Exercise is the planned, structured and repeated physical activity performed with the aim to improve performance, fitness and/or health (Bouchard, Blair, & Haskell, 2007). The term physical activity includes occupational physical activity, transport physical activity, housework and leisure time physical activity, whereas exercise refers to leisure time physical activity. Physical activity therefore includes all the terms exercise, work out and sports. In this chapter, the terms physical activity and exercise will be used interchangeably.

1.2 General effects of physical activity

Effects of physical activity can be divided into acute effects and long term effects. The acute effects include physical responses such as increased ventilation and breathing frequency, increased heart rate, stroke volume, systolic blood pressure, body temperature, and reduction in blood lipoproteins and glucose (Bouchard, et al., 2007). The immediate elevations in levels of endorphins, serotonin and dopamine are suggested as a reason why many report a positive impact of physical activity on mood, positive and negative affects

(Martinsen, 2005). These effects are temporary, but persistent physical activity behavior will among others positively affect circulatory and respiratory factors, metabolism, bone mass, and regulation of blood glucose (Pedersen & Saltin, 2006). Physical activity has also shown positive impact on psychological factors such as sleep quality, self esteem, self efficacy and well-being (Meyer & Broocks, 2000).

1.3 Physical activity recommendations

The most recent updates were published by American College of Sports Medicine (ACSM) and The American Heart Association published in 2007 (Haskell et al., 2007). These recommendations state that healthy adults need to perform at least 5 x 30 minutes of moderate intensity physical activity or 3 x 20 min of vigorous intensity physical activity per week to maintain health. For additional health benefits, up to 60 minutes of moderate-to-vigorous intensity physical activity per day is recommended. In addition, the ACSM (2009) published guidelines regarding strength training which state that strength training should be performed at least twice per week with different loading depending upon the main goal of the strength training. For example, individuals who want to increase maximum muscle strength need to perform fewer repetitions with higher loading (e.g. four repetitions of 90% of 1 repetition maximum, 1RM) compared to individuals whose main goal is hypertrophy (e.g. 8-12 repetitions of 80% of 1RM).

For individuals who are overweight or obese, the recommendations for healthy adults are insufficient to achieve significant weight loss. With moderate, but not severe, nutritional restrictions it is possible for obese individuals to achieve adequate weight loss, and maintenance of this weight loss, with about 250 minutes per week of moderate intensity physical activity (Donnelly et al., 2009). Other studies have suggested that the duration of the physical activity can be reduced with increased intensity, but there is a need for studies to examine this by randomized controlled trials with follow up design.

In 2009, Handbook of Activity was published by the Norwegian Directorate of Health (Bahr, 2009). In this handbook, recommendations for physical activity in prevention and treatment of a list of different diseases are provided. Unfortunately, as of today there are inadequate levels of knowledge regarding the effects of physical activity in prevention and treatment of eating disorders, therefore eating disorders are not included in this handbook. Hopefully, the level of knowledge will increase within the next years, and it will then be easier to make recommendations for physical activity in treatment of the different types of eating disorders.

1.4 Physical activity among patients with BN

Several studies have examined physical activity among females with and without eating disorders including BN. Pirke et al. (1991) found no differences in minutes per day of physical activity reported through a physical activity diary. However, the lack of difference can be due to a type II error because the sample size was quite small (BN patients, n=8, controls, n=11). This lack of difference in weekly duration of physical activity among BN patients and controls was also found in Sundgot-Borgen et al. (1998). This study included a larger sample size compared to Pirke et al. (1991), however use of parametric statistics on non-parametric data can have influenced on whether the statistical analysis showed significance differences or not. In a study by our research group, we assessed physical activity both objectively through an accelerometer, and through self report by a seven-days physical activity diary (Bratland-Sanda et al., 2010a). We discovered a mean higher amount of weekly physical activity among female inpatients across both anorexia nervosa (AN), BN and eating disorders not otherwise specified (EDNOS) compared to non-clinical age-matched controls. Despite this difference, the patient sample showed a large heterogeneity when it comes to weekly amount of physical activity. Although a high mean physical activity level, almost 10 percent of the patients were considered physically inactive (Bratland-Sanda, 2010).

Another important aspect with the self report methods used in the studies by Pirke et al. (1991) and Sundgot-Borgen et al. (1998) is the possibility for response bias. Our study (Bratland-Sanda et al., 2010a) discovered that adult inpatient females with longstanding eating disorders, included BN and atypical BN, tended to underreport physical activity when it was compared to objectively assessed physical activity through a motion sensor or accelerometer. This discrepancy between self reported and objectively assessed physical activity was not found among females without eating disorders. We believe that this underreport can be deliberate due to fear of restrictions of the physical activity or fear of needing to increase energy intake. On the other hand, there is a possibility that the patients define and interpret the term "physical activity" different from us as researchers and clinicians. As previously mentioned, the definition of physical activity include all human movement produced by skeletal muscles, and therefore factors such as intensity and/or duration of the physical activity is irrelevant. However, a clinical experience is that patients with eating disorders, including BN, only consider the very vigorous intensity activity to be defined as physical activity or exercise. To these patients, incidental physical activity (i.e. the physical activity performed as part of the daily routine such as household activities such as vacuuming, or walking as a transport activity) does not count as physical activity. This interpretation of the term physical activity was illustrated by the quote of one of our patients participating in the study: *"I'm not physically active – I only go for walks."* (Bratland-Sanda et al., 2010a:91). This patient, diagnosed with BN, reported that she went for walks every day, and these walks lasted approximately one hour each. Despite this, she was convinced that this was not enough to be defined as physically active. This case is an example of how the underreporting can be unintentional.

In a sample of 29 adult female inpatients with longstanding BN, 39% reported to perform aerobic endurance activities only (e.g. running, walking, cycling and swimming), whereas 50% reported to perform both aerobic and non-aerobic activity forms including strength training (see Figure 1).

2. Motivation for exercise in BN

The motives for being physically active can vary over time and from person to person. The motives are influenced by factors such as age, BMI, mood, personality, knowledge and attitudes (Dishman, Sallis, & Orenstein, 1985). The motives can be extrinsic, intrinsic or a combination of these. In females from both the general population and from eating disordered populations, weight control and/or regulation are perceived as very important reasons for physical activity and exercise (Furnham, Badmin, & Sneade, 2002; Mond & Calogero, 2009). Other motives and reasons for physical activity and exercise are physical fitness, health, well-being, regulation of mood and affects, and socializing (Cash, Novy, & Grant, 1994; Plonczynski, 2000).

Bratland-Sanda et al. (2010a) found no differences in importance of exercise as a weight regulator between patients with eating disorders and age-matched non-clinical controls.

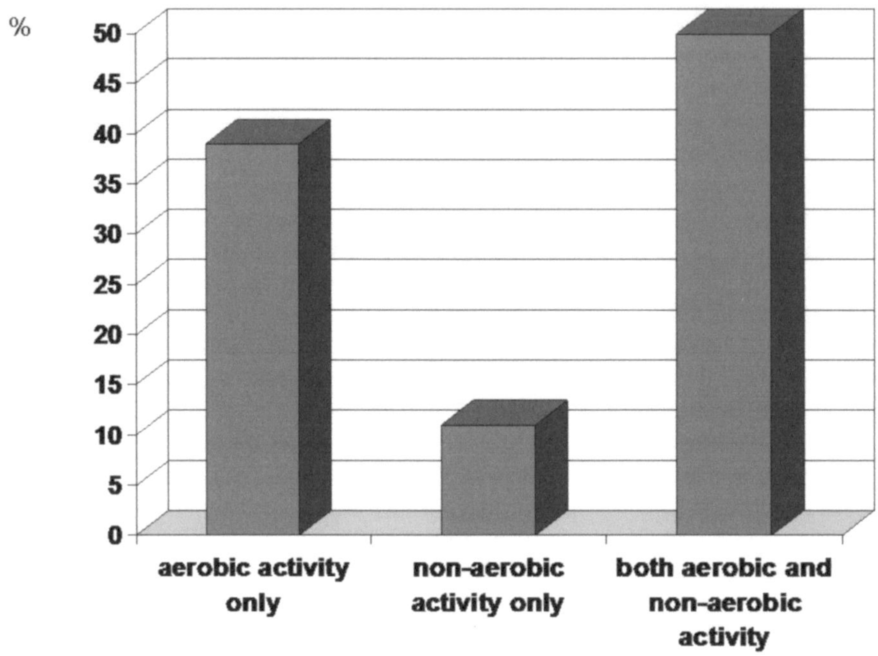

Fig. 1. Frequency of reported aerobic (e.g. running, walking, swimming, cycling) and non-aerobic (e.g. strength training, yoga, pilates) physical activities among a sample of adult female inpatients with bulimia nervosa.

Interestingly, differences did occur in importance of exercise to enhance fitness and health (perceived as less important among the patients) and importance of exercise to regulate negative affects (perceived as more important among the patients). The use of physical activity and exercise as an affect regulator did only occur for regulation of negative affects, no differences in perceived importance of exercise to regulate positive affects was found between patients and controls. One possible explanation for this finding is the high levels of negative affects such as anxiety, depression, shame, guilt etc. among the patients, and therefore the main focus is to down regulate these affects rather than to improve positive affects and well-being. It is important to note that our study was carried out on patients with longstanding eating disorders, and that motives for physical activity and exercise might change during different phases of the disorder. It can be hypothesized that body weight and shape are more important reasons for exercise among patients with short duration of the eating disorders compared to the longstanding eating disorder patients. Future studies need to address this.

3. Excessive exercise and exercise abuse in BN

3.1 When there is too much of a good thing: definition of excessive exercise and exercise dependence

There is no consensus on how to define excessive exercise and exercise dependence. And often these terms, in addition to compulsive exercise, are used interchangeably. In the DSM-IV, excessive exercise is defined under the diagnosis of BN. According to this definition, exercise becomes excessive when it makes a significant negative impact on other aspects of life, e.g. work, social life and/or family, when it is performed within inappropriate timing and/or setting, and/or the exercise is continued despite injuries, illness or severe complications (APA,1994). Compulsive or obligatory exercise refers to an individual's feeling of being forced to exercise when the motive is no longer performance enhancement, but rather avoidance of the negative feelings that occur with exercise deprivation (Draeger, Yates, & Crowell, 2005). Exercise dependence is defined as the drive to perform leisure-time exercise, and that this drive results in uncontrolled excessive exercise behavior with physiological and/or psychological symptoms of exercise deprivation. The physical withdrawal symptoms are key features of this behavior, and these symptoms did not occur before the exercise behavior pattern started (Hamer & Karageorghis, 2007; Hausenblas & Symons Downs, 2002). The reason why there are several different terms used on what seems to be the same issue, is that destructive and unhealthy exercising has been examined using different disorders and concepts from the field of psychiatry. Mechanisms of substance dependence have been used to explain exercise dependence, and obsessive-compulsiveness has been used to explain compulsive exercising.

To make the concepts of excessive exercise, compulsive exercise and exercise dependence clearer, the differences are pointed out in Table 1.

	Dimension	Main issue	Example
Excessive exercise	Quantitative only (i.e. duration, intensity and frequency)	Too much exercise, but the motives for the exercise can vary. The motives do not have to be compulsive.	BN patients who perform a high amount exercise, but the motive can be to enhance performance in a certain type of sport.
Compulsive exercise	Qualitative only (i.e. motivation and attitudes)	Compulsive motives and behavior, and expression of a need to follow rituals. The behavior does not have to be excessive in amount	BN patients who have to perform 200 sit ups before getting out of bed in the morning. If interrupted, he/she needs to do the whole procedure from the start.
Exercise dependence	Quantitative + qualitative	Avoid withdrawal symptoms.	A BN patient who constantly but unintentionally increases amount of exercise because of increased tolerance, lacks control of the exercise behavior, experiences withdrawal symptoms with exercise deprivation, exercise despite injury and/or illness and that the exercise interfere with other aspects of life.

BN: bulimia nervosa.

Table 1. Differences between the concepts of excessive exercise, compulsive exercise and exercise dependence.

Especially the term exercise dependence has been discussed to be both positive and negative. Some argue that exercise dependence is a positive type of dependence (Morgan, 1979), whereas others believe that the development of a dependency is in itself negative. Cockerill & Riddington (1996) divided between healthy commitment to exercise and a negative dependence to exercise. According to these definitions, the individuals with a healthy commitment to exercise schedule the exercise routines to the more important aspects of life (e.g. work and family life), whereas the individuals with a negative dependency to exercise schedule the rest of their lives around the exercise routines (Cockerill & Riddington, 1996).

A study from 2005 examined whether compulsive exercise would be a better term than excessive exercise for the exercise performed as weight compensatory behavior (Adkins & Keel, 2005). Using a sample of 265 female and male undergraduate students, they found that compulsive exercise score positively predicted disordered eating, whereas quantity of exercise was a negative predictor of disordered eating. They therefore argue that compulsive exercise better describe exercise as a symptom of BN. Unfortunately, this study included a non-clinical sample, and there is a possibility that findings could have been otherwise with a clinical sample of patients with BN.

3.2 Prevalence of exercise dependence among patients with BN

Studies which have examined prevalence of exercise dependence in patients with BN are listed in Table 2. As the table shows, prevalence of exercise dependence in BN ranges from 17% to 57%. This large range can be explained by different definitions of the term exercise dependence, different assessment methods, age of the patient and duration of illness. It is believed that prevalence of exercise dependence is higher among patients in the acute phase of the disorder, and therefore a higher frequency of patients with shorter duration of the illness is classified as exercise dependent (Davis et al., 1997).

3.3 Characteristics of exercise dependence: high intensity activity and affect regulation

Exercise dependent patients show more severe eating disorders psychopathology, more symptoms of anxiety and depression, longer duration of treatment, poorer prognosis for recovery, and higher risk of relapse compared to non-dependent patients (Bratland-Sanda et al., 2010b; Brewerton, et al., 1995; Calogero & Pedrotty, 2004; DalleGrave, et al., 2008; Penas-Lledo, et al., 2002; Shroff, et al., 2006; Strober, Freeman, & Morrell, 1997). Bratland-Sanda et al. (2011) examined explanatory factors for exercise dependence among patients with eating disorders and non-clinical controls. In this study, weekly amount of vigorous intensity physical activity and importance of exercising for regulation of negative affects explained 78% of the variance in exercise dependence score among the patients. Among the non-clinical controls, these two variables explained 53% of the variance.

Affect regulation is the process with the aim of decreasing negative affects and increasing positive affects (Larsen, Prizmic, Baumeister, & Vohs, 2004). Negative affect regulation can both indicate down-regulation of negative affects such as depression and anxiety, and maladaptive affect regulation strategies (Fonagy, Gergely, Jurist, & Target, 2002). Eating disorder can in itself be viewed as a maladaptive affect regulation strategy, because eating disorders symptoms such as bingeing, purging and/or starvation can function as a way to suppress and/or avoid difficult emotions and affects (Harrison, Sullivan, Tchanturia, & Treasure, 2009). Physical activity is an example of a strategy that can be positive for regulation

Study	Patient population (n)	Age	Prevalence
Davis et al. (1994)	AN, BN (n=45)	24.6 (4.8)	AN: 78%
Brewerton et al. (1995)	AN (n=18) BN (n=71)	N/A	AN: 39% BN: 23%
Davis et al.(1997)	AN, BN (n=127)	27.7 (7.8)	AN: 81% BN: 57%
Solenberger (2001)	AN (n=115) BN (n=38) EDNOS (n=56)	20.8 (7.2)	AN: 54% BN: 39% EDNOS: 46%
Penas-Lledo et al. (2002)	AN (n=63) BN (n=61)	18.8 (5.9)	AN: 46% BN: 46%
Abraham et al. (2006)	AN, BN, EDNOS (n=212)	Range: 16-40	AN, BN, EDNOS: 17%
Shroff et al. (Shroff et al., 2006)	AN, BN, EDNOS (n=1857)	26.3 (7.7)	AN: 44% BN: 21% EDNOS: 21%
DalleGrave et al. (2008)	AN, BN, EDNOS (n=165)	26.0 (7.8)	R-AN: 80% B-AN: 43% BN: 39% EDNOS: 32%
Bratland-Sanda (2010b)	AN (n=4) BN (n=17) EDNOS (n=17)	30.1 (8.5)	AN: 50% BN: 6% EDNOS: 47%

AN: anorexia nervosa. BN: bulimia nervosa. EDNOS: eating disorders not otherwise specified.
N/A: not available.

Table 2. Selected studies examining prevalence of excessive exercise, compulsive exercise and/or exercise dependence among patients with bulimia nervosa.

of negative affects into a certain level. When the amounts of physical activity or exercise get excessive, and/or the behavior is compulsive, then this strategy turns maladaptive.

Vigorous intensity physical activity is also a typical sign of exercise dependence. When a female inpatient with EDNOS was asked about her vigorous intensity physical activity, she said: *"I can't walk away from the anxiety; I have to run from it."* This quote is in my opinion a valuable illustration of the use of physical activity to reduce negative affects, and that sometimes the physical activity has to be of certain intensity for the individual to achieve the intended effect. Therefore, it is a paradox that vigorous intensity physical activity performed in excessive amounts actually can worsen mood (Lind, Ekkekakis, & Vazou, 2008). Why the exercise dependent individuals prefer vigorous intensity physical activity is still not explored adequately. It can however be hypothesized that the vigorous intensity physical activity results in an acute suppression of the negative affects, and that this effect is only temporary. In that way, the level of negative affects can in fact end up being worse after the physical activity session than it was before.

3.4 Management of exercise dependence

As of today, there is no consensus on how to manage and treat exercise dependence. Beumont et al. (1994) and Calogero & Pedrotty (2004) found promising results when using supervised and health related physical activity in treatment of excessive amounts of exercise and exercise dependence. Other strategies used are motivational interview, cognitive behavioral therapy and psycho-education (Long & Hollin, 1995; Mavissakalian, 1982; Stunkard, 1960).

4. Exercise as a beneficial part of treatment for BN

Although physical activity can be performed with compulsivity and in excessive amounts, properly dosed physical activity can also be beneficial as a part of the treatment for BN. Sundgot-Borgen et al. (2002) randomly assigned young adult females with BN to exercise, cognitive behavioral therapy, nutritional counselling or waiting list control. The exercise program was superior to cognitive behavior therapy and nutritional counselling in improving drive for thinness, body composition and aerobic fitness, and in reducing binge/purge episodes. Unfortunately, this is to my knowledge the only publication that has examined the effect of exercise in treatment of BN using a randomized controlled trial design. It is therefore necessary to carry out more studies to replicate this finding.

Studies on other eating disorders such as binge eating disorder and anorexia nervosa have found physical activity to be beneficial in reducing co morbidity of depression and anxiety, and in enhancing quality of life (Hausenblas, Cook, & Chittester, 2008). In addition, physical activity can help the patients improve social bonding and relations. For patients who undergo heavy psychotherapy etc., the physical activity can be a nice distraction and time off from these exhausting and mentally painful processes. A clinical and practical experience is that the activity needs to be pleasurable and non-competitive. There is a need for studies that examine if a certain type of exercise (e.g. endurance training, strength training, pilates or yoga) is superior to others. Important outcome variables are change in eating disorder psychopathology, general psychopathology, body dissatisfaction and image, self esteem, quality of life, physical fitness, body composition, bone health, exercise dependence and motives for physical activity. As mentioned, we found about 10 percent of the patients to be insufficiently physically active (Bratland-Sanda, 2010), and a significant number of patients with BN are overweight or obese. Therefore, these patients need to increase physical activity level. This issue of inactivity among patients needs to be thoroughly emphasized during the treatment period. However, it must be done in a way that will enhance health and enjoyment without increasing the focus upon body weight and shape. It is therefore my recommendation that personnel with education in exercise physiology and exercise psychology must be in charge for the physical activity as part of BN treatment.

4.1 Contraindications to physical activity and exercise among patients with BN

There are several medical complications related to BN, among others oral, gastrointestinal and electrolyte complications (Mehler, 2011). Especially the electrolyte abnormalities are important to take into consideration when considering physical activity among the patients. The levels of e.g. sodium and chloride can decrease or increase dependent of type of purging method (Mehler, 2011). With both vomiting, use of laxatives and use of diuretics, the levels of potassium in serum and urine will decrease. Low potassium levels, also referred to as hypokalemia, have been found in approximately 5% of the BN population, and this condition can lead to e.g. cardiac arrhythmias. During physical activity, such lethal cardiac arrhythmias can occur (Bouchard, et al., 2007).

5. Future research

Future studies need to examine the mechanisms behind exercise dependence, and different treatment options for exercise dependence. Effects of different types of physical activities in treatment of BN among both male and female patient populations need to be addressed.

6. Conclusion

Physical activity has a number of physiological and psychological effects, and it has been shown effective as a preventive and therapeutic variable in diseases such as type 2 diabetes, cardiovascular disease, osteoporosis, depression, anxiety and certain types of cancer. Among patients with BN, the physical activity is a two-edged sword. On one hand, up to about 50% of patients with BN are classified as exercise dependent, and these patients do need to reduce the amounts of weekly physical activity. On the other hand, a randomized controlled trial found an exercise program superior to nutritional counselling and cognitive behavior therapy among young adult females with BN. Future studies need to further address the possible preventive and therapeutic effects of physical activity in this patient population.

7. References

Abraham, S. F., Pettigrew, B., Boyd, C., & Russell, J. (2006). Predictors of functional and exercise amenorrhoea among eating and exercise disordered patients. *Hum.Reprod., 21*(1), 257-261.

ACSM. (2009). American College of Sports Medicine position stand. Progression models in resistance training for healthy adults. *Med Sci Sports Exerc, 41*(3), 687-708. doi: 10.1249/MSS.0b013e3181915670

Adkins, E. C., & Keel, P. K. (2005). Does "excessive" or "compulsive" best describe exercise as a symptom of bulimia nervosa? *Int.J Eat.Disord., 38*(1), 24-29.

American Psychiatric, A. (1994). *Diagnostic and Statistical Manual of Mental Disorders (DSM-IV)*. Washington DC: APA.

Bahr, R. (2009). *Aktivitetshftndboken: fysisk aktivitet i forebygging og behandling*. Oslo: Helsedirektoratet.

Beumont, P. J., Arthur, B., Russell, J. D., & Touyz, S. W. (1994). Excessive physical activity in dieting disorder patients: proposals for a supervised exercise program. *Int.J Eat.Disord, 15*(1), 21-36.

Bouchard, C., Blair, S. N., & Haskell, W. L. (2007). *Physical activity and health*. Champaign, Il.: Human Kinetics.

Bratland-Sanda, S. (2010). *Physical activity in female inpatients with longstanding eating disorders*. PhD, Norwegian school of sport sciences, Oslo.

Bratland-Sanda, S., Martinsen, E. W., Rosenvinge, J. H., Ro, O., Hoffart, A., & Sundgot-Borgen, J. (2011). Exercise dependence score in patients with longstanding eating disorders and controls: the importance of affect regulation and physical activity intensity. *Eur Eat Disord Rev, in press.*

Bratland-Sanda, S., Sundgot-Borgen, J., Ro, O., Rosenvinge, J. H., Hoffart, A., & Martinsen, E. W. (2010a). "I'm not physically active - I only go for walks": physical activity in patients with longstanding eating disorders. *Int J Eat Disord, 43*(1), 88-92.

Bratland-Sanda, S., Sundgot-Borgen, J., Ro, O., Rosenvinge, J. H., Hoffart, A., & Martinsen, E. W. (2010b). Physical activity and exercise dependence during inpatient treatment of longstanding eating disorders: an exploratory study of excessive and non-excessive exercisers. *Int J Eat Disord, 43*(3), 266-273.

Brewerton, T. D., Stellefson, E. J., Hibbs, N., Hodges, E. L., & Cochrane, C. E. (1995). Comparison of eating disorder patients with and without compulsive exercising. *Int.J.Eat.Disord., 17*(4), 413-416.

Calogero, R. M., & Pedrotty, K. N. (2004). The practice and process of healthy exercise: an investigation of the treatment of exercise abuse in women with eating disorders. *Eat Disord, 12*(4), 273-291.

Cash, T. F., Novy, P. L., & Grant, J. R. (1994). Why do women exercise? Factor analysis and further validation of the Reasons for Exercise Inventory. *Percept.Mot.Skills, 78*(2), 539-544.

Caspersen, C. J., Powell, K. E., & Christenson, G. M. (1985). Physical activity, exercise, and physical fitness: definitions and distinctions for health-related research. *Public Health Rep., 100*(2), 126-131.

Cockerill, I. M., & Riddington, M. E. (1996). Exercise dependence and associated disorders: a review. *Counselling Psychol Quarterly, 9*(2), 119-130.

DalleGrave, R., Calugi, S., & Marchesini, G. (2008). Compulsive exercise to control shape or weight in eating disorders: prevalence, associated features, and treatment outcome. *Compr.Psychiatry, 49*(4), 346-352.

Davis, C., Katzman, D. K., Kaptein, S., Kirsh, C., Brewer, H., Kalmbach, K., . . . Kaplan, A. S. (1997). The prevalence of high-level exercise in the eating disorders: etiological implications. *Compr.Psychiatry, 38*(6), 321-326.

Davis, C., Kennedy, S. H., Ravelski, E., & Dionne, M. (1994). The role of physical activity in the development and maintenance of eating disorders. *Psychol Med., 24*(4), 957-967.

Dishman, R. K., Sallis, J. F., & Orenstein, D. R. (1985). The determinants of physical activity and exercise. *Public Health Rep., 100*(2), 158-171.

Donnelly, J. E., Blair, S. N., Jakicic, J. M., Manore, M. M., Rankin, J. W., & Smith, B. K. (2009). American College of Sports Medicine Position Stand. Appropriate physical activity intervention strategies for weight loss and prevention of weight regain for adults. *Med Sci Sports Exerc, 41*(2), 459-471. doi: 10.1249/MSS.0b013e3181949333

Draeger, J., Yates, A., & Crowell, D. (2005). The obligatory exerciser. Assessing an overcommitment to exercise. *The Physician and Sports Medicine, 33*(6).

Fonagy, P., Gergely, G., Jurist, E. L., & Target, M. (2002). *Affectregulation, Mentalization, and the Development of the Self.* New York: Other Press.

Furnham, A., Badmin, N., & Sneade, I. (2002). Body image dissatisfaction: gender differences in eating attitudes, self-esteem, and reasons for exercise. *J Psychol, 136*(6), 581-596.

Hamer, M., & Karageorghis, C. I. (2007). Psychobiological mechanisms of exercise dependence. *Sports Med, 37*(6), 477-484.

Harrison, A., Sullivan, S., Tchanturia, K., & Treasure, J. (2009). Emotion recognition and regulation in anorexia nervosa. *Clin Psychol Psychother, 16*(4), 348-356.

Haskell, W. L., Lee, I. M., Pate, R. R., Powell, K. E., Blair, S. N., Franklin, B. A., . . . Bauman, A. (2007). Physical activity and public health: updated recommendation for adults from the American College of Sports Medicine and the American Heart Association. *Med Sci.Sports Exerc, 39*(8), 1423-1434.

Hausenblas, H. A., Cook, B. J., & Chittester, N. I. (2008). Can exercise treat eating disorders? *Exerc Sport Sci.Rev, 36*(1), 43-47.

Hausenblas, H. A., & Symons Downs, D. (2002). Exercise dependence: a systematic review. *Psychol Sports Exerc, 3*, 89-123.

Larsen, R. J., Prizmic, Z., Baumeister, R. F., & Vohs, K. D. (2004). Affect regulation *Handbook of self-regulation: research, theory, and application* (pp. 40-61). New York: The Guilford Press.

Lind, E., Ekkekakis, P., & Vazou, S. (2008). The affective impact of exercise intensity that slightly exceeds the preferred level: 'pain' for no additional 'gain'. *J Health Psychol, 13*(4), 464-468.

Long, C., & Hollin, C. R. (1995). Assessment and management of eating disordered patient who over-exercise: a four-year follow-up of six single case studies. *J Mental Health, 4*, 309-316.

Martinsen, E. W. (2005). Exercise and depression. *Int J Sport Exerc Psychol, 4*, 469-483.

Mavissakalian, M. (1982). Anorexia nervosa treated with response prevention and prolonged exposure. *Behav Res Ther., 20*(1), 27-31.

Mehler, P. S. (2011). Medical complications of bulimia nervosa and their treatments. *Int J Eat Disord, 44*(2), 95-104. doi: 10.1002/eat.20825

Meyer, T., & Broocks, A. (2000). Therapeutic impact of exercise on psychiatric diseases: guidelines for exercise testing and prescription. *Sports Med, 30*(4), 269-279.

Mond, J. M., & Calogero, R. M. (2009). Excessive exercise in eating disorder patients and in healthy women. *Aust.N.Z.J Psychiatry, 43*(3), 227-234.

Morgan, W. P. (1979). Negative addiction in runners. *The Physician and Sports Medicine, 7*, 57-71.

Pedersen, B. K., & Saltin, B. (2006). Evidence for prescribing exercise as therapy in chronic disease. *Scand.J Med Sci.Sports, 16 Suppl 1*, 3-63.

Penas-Lledo, E., Vaz Leal, F. J., & Waller, G. (2002). Excessive exercise in anorexia nervosa and bulimia nervosa: relation to eating characteristics and general psychopathology. *Int.J Eat.Disord., 31*(4), 370-375.

Pirke, K. M., Trimborn, P., Platte, P., & Fichter, M. (1991). Average total energy expenditure in anorexia nervosa, bulimia nervosa, and healthy young women. *Biol.Psychiatry, 30*(7), 711-718.

Plonczynski, D. (2000). Measurement of motivation for exercise. *Health.Ed.Res., 15*(6), 695-705.

Shroff, H., Reba, L., Thornton, L. M., Tozzi, F., Klump, K. L., Berrettini, W. H., . . . Bulik, C. M. (2006). Features associated with excessive exercise in women with eating disorders. *Int.J Eat Disord, 39*(6), 454-461.

Solenberger, S. E. (2001). Exercise and eating disorders: a 3-year inpatient hospital record analysis. *Eat.Behav., 2*(2), 151-168.

Strober, M., Freeman, R., & Morrell, W. (1997). The long-term course of severe anorexia nervosa in adolescents: survival analysis of recovery, relapse, and outcome predictors over 10-15 years in a prospective study. *Int.J Eat Disord, 22*(4), 339-360.

Stunkard, A. J. (1960). A method of studying physical activity in man. *Am J Clin Nutr., 8*, 595-601.

Sundgot-Borgen, J., Bahr, R., Falch, J. A., & Schneider, L. S. (1998). Normal bone mass in bulimic women. *J Clin Endocrinol.Metab, 83*(9), 3144-3149.

Sundgot-Borgen, J., Rosenvinge, J. H., Bahr, R., & Schneider, L. S. (2002). The effect of exercise, cognitive therapy, and nutritional counseling in treating bulimia nervosa. *Med.Sci.Sports Exerc., 34*(2), 190-195.

12

Personality and Coping in Groups With and Without Bulimic Behaviors

Tomaz Renata[1] and Zanini Daniela S[2]
[1]*Alves Faria College*
[2]*Pontifical Catholic University of Goias*
Brazil

1. Introduction

Eating disorders have been increasing year by year, mainly due to social demands for anorexic standards of beauty (Cordás, 2004). Among the eating disorders, bulimia, described as episodes of binge eating followed by compensatory behaviors (Cordás, 2004), stands out.

Globalization and capitalism largely develop markets that explore beauty (for example, media, marketing strategies, chemical industries), and require their audience to follow a trend dictated by them (Souza & Santos, 2007). That makes Wolf (1991) postulate beauty as a monetary system similar to gold, a cult of beauty and thinness which intensified the development of eating disorders such as bulimia.

Since Hippocrates, in 467 BC, Boulos was the terminology used to describe a sick hunger. But it was in 1743, when James described binge eating as "true boulimus", and bulimic episodes as "caninus appetites", that bulimia started to be studied in its relation to health (Cordás, 2004). However, the recognition of an eating disorder called bulimia nervosa only occurred in 1979. In that year, Russell described cases of this disease linked to anorexia nervosa. Both diseases are similar and, in most cases, appear as concurrent or comorbidities. However, in bulimia there is not extreme weight loss as in anorexia (Busse, 2004).

Bulimia is characterized by an excessive consumption of food which does not aim for satiation. The DSM-IV emphasizes two factors related to binge eating: quantitative and qualitative. The quantitative factor is related to the excess of food intake, an amount of food superior than people are used to or need to consume. The qualitative factor would be the lack of control characteristic of binge eating, in which the individuals cannot stop eating. Both factors are common in the bulimia disease.

In general, after a gorging food intake, the person experiences guilt and fear of gaining weight that can trigger compensatory behaviors like self-induced vomiting, overuse of laxatives, diuretics, thyroid hormones, anorectic drugs, diets and excessive exercise in order to avoid weight gain. In addition to these behaviors there is an increased dissatisfaction with their bodies, often leading to body image distortion (Chemin & Milito, 2007).

Compensatory behaviors used by patients with bulimia generate considerable harm to their health. Among them we can mention severe changes in the central nervous system, changes in the cycle of satiation, metabolism and production of neurotransmitters (Chemin & Milito, 2007; Sicchieri, Bighetti, Borges, Santos, Ribeiro, 2006).

The causes of this disorder are not well-known. Authors like Claudino and Zanella (2005), Castilho, Gonçalves, Milk, and Cordás Segal (1995) describe a relation between bulimia and personality factors, such as impulsivity and affective instability that may be associated to the behaviors of uncontrolled binge eating and purging to avoid weight gain. Even "low self-esteem, self-negative evaluation and greater vulnerability to stress are important risk factors for developing eating disorders" (p.19).

The relationship between personality factors and bulimia is based on an understanding of the disorder from a dynamic perspective, which considered the influence of personality traits over behaviors that can be associated with bulimia (Leonidas and Santos, 2010). In this sense, the Big Five model has been the most widely used in the investigations of personality traits and its relationship to psychopathology. This model refers to the Theory of Personality Factors based on the Big Five model composed by the factors: neuroticism, extroversion, openness, agreeableness and conscientiousness (Nunes, 2005). Figure 1 describes the personality factors according to the model of the Big Five factors.

The applicability to different cultures and the easy comprehensibility of the Big Five concepts can explain the large spread of studies based on it (Tani, Greenman, Schneider & Fregoso, 2003; & Ruiz Jiménez, 2004). The Big Five model also provides a measure of personality traits that has proved to be valid in different studies, both to predict the level of physical well being, mental and social health of individuals, and to predict the usage of coping strategies (Costa & Widiger, 1993).

For example, Furtado, Falcone and Clark (2003) found, in their studies, that dysfunctional personality factors such as perfectionism and obsessive-compulsive behavior interfere negatively in the way individuals cope with stress. In fact, we can postulate that the relation between personality and health can occur in at least two pathways. In the first one, by means of a direct effect, studies have shown a direct association between neuroticism and eating disorders (Tomaz & Zanini, 2009), anxiety and depression (Forns & Zanini, 2005), among others. In the second one, by means of an indirect effect, studies have demonstrated that individuals with high neuroticism scores have stronger tendencies to use avoidance as a way of coping with their problems, and that using this type of coping strategy is related to eating disorders (Tomaz & Zanini).

Thus, one can say that avoidance coping may influence the manifestation of psychiatric diseases such as bulimia (Margis, Picon, Cosner & Silveira, 2003; Nakahara, Yoshiuchi, Yamanaka, Sasaki, Suematsu, Kuboki, 2000), and that experiencing stressful situations can lead an individual to develop psychiatric disorders, such as posttraumatic stress, and depressive and anxiety symptoms, depending on the coping strategies they used (Blumenthal, Babyak, Carney, Keefe, Davis, Lacaille, Parekh, Freedland, Trulock Palmer, 2006, Sorkin & Rook, 2006).

On the other hand, patients with eating disorders such as bulimia tend to use less adaptive coping strategies than the general population (Nakahara, Yoshiuchi, Yamanaka, Sasaki, Suematsu, Kuboki, 2000). That can be explained by the availability of individual coping resources. To Claudino and Zanella (2005) the effect that stressful events have on the process of eating disorders "(...) depends on the resources that the individual has prior to use in response, as well as the social support network that he has access to and which can function as a protective factor "(p.21).

According to the transactional theory, coping can be defined as a person's ability to cope with a stressful situation, which exceeds its own resources (Compas, 1987; Lazarus &

Big Five Factors	Low ⟷ High	
Neuroticism: evaluation of the adjustment versus emotional instability. Identifies individuals prone to psychological disorders, unrealistic ideas, excessive needs or cravings and maladaptive responses.	Quiet, relaxed, unemotional, strong, secure, self-satisfied, stable.	Worried, nervous, emotional, insecure, inadequate, hypochondriac, tense, unstable, unhappy.
Extroversion: evaluation of the amount and quality of interpersonal interactions, activity level, need for stimulation, and ability to rejoice.	Reserved, serious, closed, aloof, task-oriented, selfless, quiet, speechless, non-assertive, non-bold, non-energetic, shy.	Sociable, active, talkative, people-oriented, optimistic, playful, affectionate, assertive, bold, energetic, fearless.
Opening: evaluation of proactive activity and appraisal of the experience, tolerance and exploration, enjoyment of new experiences.	Conventional, reasonable, limited interests, non-artistic, non-analytical, non-imaginative, non-creative, non-inquisitive, non-reflective, non-sophisticated.	Curious, broad interests, creative, original, imaginative, nontraditional, curious, thoughtful, sophisticated.
Agreeableness: evaluation of the amount of interpersonal orientation over a continuum from compassion to antagonism in thoughts, feelings and actions.	Cynical, rude, suspicious, uncooperative, vengeful, ruthless, irritable, manipulative, selfish, stingy.	Generous, kind, confident, helpful, forgiving, gullible, honest, cooperative, altruistic.
Conscientiousness: evaluation of the grade of persistence, organization and motivation to achieve his/her objectives.	Aimless, unreliable, lazy, careless, negligent, relaxed, weak, hedonistic, disorganized, irresponsible, impractical.	Organized, reliable, hardworking, self-disciplined, punctual, scrupulous, neat, ambitious, persevering, responsible, practical, detail-oriented.

Fig. 1. Description of the Big Five Factors

Folkman, 1984). Coping is characterized by a dynamic process of mutual influence between person and environment and can be classified according to their focus on problem-focused strategies (seeking to modify the problem in order to solve it), and emotion-focused strategies (which seek to transform the emotions caused by the problem and not the problem itself) (Lazarus & Folkman, 1984; Pesce, Assisi, Santos & Oliveira, 2004). There are other categories to measure coping strategies such as classifying coping responses, according to their method, in cognitive responses (when using cognitive efforts to cope with a stressful situation) and behavioral responses (when using behavioral efforts to cope with a stressful situation) (Holahan, et al. 1996; Moos, 1993).

Moos (1993) built the Coping Response Inventory (CRI) linking method to focus, to conceptualize and measure coping strategies. The CRI classify coping strategies in cognitive and behavioral responses, and also in approach and avoidance coping. In the group classified as approach coping strategies are those that employ cognitive and behavioral responses as a way to solve the problem. This group is similar to that described by Lazarus and Folkman (1984) as problem-focused coping. Examples of these strategies are logical analysis, positive reappraisal, seeking guidance and problem solving (the first two refer to cognitive efforts and the last two to behavioral efforts).

In the group of avoidance strategies there are other specific strategies that can also be classified as cognitive and behavioral efforts to avoid the problem by manipulating the emotions that cause the problem without confronting the stressful situation. Again, this classification is similar to the emotion-focused coping described by Lazarus and Folkman (1984). Examples of this type of avoidance coping would be cognitive avoidance, acceptance and resignation, seeking alternative reward, and emotional discharge (again, the first two related to cognitive efforts and the last two to behavioral efforts).

Among the various factors related to eating disorders, literature has pointed to personality traits and coping strategies towards the problem as factors that may influence the occurrence, perpetuation and adherence to treatment (Binford, 2003; Gongora, Guedes, Albuquerque, Troccoli, Noriega, JJ & Guedes, 2006; Rebelo & Leal, 2007). However, the differential analysis of this influence on bulimic subjects in comparison to other groups is still unclear and could contribute to more effective interventions for this group.

This chapter discusses the relationship between personality and coping in a group of people with bulimic behavior (cases) compared with a group without bulimic behavior (controls), highlighting the implications of these differences for intervention proposals which are more suitable to the characteristics of the group studied.

2. Method

2.1 Participants

This is a case control study which included 166 participants, pre-screened in three higher education institutions in a city in central Brazil, and with no self-reported diagnosis of mental disorders. 62 of these presented bulimic behaviors, according to the Eating Attitude Test (EAT) score. This instrument has been described as effective in the identification of eating disorders (Nunes & col., 2006; Tomáz & Zanini, 2009). Therefore, those individuals with raw scores in the general EAT range above 21 were considered cases (as standardization of the instrument made by Nunes & col., 2006), as well as a raw score higher than 3,9 on the scale for bulimia, taking into account the average score of non-clinical population (2.19) plus a standard deviation (1.71). The controls are represented by 88 individuals who have not had bulimic behaviors or any other behavior consistent with the diagnostic criteria for eating disorders, and had average scores on the EAT scale for bulimia below 2.19, as well as a general index on the EAT below 21.

2.2 Instruments

The instruments were: a Brazilian experimental scale to assess personality traits based on the Big Five theory; the Coping Response Inventory - Adult Form (CRI - A) for the evaluation of the perception of the problem and coping strategies; and the Eating Attitudes Test (EAT- 26) to assess behaviors consistent with eating disorders. All instruments have satisfactory psychometric data and were published in the Brazilian literature.

The scale of personality was used to evaluate two factors in our sample: neuroticism and extraversion. This test was based on the Personality Factor Inventory created by Pasquali, Ghesti and Azevedo (1997), which measures 15 psychological characteristics. The factors are divided into 25 phrases that participants should answer based on a Likert scale ranging from 1 (extremely uncharacteristic) to 5 (extremely characteristic). The items were preceded by a paragraph that asked participants to express their degree of agreement with each statement contained in the scale. This scale presents satisfactory psychometric characteristics, as described in Tomaz and Zanini (2009).

The Coping Response Inventory-Adult Form (Moos, 1993) measures eight specific coping strategies defined as Logical analysis, Positive Reappraisal, Seeking guidance and support, Problem solving, Cognitive avoidance, Acceptance-resignation, Seeking alternative rewards, and Emotional discharge. Each specific coping strategy comprises a six-item rating using a four-point Likert-type scale, ranging from 0 (No, not at all) to 3 (Yes, fairly often). The Cronbach alpha coefficients for Brazilian subjects are acceptable and ranged from 0,68 to 0,72. Similar Cronbach alpha coefficients are described in international coping literature (Moos, 1993).

Moos (1993) classified these specific strategies on the basis of Method or Focus of coping. The focus reflects the approach (directly coping with problems) versus avoidance coping (coping with the emotion elicited by the problem rather than the problem). Approach is composed of Logical Analysis, Positive Reappraisal, Seeking Guidance, and Problem Solving. Avoidance is composed of Cognitive Avoidance, Acceptance Resignation, Seeking Alternative Rewards, and Emotional Discharge. The method reflects a theoretical differentiation of cognitive versus behavioral efforts to cope. Cognitive method is composed of Logical Analysis, Positive Reappraisal, Cognitive Avoidance and Acceptance Resignation. Behavioral method is composed of Seeking Guidance, Problem Solving, Seeking Alternative Rewards and Emotional Discharge. These classifications allow to consider four typologies of coping: Approach, Avoidance, Cognitive and Behavioral coping, each of them rated from 0-72.

To assess eating attitudes and behaviors characteristic of people suffering from eating disorders, we used the Eating Attitudes Test (EAT-26). This instrument has good psychometric qualities and has been used in several studies to assess behaviors related to eating disorders as well as diagnostic criteria for them (Cordás & Neves, 2000). In this study we used the reduced version, which contains 26 items, divided into three ranges: diet; bulimic behaviors; and preoccupation with food and oral control (Freitas, Appolinario & Gorenstein, 2002). Items are rated using a scale from 0 to 3, in which the responses "always," "often" and "sometimes" punctuate 3, 2 and 1, respectively, but the responses "rarely", "almost never "and" never "do not give scores. Thus, individuals who achieve a score above 21 are classified as individuals with eating disorder behaviors (Nunes, Apollinario, Abuchaim, & Coutinho, 2006).

2.3 Procedures

The study was approved by the ethics in the human research committee and followed all the ethical procedures of the APA. The instrument application occurred collectively in the participants' classroom, coordinated by the researchers in charge. Data analysis was performed using the statistical package SPSS for Windows version 19.0.

3. Results

There were no significant differences in mean scores on the personality traits of extroversion (p = 0.69) between cases (M = 1.54, SD = 0.91) and controls (M = 1.48, SD = 0, 71), as well as for trait of neuroticism (p = 0.17) for both groups (M = 1.20 and 1.42, SD = 0.99 and 0.88 for cases and controls respectively) as shown in Table 1.

Personality	Group	Means	SD	F	p.
Extroversion	Case	1,54	0,91	0,16	0,69
	Control	1,48	0,71		
Neuroticism	Case	1,20	0,99	1,88	0,17
	Control	1,42	0,88		

Table 1. Means, Standard Deviation and compared means for personality in case and control groups.

However, although no significant differences were observed between the means of the personality traits, the data demonstrated a differential influence of these on coping strategies according to the group, as shown in Table 2. Table 2 shows Spearman correlation between coping strategies and personality traits neuroticism and extraversion for case and controls.

Escalas de Coping	case		Control	
	Extroversion	Neuroticism	Extroversion	Neuroticism
Logical Analysis	,248	,075	,000	-,125
Positive Reappraisal	,284*	-,149	,287	-,117
Seeking Guidance	,361*	-,088	,323*	-,084
Problem Solving	,314*	-,197	,088	-,120
Cognitive Avoidance	-,252	-,105	,038	-,114
Acceptance/Resignation	-,106	,274	,157	-,077
Seeking Alternative Reward	,356*	-,155	,314*	-,179
Emotional Descharge	,052	,086	,137	-,051

* Correlation is significant at the 0.05 level (2-tailed).

Table 2. Spearman correlation between coping strategies and personality traits neuroticism and extraversion for case and controls.

In the case group, the personality trait of extroversion is associated with coping strategies such as positive reappraisal (r = 0.28, p <0.05), social support (r = 0.36, p <0.05), problem solving (r = 0.31, p <0.05) and seeking alternative reward (r = 0.36, p <0.05). In the control group, however, the extroversion trait is only associated with coping strategies as social support (r = 0.32, p <0.05) and seeking alternative reward (r = 0.31, p <0.05),.
Table 3 shows data from compared mean between case and control groups for problem appraisal.

Appraisal questions	Group	Mean	SD	F	P
Previous experience with the problem	case	1,31	1,35	0,44	0,51
	control	1,46	1,30		
Knowing the problem would happened	case	1,73	1,38	0,01	0,92
	control	1,76	1,29		
Have enough time to prepare to cope with the problem	case	1,11	1,29	4,84	0,03
	control	1,55	1,13		
Thinking on the problem as a threat	case	1,84	1,30	1,17	0,28
	control	2,06	1,15		
Thinking on the problem as a challenge	case	1,73	1,34	0,76	0,39
	control	1,91	1,20		
If the problem were caused by yourself	case	1,23	1,27	1,99	0,16
	control	1,91	1,20		
If the problem were caused by other person	case	1,53	1,29	0,12	0,73
	control	1,46	1,27		
Positive consequences of facing the problem	case	1,82	1,35	0,01	0,92
	control	1,84	1,15		
If the problem were solved	case	1,18	1,32	3,30	0,08
	control	1,57	1,25		
If it were solved, is everything all right	case	1,47	1,30	4,07	0,05
	control	1,87	1,10		

Table 3. Mean, Standard Deviation and Compared mean between case and controls for problem appraisal.

The control group tends to evaluate having enough time to prepare to cope with the problem significantly more (p = 0.03) than the case group (m = 1.55 and 1.11, SD = 1.13 and 1,29 for the case and control group respectively). They also tend to evaluate that the problem was solved (p=0,08, F=3,30) and that everything is all right now (p=0,05, F=4,07) in levels higher than did the case group (m= 1,57 and 1,18, SD= 1,25 and 1,32 for control and case group respectively for if the problem was solved; m= 1,87 and 1,47, SD=1,10 and 1,30 for control and case group respectively for everything is all right now).

Table 4 shows data from Spearman correlation between personality trait and problem appraisal for case and control groups.

In the control group, the personality trait of neuroticism is associated with the appraisal of the problem as a threat. Thus, in this group, individuals with higher neuroticism personality trait tend to appraise more experiencing the problem as a threat (r = 0.20, p <0.05).

In the group of cases, however, the personality trait of extroversion was positively associated with the evaluation that the problem is already solved (r = 0.26, p <0.05) and if it is solved, things are alright (r = 0.39, p <0.01), while the personality trait neuroticism was negatively associated with the evaluation that, once the problem is solved, things will already be alright (r = - 0.31, p <0, 05). Thus, in the group case, a higher score on the personality traits of extroversion is associated with a perception that problems are solved and once solved, things are going well, while those individuals belonging to this group with the highest scores in trait neuroticism tend to evaluate that, although having solved the problem, things are not going well again.

Appraisal questions	case		Control	
	Extroversion	Neuroticism	Extroversion	NeurotiCism
Previous experience with the problem	0,22	0,11	0,95	-0,01
Knowing the problem would happen	0,28	-0,14	0,01	0,20
Having enough time to prepare to cope with the problem	0,17	-0,13	0,15	-0,01
Thinking on the problem as a threat	0,18	0,11	0,12	0,20*
Thinking on the problem as a challenge	0,25	-0,06	0,14	0,03
If the problem were caused by yourself	0,07	0,21	-0,01	-0,08
If the problem were caused by another person	-0,11	0,12	-0,08	0,00
Positive consequences of facing the problem	-0,03	-0,10	-0,03	0,08
If the problem were solved	0,26*	-0,15	0,10	-0,09
If it were solved, is everything all right?	0,39**	-0,31*	0,06	-0,14

* significant at a level of p≤ 0,05.
** significant at a level of p≤ 0,01.

Table 4. Spearman correlation between assessment of the problem and personality traits neuroticism and extraversion for case and controls.

4. Conclusion

In Psychology, the idea of an association between eating disorders and personality traits has already been demonstrated (Binford, 2003; Gongora, Guedes, Albuquerque , Troccoli, Noriega, & Guedes, 2006; Rebelo & Leal, 2007). However, this study found no significant differences between the personality traits of people with and without bulimic behaviors. Despite the fact the differences do not present statistically representative values within the averages found in this study, it can be postulated that the size of the clinical sample used may have contributed to minimize the statistical effect of this difference between the groups. Therefore studies with a larger number of subjects and using other instruments could demonstrate a significant difference, since this study uses a small sample size and a cross sectional data collection. However, beside that, data shows that bulimic subjects are less neurotic and more extroverted when compared with general population. That is of interesting especially because, in some sense, it demonstrate a common sense that obese people are more extroverted than others. That could be of interested for future studies.

Nevertheless, the data seems to indicate that, although this difference was not significant between both groups, the influence of personality traits on the perception of the problem as well as on ways of coping with problems occurs differentially. Thus, although no significant difference was observed between personality traits of both groups, this small difference seems to produce differential relations in perceptions and behaviors of individuals when dealing with their problems. The data is discussed in the light of coping and personality theories. We also discuss the need for psychological interventions based on the development of coping skills and geared towards the care of patients with bulimia.

We also discuss the need for psychological interventions directed towards the care of patients with bulimia that direct their aims to the development of coping abilities, which will widen their behavioral repertoire regarding ways of facing problems, and which may lead to changes in the ways of perceiving and relating to the environment, as well as higher assertiveness in order to develop a stronger emotional self-control and self-confidence.

5. References

Binford, R. B. (2003). Implementation and predictive capacity of CBT Coping in individuals with bulimia nervosa. Tese de doutorado não publicada, Universidade de Minnesota, Estados Unidos.

Blumenthal, J. A., Babyak, M. A., Carney, R. M., Keefe, F. J., Davis, R. D., LaCaille, R., Parekh, P. I., Freedland, K. E., Trulock, E., & Palmer, S. M. (2006). Telephone-based coping skills training for patients awaiting lung transplantation: The INSPIRE study. Journal of Consulting and Clinical Psychology, ISSN 0022-006X, 74, 535-544.

Castilho, Simone Mancini, Gonçalves, Simone Brunhani, Leite, Marcos da Costa, Segal, Adriano & Cordás, Táki Athanássios (1995). Bulimia nervosa III: disorders and personality evaluation in patients with bulimia nervosa. Jornal Brasileiro de Psiquiatria, ISSN 0047-2085, 44, 32-37.

Claudino, A. M., & Zanella, M. T. (2005). Transtornos Alimentares e Obesidade. Barueri: Manole, ISBN: 8520422675.

Compas, B. E. (1987). Coping With Stress During Childhood and Adolescence. Psychological Bulletin, ISSN 1641-7844, 101, 393-403.

Connor-Smith, J. K., & Flachsbart, C. (2007). Relations Between Personality and Coping: A Meta-Analysis. Journal of Personality and Social Psychology, ISSN 0022-3514, 93, 1080-1107.

Cordás, T. A., & Neves, J. E. P. (2000). Escalas de avaliação de transtornos alimentares. Em C. Gorenstein, L. H. S. G. Andrade & A. W. Zuardi (Orgs.), Escalas de avaliação em psiquiatria e psicofarmacologia (pp. 345-347). São Paulo: Lemos-Editorial, ISSN 0104-7795.

Cordás, T. A. (2004). Transtornos alimentares: classificação e diagnóstico. Revista de Psiquiatria Clínica, ISSN 0101-6083, 31, 154-157.

Costa, P. T., Somerfield, M. R., & McCrae, R. R. (1996). Personality and Health. En L. Pervin (Ed.). Handbook of personality theory and research. London: Guilford Press, ISBN: 1593858361.

Costa, P. T., & Widiger, T. A. (1993). Introduction. Em P. T. Costa & T. A. Widiger (Orgs.), Personality Disorders and the Five-Factor Model of Personality (pp. 1-10). Whashington, DC: American Psychological Association, ISSN: 0003-066X.

Chemin, C. & Milito, F. (2007). Transtornos Alimentares em Adolescentes. Revista Brasileira de Obesidade, Nutrição e Emagrecimento, ISSN 1981-9919, 1, 84-88.

Freitas, S., Gorenstein, C., & Appolinario, J. C. (2002). Instrumentos para a avaliação dos transtornos alimentares. Revista de Psiquiatria, ISSN 0101-8108, 24, 34-38.

Furtado, E. S., Falcone, E. M. O., & Clark, C. (2003). Avaliação do estresse e das habilidades sociais na experiência acadêmica de estudantes de medicina de uma universidade do Rio de Janeiro. Interação em Psicologia, ISSN 1981-8076 ,7, 43-51.

Gómez-Fraguela, J. A. Luengo-Martín, A. Romero-Triñanes, E. Villar-Torres P. & Sobral-Fernández, J. (2006). Estratégias de afrontamiento en el inicio de la adolescencia y su relación con el consumo de drogas y la conducta problemática. International Journal of Clinical and Health Psychology, ISSN 16972600, 6, 581-597.

Gongora, V. C., van de Staak, C. P. F., & Derksen, J. J. L. (2004). Personality Disorders, Depression and Coping Styles in the Argentinean Bulimic Patients. Journal of Personality Disorders, ISSN 0885-579X ,18, 272-285.

Gregor, M. M. (2005). The effect of acceptance and nonacceptance based coping strategies on symptom severity in the Eating Attitudes Test (EAT). Tese de Doutorado não publicada, Faculty of the Chicago School of Professional Psychology, Chicago.

Griffith, M. A., Dubow, E. F., & Ippolito, M. F. (2000). Developmental and cross-situational differences in adolescent's coping strategies. Journal of Youth and Adolescence, ISSN 0047-2891, 29, 183-197.

Guedea, M. T. D., Albuquerque, F. J. B., Tróccoli, B. T., Noriega, J. A. V., Seabra, M. A. B., & Guedea, R. L. D. (2006). Relação do bem-estar subjetivo, estratégias de enfrentamento e apoio social em idosos. Psicologia: Reflexão e Crítica, ISSN 0102-7972, 19, 301-308.

Holahan, C. J., Moos, R. H., & Schaefer, J. A. (1996). Coping, Stress Resistance, and Growth: Conceptualization adaptive functioning. Em M . Zeidner & N. S. Endler, (Orgs.), Handbook of Coping: theory, research, applications (pp. 24-43). New York- EUA: John Wiley & Sons, ISBN 978-0-471-59946-3.

Hutz, C. S., & Nunes, C. H. S. S. (2001). Escala fatorial de neuroticismo. São Paulo, SP: Casa do Psicólogo.

Lazarus , R. S., & Folkman, S. (1984). Stress, Appraisal and Coping. New York: Springer, ISBN 0826141919.

Leonidas, C., & Santos, M. A. D. (2010). A Avaliação da Imagem Corporal e Atitudes Alimentares de Pacientes com Anorexia Nervosa. Aconselhamento na Saúde: perspectivas integradoras, ISBN/ISSN 0874.0283, 1, 261-277.

Margis, R., Picon, P., Cosner, A. F., & Silveira, R. O. (2003). Relação entre estressores, estresse e ansiedade. Revista de Psiquiatria RS, ISSN 0101-8108, 25, 65-74.

Moos, R. H. (1993). Coping Response Inventory Adult Form - ProfessionalManual. Odessa, Flórida: PAR Psychological Assessment Resources, Inc, ISBN 0911907068.

Nakahara R; Yoshiuchi K; Yamanaka G; Sasaki T; Suematsu H & Kuboki T. (2000). Coping skills in Japanese women with eating disorders. Psychological Reports, ISSN 0033-2941, 87, 741-746.

Nunes, C. H. S. S. (2005). Construção, normatização e validação das escalas de socialização e extroversão no modelo dos Cinco Grandes Fatores. Tese de Doutorado não publicada, Instituto de Psicologia, Universidade Federal do Rio Grande do Sul, Porto Alegre.

Nunes, C. H. S. S., & Hutz, C. S. (2007). Construção e validação da escala fatorial de socialização no modelo dos Cinco Grandes Fatores de Personalidade. Psicologia: Reflexão e Crítica, ISSN 0102-7972, 20, 20-25.

Nunes, M. A. A., Apolinário, J. C., Abuchaim, A. L. G., & Coutinho, W. (2006). Transtornos alimentares e obesidade. Porto Alegre: Artmed, ISBN 9788536306773.

Pasquali, L., Azevedo, A. M., & Ghesti, I. (1997). Manual Técnico do Inventário Fatorial de Personalidade. São Paulo: Casa do Psicólogo, ISBN: 8585141913.

Pesce, R. P., Assis, S. G., Santos N., & Oliveira, R. V. C. (2004). Risco e proteção: em busca de um equilíbrio promotor de resiliência. Psicologia: Teoria e Pesquisa, ISSN 0102-3772, 20, 135-143.

Rebelo, A., & Leal, I. (2007). Fatores de Personalidade e Comportamento Alimentar em Mulheres Portuguesas com Obesidade Mórbida: Estudo Exploratório. Análise Psicológica, ISSN 0870-8231, 3, 467-477.

Rowe, M. M. (2006). Four-year Longitudinal Study of Behavioral Changes in Coping With Stress. American Journal Health Behavior, ISSN 1945-7357, 30, 602-612.

Ruiz, V. M., & Jiménez, J. A. (2004). Estructura de la personalidad: Ortogonalidad versus oblicuidad. Anales de Psicología, ISSN 1695-2294, 20, 1-13.

Sicchieri, J. M. F., Bighetti, F., Borges, N. J. B. G., Santos, J. E. D., Ribeiro, & R. P. P. (2006). Manejo Nutricional nos Transtornos Alimentares. Simpósio Transtornos Alimentares: Anorexia e Bulimia Nervosas, ISSN 1676-7314, 39 (3): 371-4.

Souza, L. V., & Santos, M. A. (2007). Anorexia e bulimia: Conversando com as famílias. São Paulo: Vetor.

Sorkin, D. H., & Rook, K. S. (2006). Dealing With Negative Social Exchanges in Later Life: Coping Response, Goals, and Effectiveness. Psychology and Aging, ISSN: 0882-7974, 21, 715-725.

Tani, F., Greenman, P. S., Schneider, B. H., & Fregoso, M. (2003). Bullying and the Big Five: A study of childhood personality and participant roles in bullying incidents. School Psychology International, ISSN: 1461-7374, 24, 131-146.

Tobin, D. L. (2004). Terapia de Estratégias para Combater a Bulimia Nervosa. São Paulo: Roca, ISBN: 85- 7241-485-1.

Tomaz, R., & Zanini, D. S. (2009). Personalidade e Coping em Pacientes com Transtornos Alimentares e Obesidade. Psicologia: Reflexão e Crítica. ISSN 0102-7972, 22, 447-454.